TUMOR ANGIOGENESIS

Edited by **Sophia Ran**

Tumor Angiogenesis
Edited by Sophia Ran

Published by InTech
Janeza Trdine 9, 51000 Rijeka, Croatia

Publishing Process Manager Molly Kaliman

Technical Editor Teodora Smiljanic

Cover Designer InTech Design Team

Additional hard copies can be obtained from orders@intechopen.com

Tumor Angiogenesis, Edited by Sophia Ran
p. cm.
ISBN 978-953-51-0009-6

Meet the editor

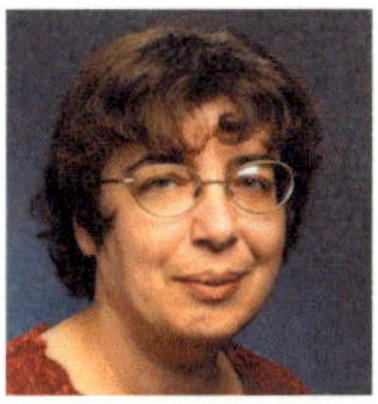

Dr Sophia Ran received her Ph.D. degree in Biochemistry in 1989 from the Weizmann Institute in Israel. She completed postgraduate training in the University of Alabama at Birmingham, USA, and the Hospital for Sick Children, Canada. After working three years in a pharmaceutical company on developing anti-cancer drugs, she moved to the Southwestern Medical Center in Dallas, Texas, to develop new agents targeting tumor vessels. In 2003, she moved to Southern Illinois University where she is currently an Associate Professor in the Department of Medical Microbiology, Immunology and Cell Biology. Her major research interests are tumor vessels and metastasis. She is an author of 23 US and 69 international patents as well as 43 scientific papers related mainly to tumor angiogenesis, lymphangiogenesis, anti-cancer therapies and metastasis. Dr. Ran is a member of Research Advisory Board of American Cancer Society in the Illinois Division and an associate editor of Frontiers in Vascular Physiology, ISRN Oncology and OJPathology. She served as a grant reviewer for NIH, ACS, the US Army, the Cancer Research Council in England, the Italian Ministry of Health, the Swiss Cancer League and the Swiss National Foundation.

Contents

Preface

Angiogenesis is the main process responsible for formation of new tumor blood that play an essential role in expansion of the tumor mass and dissemination of metastatic cells. Tumor angiogenesis significantly differs from the tightly controlled normal neovascularization driven by physiological needs. This is because the tumor environment contains excessive levels of vascular endothelial growth factor-A (VEGF-A) as well as many other pro-angiogenic factors that are produced by neoplastic, stromal, and infiltrating immune cells. This imbalance of pro-angiogenic *versus* anti-angiogenic factors promotes generation of numerous but abnormal blood vessels that exhibit severe structural and functional defects. The chaotic and poorly-perfused tumor vascular network creates a chronically inflamed site that promotes thrombosis, and impedes drug delivery, causing further complications to the cancer patient. Most importantly, the structural and functional abnormalities of tumor vessels promote hematogenous metastasis, which is the main cause for decreased survival of patients with solid tumors. It is, therefore, not surprising that tumor angiogenesis is regarded as an important target for developing anti-cancer strategies with many studies focused on mechanisms of the tumor blood vessel formation and their impact on tumor pathology and progression. This book covers a variety of topics related to the biology of tumor vasculature. This includes reviews on VEGF-A-dependent and independent mechanisms controlling the formation of new vessels; contribution of inflammatory cells and platelets to tumor neovascularization; identification of new molecular targets for inhibition of tumor angiogenesis; and potential clinical use of novel anti-angiogenic therapies based on heparin-like compounds and Chinese herbal extracts. The book covers also two emerging subjects in the field: a recently developed zebrafish model of tumor angiogenesis, and microRNA regulation of blood vessel formation at the tumor site. Collectively, the chapters in the book provide a current update on central findings in the tumor angiogenesis field, while highlighting potential targets for inhibition. We hope that this book will be useful for oncologists, cancer basic researchers, and biologists with interests in vascular and endothelial cell behavior in the context of cancer.

Sophia Ran, Ph.D.
Associate Professor
Southern Illinois University, School of Medicine
Springfield, IL
USA

1

Heparin-Like Drugs with Antiangiogenic Activity

María Rosa Aguilar, Luis García-Fernández,
Raquel Palao-Suay and Julio San Román
Biomaterials Group, Polymeric Nanomaterials and Biomaterials Department,
Institute of Polymer Science and Technology (CSIC), Madrid
Biomedical Research Networking Centre in Bioengineering,
Biomaterials and Nanomedicine (CIBER-BBN)
Spain

1. Introduction

The process of angiogenesis consists in the sprouting of new blood vessels from existing ones. This is a natural process that occurs in the human body and is essential for organ growth and repair. In the embryonic stage, the blood vessels provide the necessary oxygen, nutrients and instructive trophic signals to promote organ morphogenesis (Coultas et al., 2005). After birth the angiogenic process only contributes to organ growth and during adulthood the angiogenic process only occurs in the placenta during the pregnancy and in the cycling ovary, while most blood vessels remain quiescent. However the angiogenic activity could be reactivate because endothelial cells retain their angiogenic activity in response to a physiological stimulus (wound healing and repair) (Alitalo et al., 2005).

This angiogenic activity is also critical in the development of solid tumors and metastasis (Ferrara, 2004; Folkman, 1990). Generally, a solid tumor expands until 1-2 mm^3 is reached. At this point vascularization is required in order to ensure a supply of nutrients, oxygen, growth factors and proteolytic enzymes to the tumor (Folkman, 1990). To activate the angiogenic activity of endothelial cells, the tumor switches to an angiogenic phenotype and recruits blood vessels from the surrounding tissue, developing a dense vasculature that provides nutrients to the cancerous tissue (Figure 1). Numerous proangiogenic proteins are involved in tumor angiogenesis.

Two of the most important families of pro-angiogenic proteins are the vascular endothelial growth factors (VEGF) and the fibroblast growth factors (FGF) (Garcia-Fernandez et al., 2010c). Most of these GF isoforms (this is not the case of the smallest isoform of VEGF-A (V121), that does not present a heparin-binding domain) need to interact with heparan sulfate proteoglycans molecules (HSPG) in order to recognize their specific tyrosine kinase receptor on cell membrane and activate the angiogenic process. These cell surface molecules are low affinity receptors that do not transmit a biological response, but are essential for these growth factors to recognize their union site to the signaling receptor (FGFR or VEGFR). Therefore, disruption of the interaction of these growth factors (GF) with cell surface HSPG seems an evident target for angiogenesis (Folkman, 1971; Folkman, 1990; Folkman, 1995).

HSPGs are heparin-like molecules that favor the pro-angiogenic proteins oligomerization (Figure 1), which is necessary for the interaction with the endothelial cells membrane receptors. Heparin is a natural polysaccharide composed of alternating units of sulphated glucuronic acid and glucosamine derivatives, it presents anticoagulant activity and interacts with the most important pro-angiogenic proteins in tumor angiogenesis (*e.g.* different isoforms of FGF and VEGF) (Fernández-Tornero et al., 2003; Lindahl et al., 1994).

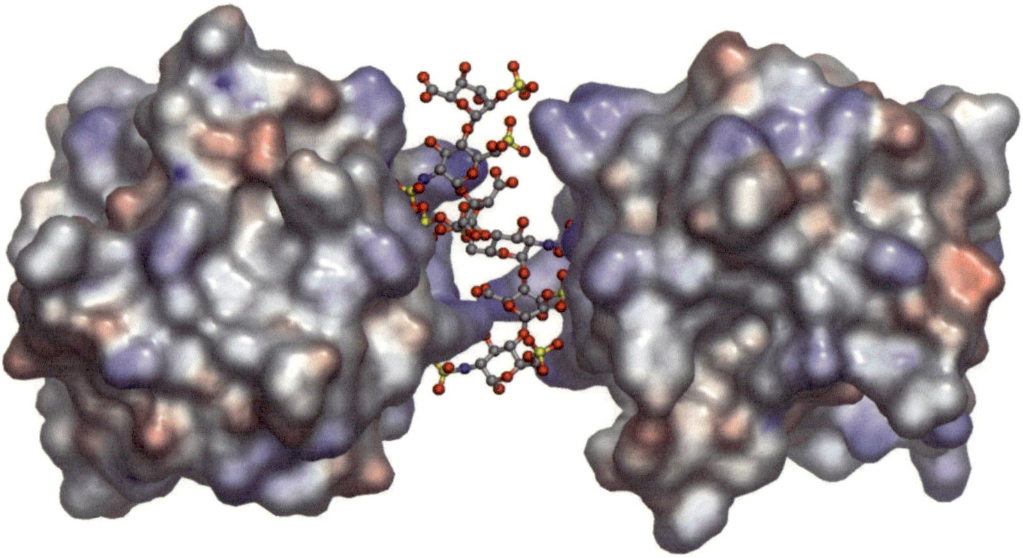

Fig. 1. Structure of a heparin-linked biologically active dimer of acidic fibroblast growth factor. Heparin is shown as stick-and-ball model (carbon: grey; oxygen: red; sulfur: yellow; nitrogen: blue). The figure was generated and the surfaces colored according the electrostatic potential (red, negative; blue, positive) using OpenAstexViewer (3.0; Astex Therapeutics Ltd.) and its internal parameters. PDB ID: 1AXM (DiGabriele et al., 1998).

The interaction between heparin and "heparin binding-proteins" (those that present a heparin-binding domain) regulates most of the biological properties of this sulfated glycosaminoglycan (GAG). However, angiogenesis is a complicated process regulated by numerous biologically active molecules and through different pathways that cannot be explained without each other (Figure 2). The ideal heparin-like drug to be designed for the treatment of tumor angiogenesis not only will interact with angiogenic growth factors (FGF-1, FGF-2, VEGF...) reducing their functional activity, but also will inhibit heparanase preventing the release of these growth factors from the extracellular matrix (ECM) and stimulate tissue factor pathway inhibitor (TFPI) conferring an antimetastatic character to the molecules. Heparanase is an endo-β-D-glucuronidase capable of cleaving the heparan sulfate (HS) side chains of HSPG, playing a key role in ECM-remodelling and heparin-binding release, and TFPI is a potent anticoagulant and antiangiogenic endogenous polypeptide.

In this chapter, the most recent studies for the design of heparin-like drugs will be reviewed starting with the effect of different heparinoids (low molecular weight heparins (LMWH) and chemically modified heparins) and finishing with the activity of synthetic antiangiogenic molecules. Many of these studies demonstrate that the biological activity of these heparin-like drugs depends on composition (charge density), microstructure (charge distribution), molecular weight, and the supramolecular organization (charge orientation) of the polymers (Garcia-Fernandez et al., 2010b; Garcia-Fernandez et al., 2010c). Most of the clinically investigated therapies target VEGF or one of its receptors (*e.g.* Bevacizumab or Avastin, a recombinant humanized monoclonal IgG1 (anti-VEGF-A) antibody) (Wahl et al., 2011), however the development of new compounds that interact with pro-angiogenic molecules through heparin-binding domains is a good strategy to obtain new therapeutics with synergistic inhibitory effect of not one but several pro-angiogenic molecules (broad-spectrum angiogenesis inhibitors).

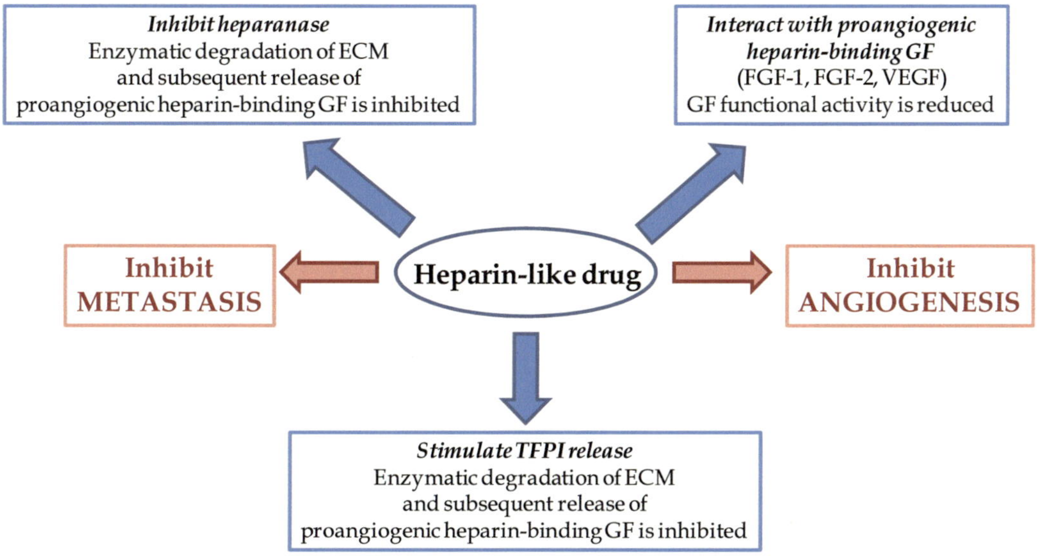

Fig. 2. Possible effects of heparin-like drugs for the treatment of tumor angiogenesis: interaction with proangiogenic heparing-binding growth factors, inhibition of heparanase and stimulation of TFPI release.

2. Heparin species (heparinoids)

Heparin presents very interesting pharmacological actions including antitumor and antimetastatic activity, however its use as anticancer agent has been limited due to the high risk of bleeding complications because of its anticoagulant and antithrombotic properties. Several efforts have been performed in the last decades in order to mimic and specifically modulate the biological action of heparin by exogenous heparin species (*i.e.* unfractionated heparin, LMWH, heparin oligosaccharides, chemically modified heparins and biotechnologically obtained heparins). Fortunately, heparin modification allowed the creation of new heparinoids with non-anticoagulant activity but antiheparanase activity and ability to interact selectively with proangiogenic growth factors. As it will be demonstrated molecular weight, charge density and charge distribution of heparin play a key role in its biological activity.

2.1 Low molecular weight heparins (LMWH)

LMWH are derived from unfractionated heparin (UFH) by chemical or controlled enzymatic depolymerization and present a lower mean molecular weight between 3 and 6 kDa and

chain lengths of 12 to 18 saccharide units. LMWHs have been available in Europe since the mid-1980s. In 1993 the first LMWH was approved in the United States for the treatment of venous thrombus (Grande & Caparro, 2005; Kakkar, 2004).
Since are prepared by different methods of depolymerization, they differ to some extent in pharmacokinetic properties and anticoagulant profile, and may not be clinically interchangeable (Hirsh et al., 2001; Norrby, 2006).
LMWH present important advantages if compared to UFH: enhanced bioavailability after subcutaneous administration, prolonged half-life and more interesting pharmacokinetic properties, reduced thrombocytopenia and a more predictable dose response (Grande & Caparro, 2005; Khorana et al., 2003).

Generation heparin	**Name**	**Commercial name**	**Method of preparation**	**Mean molecular weight (Da)**	**References**
First generation heparin	Tinzaparin	Innohep	Heparinase depolymerization	6.500	(Amirkhosravi et al., 2003; Gasowska et al., 2009; Mousa & Mohamed, 2004a; Mousa & Mohamed, 2004b; Mousa & Petersen, 2009; Norrby, 2006)
	Dalteparin	Fragmin	Nitrous acid depolymerization	6.000	(Khorana et al., 2003; Marchetti et al., 2008; Norrby, 2006; Norrby & Nordenhem, 2010; Takahashi et al., 2005)
	Enoxaparin	Clexane	Benzylation and alkaline hydrolysis	4.500	(Khorana et al., 2003; Marchetti et al., 2008; Norrby, 2000; Norrby, 2006)
	Nadroparin	Fraxiparin	Nitrous acid depolymerization	4.500	(Debergh et al., 2010; Khorana et al., 2003; Norrby, 2000)
	Reviparin	Clivarine	Nitrous acid depolymerization	4.500	(Collen et al., 2000; Gasowska et al., 2009; Mousa & Petersen, 2009; Norrby, 2006)
Second generation heparin	Bemiparin	Badyket	Chemical β-elimination depolymerization	3.500	(Depasse et al., 2003; Dogan et al., 2011; Jeske et al., 2011; Perez-Ruiz et al., 2002; Vignoli et al., 2011; Westmuckett et al., 2001)
	ULMWH (RO-14)	---	Chemical β-elimination depolymerization	2.200	(Vignoli et al., 2011)

Table 1. LMWH and ULWMW with antiangiogenic activity.

These advantages have led to their increasing use in the treatment of cancer as angiogenesis inhibitors. Clinical studies suggest a significant mortality reduction in cancer patients receiving different heparin fractions for the treatment of venous thromboembolism versus those receiving UFH (Akl et al., 2008). However, conflicting data have been presented in different clinical studies and at present there is not approved use of LMWH for survival gain in cancer patients without a need for venous thromboembolism prophylaxis or treatment (Kakkar, 2004; Kwaan et al., 2009; Mousa & Petersen, 2009; Norrby, 2006; Sideras

et al., 2006; Thodiyil & Kakkar, 2002). Therefore, the potential role of LMWH heparin requires additional clinical evaluation. In particular, these studies should focus on identifying which type and stage of cancer that are most likely to respond to this form of therapy, as well as on optimizing the dose and duration of treatment (Robert, 2010).
As mentioned in the introduction, angiogenesis is a complex multistep process involving activation, proliferation and migration of endothelial cells, degradation of ECM by proteolytic enzymes (*e.g.* heparanase) and formation of the capillary vessel lumen (Marchetti et al., 2008). Moreover, tissue factor (TF) and its natural inhibitor (TFPI) are also important heparin-binding proteins that perform well-recognized roles in the regulation of angiogenesis, tumor growth and metastasis (Bobek & Kobarik, 2004; Borsig, 2010; Debergh et al., 2010; Norrby, 2006). LMWH may influence angiogenesis through modulation of the expression of angiogenic growth factors (VEGF and bFGF) and their inhibitors (Dogan et al., 2011; Gasowska et al., 2009; Mousa & Petersen, 2009).
LMWH can be classified according to their molecular weight into first generation and second generation, as show in table 1 (Hirsh et al., 2001; Vignoli et al., 2011).

2.1.1 First generation heparins
First generation LMWH present an average molecular weight between 4 and 6 kDa and both antiangiogenic and anticoagulant properties (Hirsh et al., 2001; Mousa & Petersen, 2009; Vignoli et al., 2011). Representative examples are dalteparin, tinzaparin, enoxaparin, nadroparin and other heparin fractions in the range of this mean molecular weight. In addition to differences in average molecular sizes, these LMWH differ on sulfation density and distribution of the sulfate groups along the macromolecular chains due to the manufacturing process. These differences influence to their antiangiogenic potentials and the possible anticancer mechanism (Norrby, 2006).
The main mechanism underling the antiangiogenic effect of the LMWHs is based on their interaction with the heparin-binding site of VEGF and bFGF and the subsequent inhibition of their cellular receptors (VEGFR and FGFR) (Bobek & Kovarik, 2004; Debergh et al., 2010; Gasowska et al., 2009; Mousa & Petersen, 2009).
Norrby and Nordenhem investigated if *dalteparin* (Fragmin, 6kDa), epirubicin as an important chemotherapeutic agent or a combination of these two drugs modulated angiogenesis *in vivo* by rat mesentery assay (Norrby & Nordenhem, 2010). Heparins were administrated by subcutaneous infusion at different concentration during 14 days. In these conditions, the effects on VEGF-mediated angiogenesis were measured. Dalteparin significantly stimulated angiogenesis in an inversely dose-dependent manner. The lowest concentration of 27 IU/kg/day produced the maximum increase the microvascular length (MVL) by 25% and total microvascular length (TMVL) by 71%. On the other hand, epirubicin did not significantly affect angiogenesis. However, concurrent treatment with the two drugs significantly inhibited angiogenesis. Particularly, the MVL decreased by 24% and the TMVL by 45%, using injection of epirubicin at 3 mg/kg/week and dalteparin at 80 IU/kg/day. This appears to be the first demonstration that LMWH in its own is able to increase angiogenesis *in vivo*. Recently, it was reported that UFH and dalteparin exerted similar effects on angiogenesis using the Matrigel plug assay in mice (Takahashi et al., 2005). On the other hand, Marchetti *et al.* studied how LMWHs affected the angiogenic potential of human microvascular endothelial cells (hMVEC) promoted by different tumor cells as well as growth factors (VEGF and FGF-2). *Dalteparin,* and *enoxaparin* (Clexane, 4.5 kDa) were

selected on the basis of their different molecular weight range and manufacture process, as these characteristics are thought to affect their pharmacokinetic and biological properties (Hirsh et al., 2001). The angiogenesis inhibition was evaluated by *in vitro* capillary-like tube formation assay in Matrigel. The results demonstrated both LMWHs significantly inhibited microvascular endothelial cells capillary-like tube formation when induced by human breast cancer and leukemia cells, while a lower inhibitory effect was observed with UFH (100% inhibited by enoxaparin, 70-90% by dalteparin and only 25-33% by UHF, depending on the considered growth factor). These results indicated that these heparins played an important role in VEGF mediated capillary formation (Marchetti et al., 2008).

Recent clinical studies have shown the effect of dalteparin in the treatment of patients with cancer. In the Fragmin Advanced Malignancy Outcome Study (FAMOUS) 385 patients with advanced solid tumor malignancy were randomly assigned either a once-daily subcutaneous injection of the dalteparin in a dose of 5000 units or placebo for 1 year. The study demonstrated a 5% survival advantage at 1 year in favour of the advanced cancer patients who received dalteparin. These findings have been further confirmed in other clinical trials (Bick, 2006; Kakkar, 2004; Kakkar et al., 2004; Kwaan et al., 2009).

The differential effects of LMWHs compared to UFH on angiogenesis seem to be depending on the size of the molecule and number of saccharide units. It has been shown that LMWH, in contrast to UFH, can reduce binding of growth factors to their receptors. Based on these findings, the lower mean molecular weight of enoxaparin compared to dalteparin should be responsible for the higher inhibitory effect of capillary tube formation (Khorana et al., 2003; Marchetti et al., 2008).

Similarly, Khorana *et al.* demonstrated that molecules with a molecular weight in the range of 3-6 kDa or more than 8 saccharide units maximally inhibited angiogenesis in a Matrigel assay using human umbilical vein endothelial cells (HUVECs). Specifically, fraction of 6 and 3 kDa inhibited FGF-proliferation by 94 and 60%, respectively. However, the measure of heparin fractions of lower molecular weight, as 2.4, 1.7 and 1.2 kDa, showed no significantly inhibition of proliferation. Moreover, the time of action and the concentration of heparin fraction were optimized, determining that the maximum capacity inhibition of 6 kDa fraction was at 72 hours and 5 μg/ml.

On the other hand, the results showed that heparins fractions with the same range of molecular weight also reduced tube formation through the organization into tubular structures (3 and 6 kDa heparin fractions decreased the formation of capillary-like tube structures between 58 and 78%, respectively). Chain length and molecular weight significantly affect other functional properties such as bioavailability after subcutaneous administration, half-life, binding proteins or anticoagulant activities.

Norrby *et al.* studied the effect of heparin fractions on the microcapillary sprouting in angiogenesis mediated by VEGF using a rat mesenteric window assay. Heparin fragments with molecular weight of 2.5 to 5 kDa reduced the number of microvessel and branching points per unit tissue volume more effectively than 16.4 kDa fraction (Norrby, 2000). On the other hand, FGF-mediated angiogenesis was more intensely suppressed by 2.6 kDa fraction compared with 4 fractions of higher molecular weight. The heparins fraction in this study varied in charge density and anticoagulant activity (Khorana et al., 2003). In this sense, it is important to emphasize that the anticoagulant properties of heparins are related to chain length, as reflected by the increased anti-Xa/anti-IIa activity of LMWHs (Figure 3) (Bobek & Kovarik, 2004; Grande & Caparro, 2005; Hirsh et al., 2001). Other authors demonstrated that heparin fragments with less than 18 saccharides hinder the activity of VEGF and those with less than 10 saccharides reduce bFGF activity (Bobek & Kovarik, 2004; Debergh et al., 2010; Dogan et al., 2011).

Debergh *et al.* studied the effects of *nadroparin* (Fraxiparin, 4.5 kDa) on tumor-associated angiogenesis, using a dorsal skinfold window chamber model in the Syrian hamster. Active angiogenesis was observed in control animals, however nadroparin inhibited tumor-associated angiogenesis and normalized microvessel structure in this immunocompetent tumor model (Debergh et al., 2010).

Klerk *et al.* evaluated the effect of nadroparin on survival in patients with advanced malignancy based on time from random assignment to death. At 6 months the survival was 61% in the nadroparin group versus 56% in the placebo group indicating that a brief 6-week course of subcutaneous nadroparin favourably influences the survival in patients with advanced solid malignancy (Klerk et al., 2005; Kwaan et al., 2009).

It is important to consider that angiogenesis is a multi-step process. Tumoral cells activate blood coagulation involving procoagulant factors, such as the tissue factor (TF). TFPI is a natural inhibitor of this procoagulant factor that suppresses a number of steps in the angiogenic process. TFPI is a heparin-binding protein. Particularly, LMWH suppress the activity of the TF and release of TFPI which appear to inhibit tumor growth (Amirkhosravi et al., 2003; Bobek & Kovarik, 2004; Gasowska et al., 2009; Kuczka et al., 2009; Mousa & Petersen, 2009; Vignoli et al., 2006). Recent studies demonstrated that the inhibition of angiogenesis through the TFPI release is dependent on the molecular size of the heparin used. *Tinzaparin* (Innohep, 6.5 kDa) is especially effective at releasing TFPI (Amirkhosravi et al., 2003; Hirsh et al., 2001). Preclinical *in vitro* studies have shown that the higher the molecular weight and degree of sulfation of tinzaparin fractions, the higher the angiogenesis inhibition by control of TFPI (Mousa & Mohamed, 2004b; Mousa & Petersen, 2009; Norrby, 2006).

Several trials have confirmed clinical efficacy and tolerability of tinzaparin, including in cancer patients where tinzaparin was found more effective and as safe as warfarin (a commonly used anticoagulant) for long-term treatment (Kwaan et al., 2009). Amirkohsravi *et al.* investigated the effect of tinzaparin on long metastasis using a B16 melanoma model in experimental mice. The results indicated that administration of tinzaparin strongly inhibits tumor-associated coagulopathy and experimental metastasis. In particular, the injection of 10 mg/kg of tinzaparin significantly decreased the number of lung tumor modules from 30 with controls to only 3. Additionally, a second injection of the same dose of heparin during 14 days reduced the tumor mass by 96%. The favorable pharmacokinetic attributed to this agent compared to UFH, together with its superior ability to release TFPI for relatively long periods from vascular endothelial cells, provide a rationale for its use in oncology as a metastatic as well as an antiangiogenic agent (Amirkhosravi et al., 2003). As TF is involved in tumor angiogenesis through the regulation of VEGF expression, it could be hypothesized that heparins can interfere with the angiogenic process through TF downregulation as well (Debergh et al., 2010; Kuczka et al., 2009; Marchetti et al., 2008; Mousa & Petersen, 2009; Vignoli et al., 2006).

Other important first generation heparins are *certoparin* (6.0 kDa) (Kwaan et al., 2009; Norrby, 2006) and *reviparin* (Clivarine, 4.5 kDa) (Hirsh et al., 2001; Norrby, 2006). Tempelhoff *et al.* studied whether cancer mortality in women with previously untreated breast and pelvic cancer is reduced in those who randomly received certoparin compared to patients treated with UFH. Survival in the patients with certoparin treatment was significantly improved after 650 days for pelvic cancer. Particularly, the mortality rate was 9% in the certoparin group versus 29% in the patients with UFH treatment (Von Tempelhoff et al., 2000).

Pross *et al.* studied the influence of reviparin at different concentration (0.55, 1.10 and 2.76 mg/ml) on the intraabdominal tumor growth through *in vitro* Matrigel assay and *in vivo* experiments with rats. After application of reviparin, an important inhibition of tumor cells adhesion was observed, particularly with the highest concentration used ($1.6 \cdot 10^5$ cells were measured in the control group, whereas the number of cells were $0.36 \cdot 10^5$ with the reviparin). Moreover, the invasive potential was reduced to more than 50% for all concentrations of heparin. On the other hand, a combination of peritoneal and subcutaneous administration of reviparin reduced tumor growth in rats to higher concentrations of 4 mg/ml (Mousa & Petersen, 2009; Norrby, 2006; Pross et al., 2003).

Collen *et al.* evaluated the effects of reviparin and UFH on growth factor-induced proliferation and the formation of capillary-like tubular structures by hMVEC. Reviparin inhibited the proliferation of hMVEC induced by angiogenic factors bFGF and VEGF and affected fibrin matrix formation. Particularly, reviparin enabled the formation of more rigid and fine fibrin fibers, whereas UFH caused the formation of thick and porous fibers. These results may indicate a novel mechanism by which LMWHs affect tumor angiogenesis. However, contradictory results have been described in recent studies (Bobek & Kovarik, 2004; Collen et al., 2000; Gasowska et al., 2009; Norrby, 2006).

2.1.2 Second generation heparins

Recently, the second generation LMWHs is being investigated. These new generation of heparins are characterized by a lower mean molecular weight, a more precisely defined composition of polysaccharidic chains and better anti-Xa/anti-IIa ratio. The first generation LMWHs had between 25 and 50% of fragments with 18 or more saccharides. However, the new generation of heparins contains a significant lower percentage of long chains, improving their therapeutic action and reduce the problems of coagulation and bleeding. Moreover, these properties may lead to a more favorable behavior as regards the efficacy / safety ratio. The comparison of the properties of first and second generation heparins is shown in Figure 3 (Norrby, 2006).

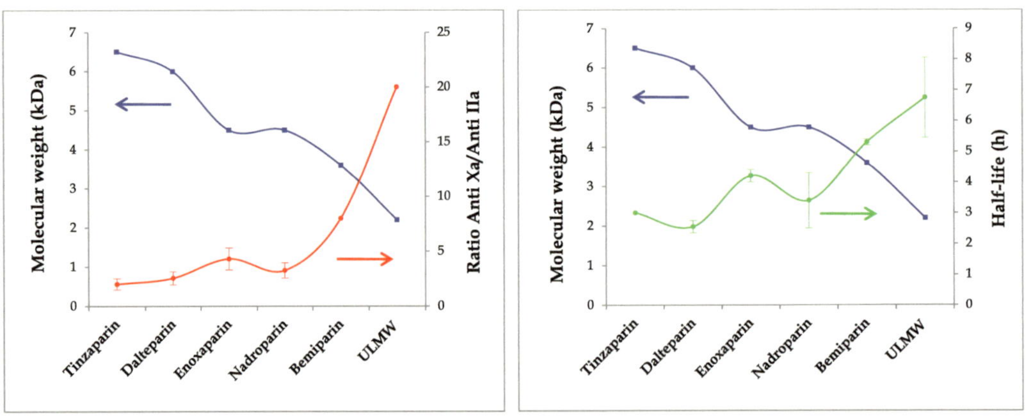

Fig. 3. Molecular weight vs antiXa/antiIIa ratio and molecular weight vs half-life.

Bemiparin (Badyket, 3.5 kDa) (Balibrea et al., 2007; Dogan et al., 2011; Jeske et al., 2011; Vignoli et al., 2011) has been available in Europe for 10 years but only recently has been evaluated in clinical trials to determine its angionenic potential in patients with cancer. The efficacy of bemiparin administration in patients limited small cell lung cancer was evaluated in the ABEL study. Randomized patients received homogeneous treatment with chemotherapy or standard treatment plus bemiparin during 26 weeks. The administration of bemiparin significantly improved the clinical outcome in patients with cancer. Particularly, after several months of treatment, 77% of the bemiparin group patients were alive compared to 20% of the control group. Moreover, significant survival advantages have been demonstrated when this molecule was co-administrated with chemotherapeutic agents.

Ultralow molecular weight heparins (ULMWH), such as *RO-14*, (2.2kDa) are currently in clinical developmental phase. The aim of these early studies is to evaluate the safety and pharmacodynamic profile of ULMWH. Rico *et al.* conducted a complete randomized study with two cohorts of volunteers to determine the pharmacodynamic properties of RO-14. The results indicated that RO-14 has a good anti-Xa activity (80-140 IU/mg), a higher half-life than other marketed LMWH (between 5 and 8 hours compared with 2 - 4 hours for dalteparin, enoxaparin or tinzaparin) and is characterized by its non-anti-IIa activity (< 10 IU/mg versus 58 IU/mg of dalteparin, for example) (Rico et al., 2011).

Since the antiangiogenic properties of heparin fractions depend on the average molecular weight and the composition of their polysaccharidic chains, it is necessary to evaluate the angiogenesis effect of the second generation heparins. According to recent studies, bemiparin and RO-14 appear to be effective in preventing and inhibiting angiogenesis in *in vitro* assays (Bosch et al., 2010).

Vignoli *et al.* determined the angiogenesis inhibition of the bemiparin and RO-14 by *in vitro* capillary-like tube formation assay in Matrigel. The experiments were performed using tumor-cell-conditioned media (TCM) from different tumor cell lines as well as growth factors (VEGF and FGF-2). In these conditions, heparins decreased tube formation induced by TCM, between 82 - 100% at 10 IU/ depending on the tumor cell line used. Moreover, capillary-like tube formation induced by growth factors was 100% inhibited at the highest concentration of heparin used. These complete results indicate a possible role of these molecules as adjuvant drugs in cancer treatment and suggest that the antiangiogenic inhibition can be remained by heparins with a lower molecular weight and shorter polysaccharidic chains (Vignoli et al., 2010; Vignoli et al., 2007; Vignoli et al., 2011).

Different authors have shown that bemiparin increases the release and activity of TFPI from endothelial cells (Planès, 2003; Sánchez-Ferrer, 2010; Vignoli et al., 2011). In addition, recent studies have demonstrated that bemiparin has a better control over this factor compared to UFH and first generation heparins such as dalteparin. (Perez-Ruiz et al., 2002; Westmuckett et al., 2001)

Westmuckett *et al.* studied the release and expression of TFPI in endothelial cells under static conditions and arterial sheer stress with the therapeutic action of bemiparin compared with dalteparin and UFH. In all experiments, bemiparin showed the most important cellular TFPI activity. On the other hand, the three types of heparin enhanced the expression of TFPI by 60 to 120% under static conditions and this increase only was possible with bemiparin under arterial stress. Perez-Ruiz *et al.* compared the TF activity of bemiparin and UFH using human umbilical vein endothelial cells (HUVEC). Samples were prepared with the addition of heparins at 1 or 10 IU/ml and measured after 2, 6, and 24 hours. Only both concentrations of UFH produced a significant enhance of TF expression.

However, conflicting data have been presented in different studies. Depasse *et al.* studied the TFPI release profiles of bemiparin and tinzaparin through their subcutaneous administration to randomized volunteers. These parameters were performed by using ELISA total and free TFPI kits. The results indicated that bemiparin experimented more rapid and potent antithrombotic (antiXa) activity but the TFPI release was significantly lower than with tinziparin. Particularly, the mean maximum free TFPI was 70 ng/ml after the injection of tinzaparin but only 30 ng/ml in the case of bemiparin. The differences in the average molecular weight and sulfation degree may influence these behaviours (Depasse et al., 2003).

Recent studies compare the angiogenic effect of the bemiparin with others first generation LMWH in the chick embryo chorioallantoic membrane (CAM) model. This *in vivo* study used different concentrations of heparins (1, 10, and 100 IU/10 μl) and measured the decrease of vessel formation using stereoscopic microscope. The results demonstrated that bemiparin, enoxaparin, nadroparin and tinzaparin have antiangiogenic effects on CAM, being more significant in high concentrations (100 IU/10 μl). Moreover, nadroparin and tinzaparin have also substantial antiangiogenic effects at the moderate concentration of 10 IU/10 μl as a result of their higher antiangiogenic potential. A possible categorization of LMWHs in this context would facilitate the choice of drug that would be used in further experimental and clinical research (Dogan et al., 2011).

Actually, new ULMWHs are investigated as *semuloparin* (2.5 kDa) with a half-life of 16-20 hours that allows one daily subcutaneous injection. It is produced using a novel depolymerization reaction with high selectivity. Jeske *et al.* compared the biological activity of semuloparin and bemiparin through coagulation and pharmacological assays. The results of this study indicated that the differences in the oligosaccharide composition and manufacturing process may influence biological activity such as protein interactions with growth factors. Moreover, these differences may translate into a different clinical safety-efficacy profile (Jeske et al., 2011).

2.2 Chemically modified heparins

Chemical modification of heparin has become a potent strategy to obtain new compounds with different biological properties from the original GAG. This is possible because of the presence of multiple functional groups susceptible of chemical modification. Heparin is a linear, polysulfated and polydispersed polysaccharide composed of β-D-glucopyranosiduronic acid (glucuronic acid, GlnA) or α-L-idopyranosiduronic acid (iduronic acid, IdoA) and *N*-acetyl or *N*-sulfo D-glucosamine (GlcN) with a (1→4) linkage. These residues are variably substituted with anionic *O*-sulfo (sulfate) and *N*-sulfo (sulfoamino) groups giving the GAG a highly negatively charge (-2.7 sulfo groups / disaccharide) (Figure 4).

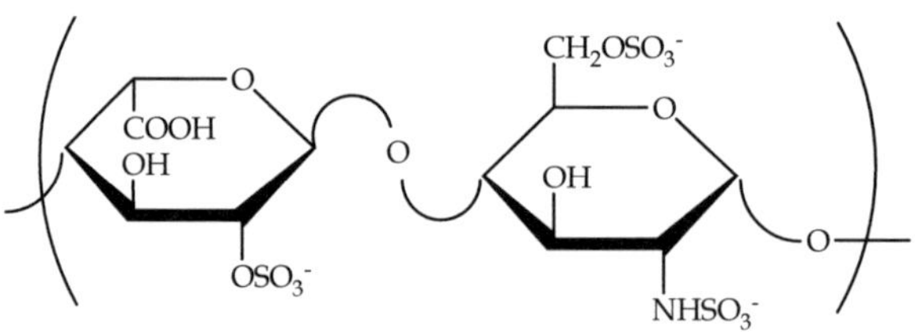

Fig. 4. Chemical structure of heparin.

Most of the attempts to modulate protein binding and biological properties of heparin have been made by the modulation of the sulfation patterns of the GAG backbone and enhance of chain flexibility of the GAG by the glycol-splitting of C2-C3 bonds of nonsulfated GlcA and IdoA residues. Both the degree of sulfation (charge density) and the appropriate distribution of *N*-sulfate and *N*-acetyl groups (charge distribution) along the heparin molecule is determinant in its biological properties. For example, the strongest protein binding was observed for 'fully sulfated' heparin and extra-sulfate groups potentiated this interaction.

Chain flexibility is thought to play a key role in heparin-protein interactions. It is conferred by IdoA-containing sequences which are considered to facilitate the appropriate orientation of substituents for the suitable interaction (Casu et al., 2002a; Casu et al., 2002b). Additional local flexibility was obtained by glycol-splitting that act as flexible joints along the heparin chain were conformation changes can be induced by the protein interaction.

Chemical modifications of heparin have been reviewed in depth by Casu *et al.* (Casu et al., 2002b) and Fernandez *et al.* (Fernåndez et al., 2006) that described the biological effect of *N*-sulfate removal, *N*-acylation of native amino groups or amino groups created after *N*-desulfation, *O*-sulfate removal, sulfation of hydroxyl groups (existing in the molecule or exposed by desulfation), acylation of unsubstituted hydroxyl groups and glycol-splitting.

Several groups have dedicated their research activity of the last decades to understand the structure-activity relationship of this molecule by its controlled chemical modification. One of the most interesting chemically modified heparins was developed by Nagi *et al.* (Naggi et al., 2005) SST0001 (= ^{100}NA-RO.H = HI2), a 100% *N*-acetylated and 25% glycol-split modified heparin (Figure 5), inhibits heparanase and presents non-anticoagulant activity and the ability to inhibit metastasis formation in various metastatic tumor animal models and activity also in human multiple myeloma models (Ritchie et al., 2011).

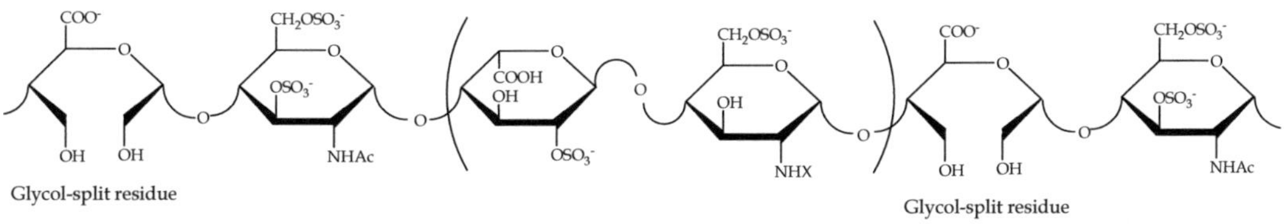

Fig. 5. Chemical structure of **SST0001 (=** ^{100}NA-RO.H = HI2), a 100% *N*-acetylated and 25% glycol-split heparin. Heparin was *N*-acetylated by time-controlled *N*-desulfation under solvolytic conditions. Glycol-split *N*-acetylated heparin was prepared by exhaustive periodate oxidation and borohydride reduction of the resulting dialdehydes.

Heparanase inhibition decreases heparin-binding growth factor release (FGF, VEGF) from ECM via HPGS degradation inhibiting the angiogenesis activity induced by these GF. Glycol-splitting causes heparin to lose affinity for antithrombin (GlcA residue in the pentasaccharide sequence of the active site for antithrombin is modified) and therefore a non-anticoagulant activity. The combination of heparanase inhibition, inhibition of ECM-bound proangiogenic growth factors release and the non-anticoagulant activity points SST0001 as potential antiangiogenic and antimetastatic agent.

Another heparinoid with negligible anticoagulant activity is ST2184 obtained by controlled nitrous acid depolymerization of undersulfated glicol-split ST1514 (Pisano et al., 2005).

2.3 Heparin-conjugates

Heparin has been conjugated to different molecules in order to obtain new drug delivery systems and scaffolds for tissue engineering with controlled angiogenic properties. In this sense, heparin has been conjugated to chemotherapeutic agents (*e.g.* paclitaxel), hydrophobic moieties (*e.g.* *N*-deoxycholyethylenediamine), thermosensitive polymers (e.g. Poloxamers) or even proteins (*e.g.* antithrombin or endostatin) in order to improve drug availability, drug targeting, heparin stability or modulate anticoagulant behaviour and angiogenic properties.

Paclitaxel is a widely used chemotherapeutic agent for the treatment of solid carcinomas. However, its clinical use is limited by its poor aqueous solubility. Several authors have been working in the preparation of new paclitaxel-heparin delivery systems with improved chemotherapy efficacy and enhanced antiangiogenic activity. In this sense, Wang *et al.* prepared amphiphilic heparin-paclitaxel prodrugs by covalent conjugation through hydrolysable bonds based on a single aminoacid spacer, either valine, leucine or phenylalanine (Y. Wang et al., 2009a; Y. Wang et al., 2009b). Heparin (hydrophilic)-paclitaxel (hydrophobic) system spontaneously self-assembled in aqueous solution forming nanoparticles with appropriate properties for drug delivery applications. These materials preserved structural integrity of paclitaxel, presented appropriate drug delivery profiles and also enhanced targeting capacity to solid tumors. Park *et al.* followed a similar strategy and conjugated heparin with paclitaxel through an amide linkage and observed comparable results (I.K. Park et al., 2010b).

A ternary conjugate *heparin-folic acid-paclitaxel*, loaded with additional paclitaxel, was developed to specifically target folate receptor that is highly expressed in several types of solid tumors, including ovarian, uterine, lung, breast, and head and neck cancers (X. Wang et al., 2009). Other ternary system that included folate has been recently developed: succinylated heparin conjugated with folate via polyethylene glycol (PEG) 1000/3000 spacers (Wang et al., 2010) or *heparin-retinoic acid-folic acid* conjugates (I.K. Park et al., 2010a). These systems displayed amphiphilic properties and formed nanoparticles capable of entrapping hydrophobic agents, such as taxol.

N-deoxycholyethylenediamine (DOCA) was covalently attached to the carboxylic acids of heparin (Park et al., 2007) or LMWH Fraxiparin (D.Y. Lee et al., 2009; J.W. Park et al., 2010) via amide formation resulting in an amphiphilic system. Heparin-DOCA derivatives presented lower anticoagulant activity, but inhibited angiogenesis both *in vitro* and in mice model and were postulated as promising drug carriers due to its amphiphilic structure. Moreover, LMWH-DOCA (D.Y. Lee et al., 2009) systems were successfully designed to be orally absorbed improving their therapeutical potential, due to DOCA (hydrophobic) enhanced the interaction between heparin and the intestinal membrane. Fraxiparin was also conjugated with *taurocholate* giving rise to helical-structured macromolecules with strong antiangiogenic activity and significant tumor growth inhibition potencial on SCC7 and MDA-MB231 human breast carcinoma cells subcutaneously injected in mice (E. Lee et al., 2009).

Tan *et al.* prepared *LMWH-endostatin* conjugates in order to obtain a synergistic effect of both endostatin (a potent endogenous angiogenesis inhibitor) and LMWH, so better antiangiogenesis and antitumor activity of the modified products was observed *in vitro* (Tan et al., 2008) and *in vivo* using the CAM assay, corneal neovascularization (CNV) assay and S_{180} tumor bearing mice (Tan et al., 2011). LMWH not only acted as a good protein modifier (the conjugates presented enhanced heat stability than endostatin, high percentage of retained activity and slight secondary structure alteration), but also played an active role in the biological activity of the resulting product.

Heparin-poloxamer-heparin conjugates were also developed giving rise to self-assembled nanoparticles with marked thermosensitivity for drug delivery (Chung et al., 2010; Tian et al., 2010).

Latent antithrombin was covalently attached to heparin and both the anticoagulant behaviour and antiangiogenic activity of the conjugate studied for its application in the treatment of the respiratory distress syndrome (Parmar et al., 2009). The conjugate exerted a selective antiproliferative effect on lung fibroblasts and the antiangiogenic effect of latent antithrombin was prevented when permanently bound to heparin. Anticoagulant activity of antithrombin was not significantly affected by the chemical modification.

2.4 Biotechnological heparins

Heparin is a heterogeneous mixture of molecules isolated from animal tissues, historically from bovine tissues and currently mostly from porcine tissues. Animal-derived pharmaceutical products represent a high risk to humans due to possible animal-to-man transmitted diseases (*e.g.* Creutzfeldt-Jacobs syndrome) and the different chemical structure and biological effect depending on the animal source, tissue and purification procedure. Moreover, heparin is a minor component in animal tissues and its purification requires high volumes of solvents and chemicals. Therefore, new routes to obtain chemically-modified heparins in high quantities and homogeneous composition were found in biotechnology (Presta et al., 2005).

K5, a bacterial polysaccharide from *Escherichia Coli*, presents the same structure as heparin biosynthetic precursor and can be tailored modified by combined chemical and enzymatic approaches giving rise to a multi-target class of biotechnological heparin/HS-like molecules. These products present different biological properties including anticoagulant/ antithrombotic, anti-AIDS and antitumor activities (antineoplastic, antiangiogenic, and antimetastatic) depending on the performed modification (Rusnati et al., 2005).

PI88 (Progen Pharmaceuticals, http://www.progen.com.au/pipeline/angiogenesis.aspx) is a phosphosulfomannanopentaose derived from the polysaccharide secreted by the yeast *P. Holstii* (Parish et al., 1999) that not only inhibits heparanase and stimulates TFPI release, but also interferes with heparin-binding growth factors inhibiting angiogenesis and metastasis. PI88 is currently being evaluated in multiple phase II clinical trials for the treatment of lung cancer (NSCLC), primary liver cancer, multiple myeloma and melanoma.

2.5 Synthetic sulfated oligosaccharides

Synthetic oligosaccharides are also under investigation as heparin-like compounds with antiangiogenic activity.

Progen Pharmaceuticals has also developed **PG500** a series of fully synthetic and fully sulfated family of single entity oligosaccharides attached to a lipophilic moiety (aglycone) at the reducing end of the molecule. These compounds inhibit FGF-1, FGF-2 and VEGF and also heparanase (Dredge et al., 2010).

Borsig *et al.* described the heparanase and selectin inhibitory effect of novel semisynthetic sulfated trimannose C-C-linked dimmers. These *sulfated hexasaccharides* mimic maltohexaose sulfate, a potent carbohydrate-based heparanase inhibitor currently subjected to phase II/III clinical trials in cancer patients (Borsig et al., 2011).

3. Synthetic heparin-like compounds

The polysulfated character of heparin suggests that polymers carring sulfonic groups could be a good strategy to sinthesize new antiangiogenic drugs.
The evolution of heparin-like synthetic drugs started in the early 90's. A polysulfonated naphthylurea (Suramin) was investigated in the inhibition of different proangiogenic factors (Danesi et al., 1993; Gagliardi et al., 1992). Based on the structure of suramin, different polysulfated and polysulfonic acid polymers were developed with capacity to interact with proangiogenic factors in similar mode to heparin (Fernández-Tornero et al., 2003; Liekens et al., 1999; Liekens et al., 1997). Actually there are different polyanionic and non-polysulfonated components under study with capacity to interact with proangiogenic factor in the same binding-site that HSPGs (Fernández et al., 2010).

3.1 Polysulfated/polysulfonated heparin-like compounds

The mechanism of action of these heparin-like drugs is based on its similarity with heparin structure. The sulfate groups of these compounds interact with different heparin-binding angiogenic factors in a similar way to heparin and inactivate it thereby preventing induction of angiogenesis.

3.1.1 Suramin

Suramin is a polysulfonated naphthylurea and an antitrypanosomal agent used since the early 1920s for the treatment of onchocerciasis and African sleeping sickness (Williamson, 1957; Williamson & Desowitz, 1956). In the early 90's suramin was investigated in the inhibition of different growth factors due to its similarity with heparin. Different researchers demonstrated the antagonism character between heparin and suramin and the capacity to inhibit different angiogenic factors by preventing their interaction with cell-surface HSPGs (Danesi et al., 1993; Gagliardi et al., 1992). This activity is due to the capacity of suramin to bind to the heparin-binding site of the proangiogenic factors via the sulfonate groups (Braddock et al., 1994; Middaugh et al., 1992).
Suramin was employed in the treatment of conventional chemotherapy unresponsive tumors (Hawkins, 1995), however high doses were necessary to achieve anti-tumor activity which developed intolerable toxicities (Collins et al., 1986; Constantopoulos et al., 1983).
In order to improve the activity of suramins and decrease its toxic-side effects, different polysulfonated naphthylureas structurally related to suramin were investigated. The results demonstrated that modifications in the backbone and the number of sufonic groups had a significant effect on angiogenesis inhibition (Manetti et al., 1998; Zamai et al., 1998). All the suramin derivatives contain the amido-*N*-methylpyrrolnaphthalenesulfonic acid group and are generally called suradistas.
Suradistas present a higher inhibition of bFGF-induced mitogenesis on fibroblasts and a higher inhibition of the neovascularization of the CAM than suramins (Hassan, 2007).

3.1.2 Pentosan polysulfate

Pentosan polysulfate (PPS) is a semi-synthetic pentasaccharide heparinoid derived from beech wood shavings. Its activity is also due to the presence of sulfonic groups that interact with different heparin-binding growth factors (Zugmaier et al., 1992). PPS has demonstrated inhibition of endothelial cell motility, tubule formation *in vitro* and capillary formation in *in vivo* assay (Nguyen et al., 1993).

PPS has been evaluated in the inhibition of cancer and Kaposi's sarcoma *in vitro* (Nakamura et al., 1992) and, also, in clinical trials phase I/II (Lush et al., 1996), but its clinical application has been limited by the high anti-coagulant activity at doses needed to inhibit the angiogenesis.

3.1.3 1,3,6-Naphthalenetrisulfonic acid

In order to decrease the toxic side-effects of suramin, different derivatives of these compounds were studied in the last years. Lozano *et al.* demonstrated that 1,3,6-naphthalenetrisulfonic acid (NTS) seem the active part of suramin (Lozano et al., 1998). In their studies showed that NTS is an effective inhibitor of the mitogenic activity of aFGF and this activity is due to the interaction with aFGF in the heparin binding-site.

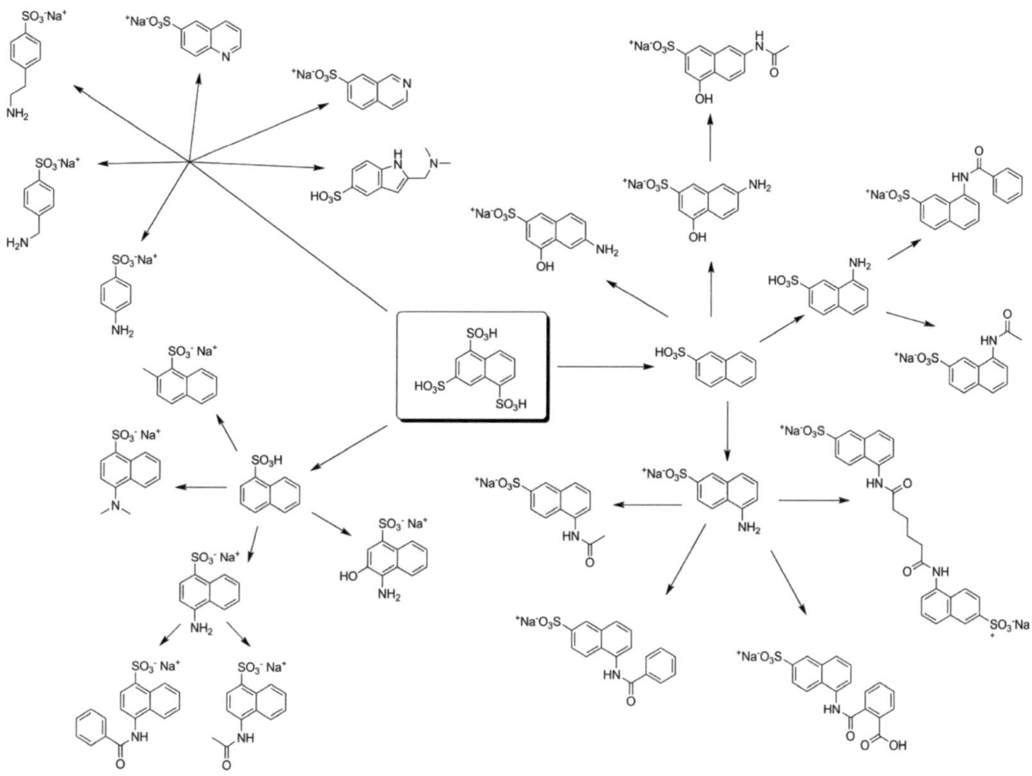

Fig. 6. NTS-based compounds studied by Fernández-Tornero *et al.*

The union of NTS to aFGF causes a displacement in the aminoacids and creates a cavity in the surface of NTS-bound aFGF. This cavity increases the solvent accessibility of this inner core and stabilizes the molecule, in this conformation the aFGF become inactive to activate the angiogenic process.

In the last years, Fernández Tornero *et al.* studied different compound derived from NTS with different numbers of sulfonic groups and substituents (Figure 6) (Fernández-Tornero et al., 2003).

5-amino-2-naphthalenesulfonic acid (ANSA) showed the best antiangiogenic activity and lower toxicity. The activity was related to the capacity to interact with heparin-binding site of FGF due to the presence of the sulfonic acid group (Figure 7). In this case ANSA binds in a 1:1 stoichiometric ratio to a positively charged cavity at the surface of FGF (some of the basic residues implicated in the interaction of this protein with heparin) by the sulfonate and the amino groups. This interaction prevents the union between FGF and heparin and inhibits the activation of angiogenic process. This compound has been recently used to synthesize new sulfonic acid-bearing polymers with antiangiogenic activity (Garcia-Fernandez et al., 2010a; Garcia-Fernandez et al., 2010b) as described in the next section.

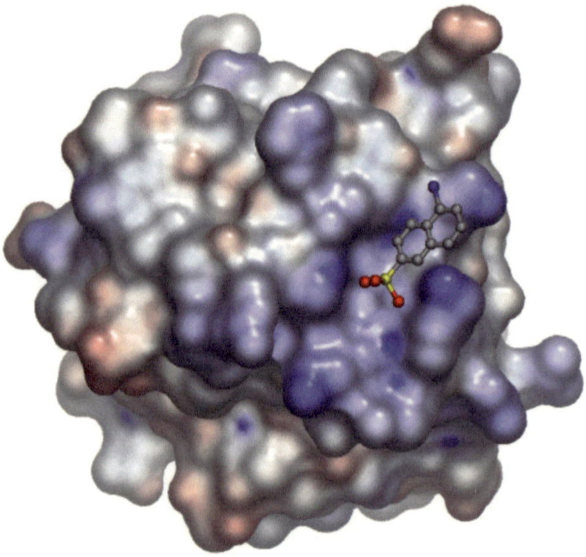

Fig. 7. A complex between acidic fibroblast growth factor and ANSA. ANSA is shown as stick-and-ball model (carbon: grey; oxygen: red; sulfur: yellow; nitrogen: blue). The figure was generated and the surfaces colored according the electrostatic potential (red, negative; blue, positive) using OpenAstexViewer (3.0; Astex Therapeutics Ltd.) and its internal parameters. PDB ID: 1HKN (Fernández-Tornero et al., 2003).

3.1.4 Sulfonic acid polymers

The synthesis of polymers with a heparin-like structure is a recent way to obtain polymers and copolymers with antiangiogenic activity. Liekens *et al.* (Bugatti et al., 2007; Liekens et al., 1999; Liekens et al., 1997) studied different sulfonic acid-bearing polymers and demonstrated their capacity to impair the binding of bFGF to HSPGs. In these studies different polymers (poly(2-acrylamido-2-methyl-1-propanesulfonic acid) (polyAMPS), poly(anetholesulfonic acid) and poly(4-styrenesulfonic acid)) showed a inhibition of the aFGF-mediated mitogenic response. The highest antiangiogenic activity was obtained for polyAMPS and the study of its intereaction with FGF showed that in the polymerization each AMPS units develops several intramolecular hydrogen bonds between adjacent acrylamido units producing a helical structure similar to heparin with the sulfonate groups spaced 9-10 Å.

In the last years García-Fernández *et al.* developed different families of new polysulfonic acid copolymers based on AMPS and a methacrylic derivative of ANSA (MANSA) (Garcia-

Fernandez et al., 2010a; Garcia-Fernandez et al., 2010b; Garcia-Fernandez et al., 2010c). Two different families of copolymers with *N*-vinylpyrrolidone (hydrophilic, VP) and butylacrylate (hydrophobic, BA) were synthesised in order to obtain different properties in aqueous media. The highest antiangiogenic activity was obtained for the hydrophobic MANSA copolymers (poly(BA-*co*-MANSA)) due to the formation of an interesting micellar morphology by self-assembling with the hydrophilic MANSA units located on the surface of the micelle. This organization provides an optimal orientation of the sulfonic acid groups for the interaction with the growth factor. This gives an increasing inhibitory bioactivity of the poly(BA-*co*-MANSA) with the concentration.

3.2 Other polyanionic compounds

Besides the molecules described above, various non-sulfated polyanionic compounds have been investigated. For example, aurintricarboxylic acid (Figure 8) showed inhibition of heparin-stimulated angiogenesis in the CAM (Gagliardi & Collins, 1994) or RG-13577 (a linear polymer of carboxylated phenol-based monomers) prevented microvessel outgrowth from rat aortic rings embedded in a collagen gel (Miao et al., 1997).

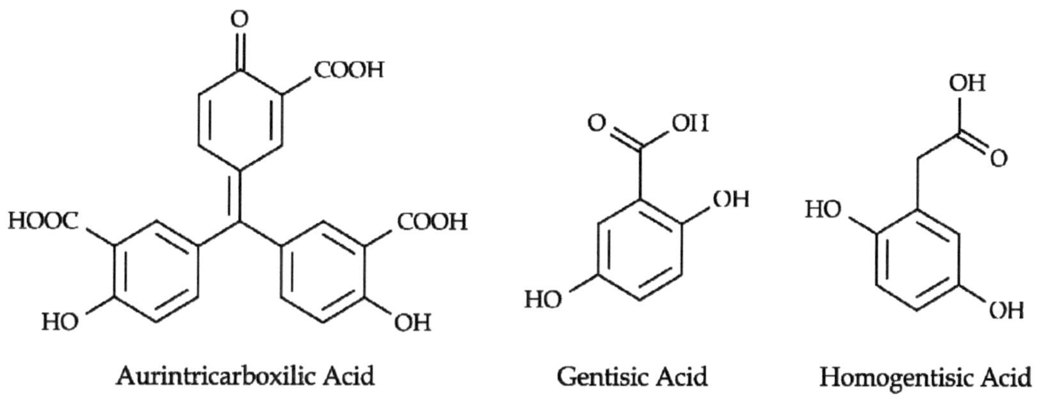

Fig. 8. Polyanionic compounds with antiangiogenic activity (aurintricarboxylic acid, gentisic acid and homogentisic acid).

But the most promising polyanionic compounds are gentisic (a widespread plant secondary metabolite, GA) and homogentisic acid (the toxic agent in alkaptonuria, HGA) (Fernández et al., 2010) (Figure 8).

These compounds present higher antiangiogenic activity than ANSA and other sulfonic compounds both *in vivo* and *in vitro*. Both, GA and HGA bind in a 1:1 stoichiometric ratio to a positively charged cavity at the surface of FGF (part of the long cationic hearing-binding site) (Figure 9).

ANSA, GA, and HGA bind to the same site, these results were unexpected because these compounds are chemically unrelated. The relative positions of the hydroxyl groups in the aromatic ring stabilized the molecules by a network of non-covalent contacts. This inactivates FGF and blocks FGF-dependent angiogenesis.

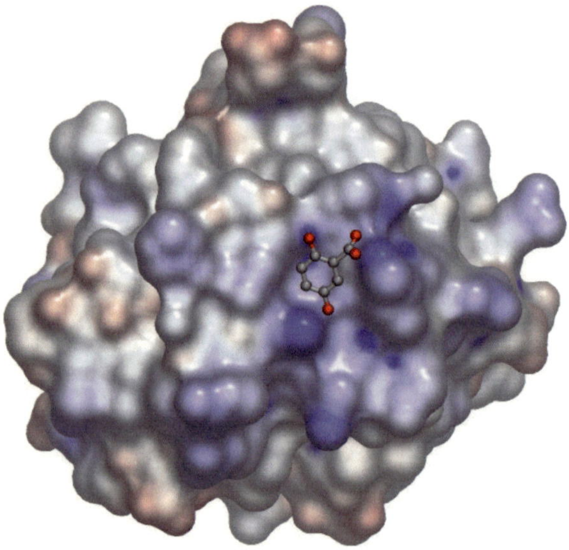

Fig. 9. A complex between acidic fibroblast growth factor and GA. GA is shown as stick-and-ball model (carbon: grey; oxygen: red). The figure was generated and the surfaces colored according the electrostatic potential (red, negative; blue, positive) using OpenAstexViewer (3.0; Astex Therapeutics Ltd.) and its internal parameters. PDB ID: 3JUT (Fernández et al., 2010).

4. Conclusions

Heparin-like molecules that inhibit proangiogenic molecules through heparin-binding domains constitute an effective tool for the design of broad-spectrum antiangiogenic drugs. Different types of these molecules were described in this chapter, *i.e.* heparin species (heparinoids, chemically modified heparins, heparin conjugates, biotechnological heparins, and synthetic sulfated oligosaccharides) and synthetic heparin-like compounds. Both offer endless possibilities for the development of optimized antiangiogenic drugs using the organic chemistry procedures.

On the one hand, numerous heparin species have demonstrated their antiangiogenic activity, however it depends on a great number of factors like molecular weight, composition (saccharide units concentration), physicochemical properties (such as flexibility), charge density (degree of sulfation) and charge distribution, chemical modification, conjugated molecule, etc. Currently, for example, it is unknown which commercial LMWH and ULMWH have the greatest antiangiogenic effect in cancer patients. Therefore, systematic experimental studies of the angiogenesis-modulating effect of heparin species and comparative and complete clinical studies are needed in the future (Debergh et al., 2010; Dogan et al., 2011; Mousa & Petersen, 2009; Norrby, 2006).

On the other hand, synthetic heparin like compounds have been developed using systematic routines in order to rationally identify the best activity/toxicity ratio. However, few of these products are currently in clinical trials and still need FDA approval.

5. References

Akl, E.A., Rohilla, S., Barba, M., Sperati, F., Terrenato, I., Muti, P., Bdair, F. & Schünemann, H.J. (2008). Anticoagulation for the initial treatment of venous thromboembolism in patients with cancer: a systematic review. *Cancer,* Vol. 113, No. 7, pp. 1685-1694

Alitalo, K., Tammela, T. & Petrova, T.V. (2005). Lymphangiogenesis in development and human disease. *Nature,* Vol. 438, No. 7070, pp. 946-953

Amirkhosravi, A., Mousa, S.A., Amaya, M. & Francis, J.L. (2003). Antimetastatic effect of tinzaparin, a low-molecular-weight heparin. *Journal of thrombosis and haemostasis : JTH,* Vol. 1, No. 9, pp. 1972-1976

Balibrea, J.L., Altimiras, J., Larruzea, I., Gómez-Outes, A., Martínez-González, J. & Rocha, E. (2007). Optimal dosing of bemiparin as prophylaxis against venous thromboembolism in surgery for cancer: An audit of practice. *International Journal of Surgery,* Vol. 5, No. 2, pp. 114-119

Bick, R.L. (2006). Cancer-associated thrombosis: Focus on extended therapy with dalteparin. *Journal of Supportive Oncology,* Vol. 4, No. 3, pp. 115-119

Bobek, V. & Kovarik, J. (2004). Antitumor and antimetastatic effect of warfarin and heparins. *Biomedicine and Pharmacotherapy,* Vol. 58, No. 4, pp. 213-219

Borsig, L. (2010). Antimetastatic activities of heparins and modified heparins. Experimental evidence. *Thrombosis Research,* Vol. 125, No. Supplement 2, pp. S66-S71

Borsig, L., Vlodavsky, I., Ishai-Michaeli, R., Torri, G. & Vismara, E. (2011). Sulfated hexasaccharides attenuate metastasis by inhibition of p-selectin and heparanase. *Neoplasia,* Vol. 13, No. 5, pp. 445-452

Bosch, M.M., Vignoli, A., Villamediana, R.L. & Prandoni, P. (2010). Bemiparin in oncology. *Drugs,* Vol. 70, No. SUPPL. 2, pp. 35-42

Braddock, P.S., Hu, D.E., Fan, T.P.D., Stratford, I.J., Harris, A.L. & Bicknell, R. (1994). A structure-activity analysis of antagonism of the growth factor and angiogenic activity of basic fibroblast growth factor by suramin and related polyanions. *British Journal of Cancer,* Vol. 69, No. 5, pp. 890-898

Bugatti, A., Urbinati, C., Ravelli, C., De Clercq, E., Liekens, S. & Rusnati, M. (2007). Heparin-mimicking sulfonic acid polymers as multitarget inhibitors of human immunodeficiency virus type 1 Tat and gp120 proteins. *Antimicrobial Agents and Chemotherapy,* Vol. 51, No. 7, pp. 2337-2345

Casu, B., Guerrini, M., Naggi, A., Perez, M., Torri, G., Ribatti, D., Carminati, P., Giannini, G., Penco, S., Pisano, C., Belleri, M., Rusnati, M. & Presta, M. (2002a). Short heparin sequences spaced by glycol-split uronate residues are antagonists of Fibroblast Growth Factor 2 and angiogenesis inhibitors. *Biochemistry,* Vol. 41, No. 33, pp. 10519-10528

Casu, B., Naggi, A. & Torri, G. (2002b). Chemical derivatization as a strategy to study structure-activity relationships of glycosaminoglycans. *Seminars in Thrombosis and Hemostasis,* Vol. 28, No. 4, pp. 335-342

Collen, A., Smorenburg, S.M., Peters, E., Lupu, F., Koolwijk, P., Van Noorden, C. & Van Hinsbergh, V.W.M. (2000). Unfractionated and low molecular weight heparin affect fibrin structure and angiogenesis in Vitro. *Cancer Research,* Vol. 60, No. 21, pp. 6196-6200

Collins, J.M., Klecker Jr, R.W. & Yarchoan, R. (1986). Clinical pharmacokinetics of suramin in patients with HTLV-III/LAV infection. *Journal of Clinical Pharmacology,* Vol. 26, No. 1, pp. 22-26

Constantopoulos, G., Rees, S., Barranger, J.A. & Brady, R.O. (1983). Suramin-induced storage disease. Mucopolysaccharidosis. *American Journal of Pathology,* Vol. 113, No. 2, pp. 266-268

Coultas, L., Chawengsaksophak, K. & Rossant, J. (2005). Endothelial cells and VEGF in vascular development. *Nature,* Vol. 438, No. 7070, pp. 937-945

Chung, Y.I., Kim, J.C., Kim, Y.H., Tae, G., Lee, S.Y., Kim, K. & Kwon, I.C. (2010). The effect of surface functionalization of PLGA nanoparticles by heparin- or chitosan-conjugated Pluronic on tumor targeting. *Journal of Controlled Release,* Vol. 143, No. 3, pp. 374-382

Danesi, R., Del Bianchi, S., Soldani, P., Campagni, A., La Roccas, R.V., Myers, C.E., Paparelli, A. & Del Tacca, M. (1993). Suramin inhibits bFGF-induced endothelial cell proliferation and angiogenesis in the chick chorioallantoic membrane. *British Journal of Cancer,* Vol. 68, No. 5, pp. 932-938

Debergh, I., Van Damme, N., Pattyn, P., Peeters, M. & Ceelen, W.P. (2010). The low-molecular-weight heparin, nadroparin, inhibits tumour angiogenesis in a rodent dorsal skinfold chamber model. *British Journal of Cancer,* Vol. 102, No. 5, pp. 837-843

Depasse, F., González de Suso, M.J., Lagoutte, I., Fontcuberta, J., Borrell, M. & Samama, M.M. (2003). Comparative study of the pharmacokinetic profiles of two LMWHs--bemiparin (3500 IU, anti-Xa) and tinzaparin (4500 IU, anti-Xa)--administered subcutaneously to healthy male volunteers. *Thrombosis Research,* Vol. 109, No. 2-3, pp. 109-117

DiGabriele, A.D., Lax, I., Chen, D.I., Svahn, C.M., Jaye, M., Schlessinger, J. & Hendrickson, W.A. (1998). Structure of a heparin-linked biologically active dimer of fibroblast growth factor. *Nature,* Vol. 393, No. 6687, pp. 812-817

Dogan, O.T., Polat, Z.A., Karahan, O., Epozturk, K., Altun, A., Akkurt, I. & Cetin, A. (2011). Antiangiogenic activities of bemiparin sodium, enoxaparin sodium, nadroparin calcium and tinzaparin sodium. *Thrombosis Research,* Vol. In Press, Corrected Proof, No. pp.

Dredge, K., Hammond, E., Davis, K., Li, C.P., Liu, L., Johnstone, K., Handley, P., Wimmer, N., Gonda, T.J., Gautam, A., Ferro, V. & Bytheway, I. (2010). The PG500 series: Novel heparan sulfate mimetics as potent angiogenesis and heparanase inhibitors for cancer therapy. *Investigational New Drugs,* Vol. 28, No. 3, pp. 276-283

Fernández-Tornero, C., Lozano, R.M., Redondo-Horcajo, M., Gómez, A.M., López, J.C., Quesada, E., Uriel, C., Valverdell, S., Cuevas, P., Romero, A. & Giménez-Gallego, G. (2003). Leads for development of new naphthalenesulfonate derivatives with enhanced antiangiogenic activity. Crystal structure of acidic fibroblast growth factor in complex with 5-amino-2-naphthalenesulfonate. *Journal of Biological Chemistry,* Vol. 278, No. 24, pp. 21774-21781

Fernández, C., Hattan, C.M. & Kerns, R.J. (2006). Semi-synthetic heparin derivatives: chemical modifications of heparin beyond chain length, sulfate substitution pattern and N-sulfo/N-acetyl groups. *Carbohydrate Research,* Vol. 341, No. 10, pp. 1253-1265

Fernández, I.S., Cuevas, P., Angulo, J., López-Navajas, P., Canales-Mayordomo, Á., González-Corrochano, R., Lozano, R.M., Valverde, S., Jiménez-Barbero, J., Romero,

A. & Giménez-Gallego, G. (2010). Gentisic acid, a compound associated with plant defense and a metabolite of aspirin, heads a new class of in vivo fibroblast growth factor inhibitors. *Journal of Biological Chemistry,* Vol. 285, No. 15, pp. 11714-11729

Ferrara, N. (2004). Vascular Endothelial Growth Factor as a Target for Anticancer Therapy. *The Oncologist,* Vol. 9, No. suppl 1, pp. 2-10

Folkman, J. (1971). Tumor angiogenesis: therapeutic implications. *New England Journal of Medicine,* Vol. 285, No. 21, pp. 1182-1186

Folkman, J. (1990). What is the evidence that tumors are angiogenesis dependent? *Journal of the National Cancer Institute,* Vol. 82, No. 1, pp. 4-6

Folkman, J. (1995). Angiogenesis in cancer, vascular, rheumatoid and other disease. *Nature Medicine,* Vol. 1, No. 1, pp. 27-31

Gagliardi, A., Hadd, H. & Collins, D.C. (1992). Inhibition of angiogenesis by suramin. *Cancer Research,* Vol. 52, No. 18, pp. 5073-5075

Gagliardi, A.R.T. & Collins, D.C. (1994). Inhibition of angiogenesis by aurintricarboxylic acid. *Anticancer Research,* Vol. 14, No. 2 A, pp. 475-479

Garcia-Fernandez, L., Aguilar, M.R., Fernandez, M.M., Lozano, R.M., Gimenez, G. & San Roman, J. (2010a). Antimitogenic Polymer Drugs Based on AMPS: Monomer Distribution−Bioactivity Relationship of Water-Soluble Macromolecules. *Biomacromolecules,* Vol. 11, No. 3, pp. 626-634

Garcia-Fernandez, L., Aguilar, M.R., Fernandez, M.M., Lozano, R.M., Gimenez, G., Valverde, S. & San Roman J. (2010b). Structure, Morphology, and Bioactivity of Biocompatible Systems Derived from Functionalized Acrylic Polymers Based on 5-Amino-2-naphthalene Sulfonic Acid. *Biomacromolecules,* Vol. 11, No. 7, pp. 1763-1772

Garcia-Fernandez, L., Halstenberg, S., Unger, R.E., Aguilar, M.R., Kirkpatrick, C.J. & San Roman, J. (2010c). Anti-angiogenic activity of heparin-like polysulfonated polymeric drugs in 3D human cell culture. *Biomaterials,* Vol. 31, No. 31, pp. 7863-7872

Gasowska, K., Naumnik, B., Klejna, K. & Mysliwiec, M. (2009). The influence of unfractionated and low-molecular weight heparins on the properties of human umbilical vein endothelial cells (HUVEC). *Folia Histochemica et Cytobiologica,* Vol. 47, No. 1, pp. 17-23

Grande, C. & Caparro, M. (2005). Use of Low-Molecular-Weight Heparins in the Treatment and Secondary Prevention of Cancer-Associated Thrombosis. *Seminars in Oncology Nursing,* Vol. 21, No. 4, Supplement 1, pp. 41-49

Hassan, H.H.A.M. (2007). Chemistry and biology of heparin mimetics that bind to fibroblast growth factors. *Mini-Reviews in Medicinal Chemistry,* Vol. 7, No. 12, pp. 1206-1235

Hawkins, M.J. (1995). Clinical trials of antiangiogenic agents. *Current Opinion in Oncology,* Vol. 7, No. 1, pp. 90-93

Hirsh, J., Warkentin, T.E., Shaughnessy, S.G., Anand, S.S., Halperin, J.L., Raschke, R., Granger, C., Ohman, E.M. & Dalen, J.E. (2001). Heparin and Low-Molecular-Weight Heparin Mechanisms of Action, Pharmacokinetics, Dosing, Monitoring, Efficacy, and Safety. *Chest,* Vol. 119, No. 1 suppl, pp. 64S-94S

Jeske, W.P., Hoppensteadt, D., Gray, A., Walenga, J.M., Cunanan, J., Myers, L., Fareed, J., Bayol, A., Rigal, H. & Viskov, C. (2011). A common standard is inappropriate for determining the potency of ultra low molecular weight heparins such as semuloparin and bemiparin. *Thrombosis Research,* Vol. 128, No. 4, pp. 361-367

Kakkar, A.K. (2004). Low- and ultra-low-molecular-weight heparins. *Best Practice and Research: Clinical Haematology,* Vol. 17, No. 1, pp. 77-87

Kakkar, A.K., Levine, M.N., Kadziola, Z., Lemoine, N.R., Low, V., Patel, H.K., Rustin, G., Thomas, M., Quigley, M. & Williamson, R.C.N. (2004). Low molecular weight heparin, therapy with dalteparin, and survival in advanced cancer: The fragmin advanced malignancy outcome study (FAMOUS). *Journal of Clinical Oncology,* Vol. 22, No. 10, pp. 1944-1948

Khorana, A.A., Sahni, A., Altland, O.D. & Francis, C.W. (2003). Heparin Inhibition of Endothelial Cell Proliferation and Organization Is Dependent on Molecular Weight. *Arteriosclerosis, Thrombosis, and Vascular Biology,* Vol. 23, No. 11, pp. 2110-2115

Klerk, C.P.W., Smorenburg, S.M., Otten, H.M., Lensing, A.W.A., Prins, M.H., Piovella, F., Prandoni, P., Bos, M.M.E.M., Richel, D.J., Van Tienhoven, G. & Büller, H.R. (2005). The effect of low molecular weight heparin on survival in patients with advanced malignancy. *Journal of Clinical Oncology,* Vol. 23, No. 10, pp. 2130-2135

Kuczka, K., Baum, K., Picard-Willems, B. & Harder, S. (2009). Long term administration of LMWH - pharmacodynamic parameters under therapeutic or prophylactic regimen of enoxaparin or tinzaparin in neurological rehabilitation patients. *Thrombosis Research,* Vol. 124, No. 5, pp. 625-630

Kwaan, H.C., Green, D., Pineo, G.F. & Hull, R.D. (2009) Effects of Anticoagulants on Cancer: Heparins. in *Coagulation in Cancer (*Rosen, S.T. ed.), Springer US. pp 259-275

Lee, D.Y., Lee, S.W., Kim, S.K., Lee, M., Chang, H.W., Moon, H.T., Byun, Y. & Kim, S.Y. (2009). Antiangiogenic activity of orally absorbable heparin derivative in different types of cancer cells. *Pharmaceutical Research,* Vol. 26, No. 12, pp. 2667-2676

Lee, E., Kim, Y.S., Bae, S.M., Kim, S.K., Jin, S., Chung, S.W., Lee, M., Moon, H.T., Jeon, O.C., Park, R.W., Kim, I.S., Byun, Y. & Kim, S.Y. (2009). Polyproline-type helical-structured low-molecular weight heparin (LMWH)-taurocholate conjugate as a new angiogenesis inhibitor. *International Journal of Cancer,* Vol. 124, No. 12, pp. 2755-2765

Liekens, S., Leali, D., Neyts, J., Esnouf, R., Rusnati, M., Dell'era, P., Maudgal, P.C., De Clercq, E. & Presta, M. (1999). Modulation of fibroblast growth factor-2 receptor binding, signaling, and mitogenic activity by heparin-mimicking polysulfonated compounds. *Molecular Pharmacology,* Vol. 56, No. 1, pp. 204-213

Liekens, S., Neyts, J., ve, B. & De Clercq, E. (1997). The sulfonic acid polymers PAMPS [Poly (2-acrylamido-2-methyl-1-propanesuifonie acid)] and related analogues are highly potent inhibitors of angiogenesis. *Oncology Research,* Vol. 9, No. 4, pp. 173-181

Lindahl, U., Lidholt, K., Spillmann, D. & Kjellen, L. (1994). More to 'heparin' than anticoagulation. *Thrombosis Research,* Vol. 75, No. 1, pp. 1-32

Lozano, R.M., Jiménez, M.Á., Santoro, J., Rico, M. & Giménez-Gallego, G. (1998). Solution structure of acidic fibroblast growth factor bound to 1,3,6-naphthalenetrisulfonate: A minimal model for the anti-tumoral action of suramins and suradistas. *Journal of Molecular Biology,* Vol. 281, No. 5, pp. 899-915

Lush, R.M., Figg, W.D., Pluda, J.M., Bitton, R., Headlee, D., Kohler, D., Reed, E., Sartor, O. & Cooper, M.R. (1996). A phase I study of pentosan polysulfate sodium in patients with advanced malignancies. *Annals of Oncology,* Vol. 7, No. 9, pp. 939-944

Manetti, F., Cappello, V., Botta, M., Corelli, F., Mongelli, N., Biasoli, G., Borgia, A.L. & Ciomei, M. (1998). Synthesis and binding mode of heterocyclic analogues of suramin inhibiting the human basic fibroblast growth factor. *Bioorganic and Medicinal Chemistry,* Vol. 6, No. 7, pp. 947-958

Marchetti, M., Vignoli, A., Russo, L., Balducci, D., Pagnoncelli, M., Barbui, T. & Falanga, A. (2008). Endothelial capillary tube formation and cell proliferation induced by tumor cells are affected by low molecular weight heparins and unfractionated heparin. *Thrombosis Research,* Vol. 121, No. 5, pp. 637-645

Miao, H.Q., Ornitz, D.M., Aingorn, E., Ben-Sasson, S.A. & Vlodavsky, I. (1997). Modulation of fibroblast growth factor-2 receptor binding, dimerization, signaling, and angiogenic activity by a synthetic heparin-mimicking polyanionic compound. *Journal of Clinical Investigation,* Vol. 99, No. 7, pp. 1565-1575

Middaugh, C.R., Mach, H., Burke, C.J., Volkin, D.B., Dabora, J.M., Tsai, P.K., Bruner, M.W., Ryan, J.A. & Marfia, K.E. (1992). Nature of the interaction of growth factors with suramin. *Biochemistry,* Vol. 31, No. 37, pp. 9016-9024

Mousa, S.A. & Mohamed, S. (2004a). Anti-angiogenic mechanisms and efficacy of the low molecular weight heparin, tinzaparin: anti-cancer efficacy. *Oncology reports,* Vol. 12, No. 4, pp. 683-688

Mousa, S.A. & Mohamed, S. (2004b). Inhibition of endothelial cell tube formation by the low molecular weight heparin, tinzaparin, is mediated by tissue factor pathway inhibitor. *Thrombosis and Haemostasis,* Vol. 92, No. 3, pp. 627-633

Mousa, S.A. & Petersen, L.J. (2009). Anti-cancer properties of low-molecular-weight heparin: Preclinical evidence. *Thrombosis and Haemostasis,* Vol. 102, No. 2, pp. 258-267

Naggi, A., Casu, B., Perez, M., Torri, G., Cassinelli, G., Penco, S., Pisano, C., Giannini, G., Ishai-Michaeli, R. & Vlodavsky, I. (2005). Modulation of the heparanase-inhibiting activity of heparin through selective desulfation, graded N-acetylation, and glycol splitting. *Journal of Biological Chemistry,* Vol. 280, No. 13, pp. 12103-12113

Nakamura, S., Sakurada, S., Zaki Salahuddin, S., Osada, Y., Tanaka, N.G., Sakamoto, N., Sekiguchi, M. & Gallo, R.C. (1992). Inhibition of development of Kaposi's sarcoma-related lesions by a bacterial cell wall complex. *Science,* Vol. 255, No. 5050, pp. 1437-1440

Nguyen, N.M., Lehr, J.E. & Pienta, K.J. (1993). Pentosan inhibits angiogenesis in vitro and suppresses prostate tumor growth in vivo. *Anticancer Research,* Vol. 13, No. 6 A, pp. 2143-2147

Norrby, K. (2000). 2.5 kDa and 5.0 kDa heparin fragments specifically inhibit microvessel sprouting and network formation in VEFG165-mediated mammalian angiogenesis. *International Journal of Experimental Pathology,* Vol. 81, No. 3, pp. 191-198

Norrby, K. (2006). Low-molecular-weight heparins and angiogenesis. *APMIS,* Vol. 114, No. 2, pp. 79-102

Norrby, K. & Nordenhem, A. (2010). Dalteparin, a low-molecular-weight heparin, promotes angiogenesis mediated by heparin-binding VEGF-A in vivo. *APMIS,* Vol. 118, No. 12, pp. 949-957

Parish, C.R., Freeman, C., Brown, K.J., Francis, D.J. & Cowden, W.B. (1999). Identification of sulfated oligosaccharide-based inhibitors of tumor growth and metastasis using novel in vitro assays for angiogenesis and heparanase activity. *Cancer Research,* Vol. 59, No. 14, pp. 3433-3441

Park, I.K., Kim, Y.J., Huh, K.M. & Lee, Y.K. (2010a). Preparation and characterization of heparin-retinoic acid-folic acid conjugates for targeted cancer therapy. *Advanced Materials Research,* Vol. 93-94, No. pp. 324-327

Park, I.K., Kim, Y.J., Tran, T.H., Huh, K.M. & Lee, Y.K. (2010b). Water-soluble heparin-PTX conjugates for cancer targeting. *Polymer,* Vol. 51, No. 15, pp. 3387-3393

Park, J.W., Jeon, O.C., Kim, S.K., Al-Hilal, T.A., Jin, S.J., Moon, H.T., Yang, V.C., Kim, S.Y. & Byun, Y. (2010). High antiangiogenic and low anticoagulant efficacy of orally active low molecular weight heparin derivatives. *Journal of Controlled Release,* Vol. 148, No. 3, pp. 317-326

Park, K., Kim, Y.S., Lee, G.Y., Nam, J.O., Lee, S.K., Park, R.W., Kim, S.Y., Kim, I.S. & Byun, Y. (2007). Antiangiogenic effect of bile acid acylated heparin derivative. *Pharmaceutical Research,* Vol. 24, No. 1, pp. 176-185

Parmar, N., Berry, L.R., Post, M. & Chan, A.K.C. (2009). Effect of covalent antithrombin-heparin complex on developmental mechanisms in the lung. *American Journal of Physiology - Lung Cellular and Molecular Physiology,* Vol. 296, No. 3, pp. L394-L403

Perez-Ruiz, A., Montes, R., Carrasco, P. & Rocha, E. (2002). Effects of a low molecular weight heparin, Bemiparin, and unfractionated heparin on hemostatic properties of endothelium. *Clinical and Applied Thrombosis/Hemostasis,* Vol. 8, No. 1, pp. 65-71

Pisano, C., Aulicino, C., Vesci, L., Casu, B., Naggi, A., Torri, G., Ribatti, D., Belleri, M., Rusnati, M. & Presta, M. (2005). Undersulfated, low-molecular-weight glycol-split heparin as an antiangiogenic VEGF antagonist. *Glycobiology,* Vol. 15, No. 2, pp. 1C-6C

Planès, A. (2003). Review of bemiparin sodium - A new second-generation low molecular weight heparin and its applications in venous thromboembolism. *Expert Opinion on Pharmacotherapy,* Vol. 4, No. 9, pp. 1551-1561

Presta, M., Oreste, P., Zoppetti, G., Belleri, M., Tanghetti, E., Leali, D., Urbinati, C., Bugatti, A., Ronca, R., Nicoli, S., Moroni, E., Stabile, H., Camozzi, M., Hernandez, G.A., Mitola, S., Dell'Era, P., Rusnati, M. & Ribatti, D. (2005). Antiangiogenic activity of semisynthetic biotechnological heparins: Low-molecular-weight-sulfated Escherichia coli K5 polysaccharide derivatives as fibroblast growth factor antagonists. *Arteriosclerosis, Thrombosis, and Vascular Biology,* Vol. 25, No. 1, pp. 71-76

Pross, M., Lippert, H., Misselwitz, F., Nestler, G., Krüger, S., Langer, H., Halangk, W. & Schulz, H.-U. (2003). Low-molecular-weight heparin (reviparin) diminishes tumor cell adhesion and invasion in vitro, and decreases intraperitoneal growth of colonadeno-carcinoma cells in rats after laparoscopy. *Thrombosis Research,* Vol. 110, No. 4, pp. 215-220

Rico, S., Antonijoan, R.M., Gich, I., Borrell, M., Fontcuberta, J., Monreal, M., Martinez-Gonzalez, J. & Barbanoj, M.J. (2011). Safety Assessment and Pharmacodynamics of a Novel Ultra Low Molecular Weight Heparin (RO-14) in Healthy Volunteers - A First-Time-In-Human Single Ascending Dose Study. *Thrombosis Research,* Vol. 127, No. 4, pp. 292-298

Ritchie, J.P., Ramani, V.C., Ren, Y., Naggi, A., Torri, G., Casu, B., Penco, S., Pisano, C., Carminati, P., Tortoreto, M., Zunino, F., Vlodavsky, I., Sanderson, R.D. & Yang, Y. (2011). SST0001, a chemically modified heparin, inhibits myeloma growth and angiogenesis via disruption of the heparanase/syndecan-1 axis. *Clinical Cancer Research,* Vol. 17, No. 6, pp. 1382-1393

Robert, F. (2010). The potential benefits of low-molecular-weight heparins in cancer patients. *Journal of Hematology and Oncology,* Vol. 3, No. 3, pp. 1-12

Rusnati, M., Oreste, P., Zoppetti, G. & Presta, M. (2005). Biotechnological engineering of heparin/heparan sulphate: A novel area of multi-target drug discovery. *Current Pharmaceutical Design,* Vol. 11, No. 19, pp. 2489-2499

Sánchez-Ferrer, C.F. (2010). Bemiparin: Pharmacological profile. *Drugs,* Vol. 70, No. SUPPL. 2, pp. 19-23

Sideras, K., Schaefer, P.L., Okuno, S.H., Sloan, J.A., Kutteh, L., Fitch, T.R., Dakhil, S.R., Levitt, R., Alberts, S.R., Morton, R.F., Rowland, K.M., Novotny, P.J. & Loprinzi, C.L. (2006). Low-molecular-weight heparin in patients with advanced cancer: A phase 3 clinical trial. *Mayo Clinic Proceedings,* Vol. 81, No. 6, pp. 758-767

Takahashi, H., Ebihara, S., Okazaki, T., Asada, M., Sasaki, H. & Yamaya, M. (2005). A comparison of the effects of unfractionated heparin, dalteparin and danaparoid on vascular endothelial growth factor-induced tumour angiogenesis and heparanase activity. *British Journal of Pharmacology,* Vol. 146, No. 3, pp. 333-343

Tan, H., Mu, G., Zhu, W., Liu, J. & Wang, F. (2011). Down-regulation of vascular endothelial growth factor and up-regulation of pigment epithelium derived factor make low molecular weight heparin-endostatin and polyethylene glycol-endostatin potential candidates for anti-angiogenesis drug. *Biological and Pharmaceutical Bulletin,* Vol. 34, No. 4, pp. 545-550

Tan, H., Yang, S., Feng, Y., Liu, C., Cao, J., Mu, G. & Wang, F. (2008). Characterization and secondary structure analysis of endostatin covalently modified by polyethylene glycol and low molecular weight heparin. *Journal of Biochemistry,* Vol. 144, No. 2, pp. 207-213

Thodiyil, P. & Kakkar, A.K. (2002). Can low-molecular-weight heparins improve outcome in patients with cancer? *Cancer Treatment Reviews,* Vol. 28, No. 3, pp. 151-155

Tian, J.L., Zhao, Y.Z., Jin, Z., Lu, C.T., Tang, Q.Q., Xiang, Q., Sun, C.Z., Zhang, L., Xu, Y.Y., Gao, H.S., Zhou, Z.C., Li, X.K. & Zhang, Y. (2010). Synthesis and characterization of Poloxamer 188-grafted heparin copolymer. *Drug Development and Industrial Pharmacy,* Vol. 36, No. 7, pp. 832-838

Vignoli, A., Marchetti, M., Balducci, D., Barbui, T. & Falanga, A. (2006). Differential effect of the low-molecular-weight heparin, dalteparin, and unfractionated heparin on microvascular endothelial cell hemostatic properties. *Haematologica,* Vol. 91, No. 2, pp. 207-214

Vignoli, A., Marchetti, M., Cantalino, E., Diani, E., Bonacina, G. & Falanga, A. (2010). Very low molecular weight heparins (LMWH) retain the capacity to inhibit endothelial cell migration and capillary-like tube formation induced by tumor cells. *Thrombosis Research,* Vol. 125, No. Supplement 2, pp. S191-S191

Vignoli, A., Marchetti, M., Cantalino, E., Russo, L., Balducci, D. & Falanga, A. (2007). Low-molecular weight heparin (LMWH) bemiparin and ultra-low-MWH RO-14 inhibit lung, breast and leukemia cancer cell-induced endothelial angiogenesis. *Thrombosis Research,* Vol. 120, No. Supplement 2, pp. S149-S149

Vignoli, A., Marchetti, M., Russo, L., Cantalino, E., Diani, E., Bonacina, G. & Falanga, A. (2011). LMWH bemiparin and ULMWH RO-14 reduce the endothelial angiogenic features elicited by leukemia, lung cancer, or breast cancer cells. *Cancer Investigation,* Vol. 29, No. 2, pp. 153-161

Von Tempelhoff, G., Harenberg, J. & Niemann, F. (2000). Effect of low molecular weight heparin (certoparin) versus unfractionated heparin on cancer survival following breast and pelvic cancer surgery: a prospective randomized double-blind trial. *International Journal of Oncology,* Vol. 16, No. 4, pp. 815-824

Wahl, O., Oswald, M., Tretzel, L., Herres, E., Arend, J. & Efferth, T. (2011). Inhibition of tumor angiogenesis by antibodies, synthetic small molecules and natural products. *Current Medicinal Chemistry,* Vol. 18, No. 21, pp. 3136-3155

Wang, X., Li, J., Wang, Y., Cho, K.J., Kim, G., Gjyrezi, A., Koenig, L., Giannakakou, P., Shin, H.J.C., Tighiouart, M., Nie, S., Chen, Z. & Shin, D.M. (2009). HFT-T, a targeting nanoparticle, enhances specific delivery of paclitaxel to folate receptor-positive tumors. *ACS Nano,* Vol. 3, No. 10, pp. 3165-3174

Wang, Y., Xiang, J. & Yao, K. (2010). Target-specific cellular uptake of taxol-loaded heparin-PEG-folate nanoparticles. *Biomacromolecules,* Vol. 11, No. 12, pp. 3531-3538

Wang, Y., Xin, D., Liu, K. & Xiang, J. (2009a). Heparin-Paclitaxel conjugates using mixed anhydride as intermediate: Synthesis, influence of polymer structure on drug release, anticoagulant activity and in vitro efficiency. *Pharmaceutical Research,* Vol. 26, No. 4, pp. 785-793

Wang, Y., Xin, D., Liu, K., Zhu, M. & Xiang, J. (2009b). Heparin-paclitaxel conjugates as drug delivery system: Synthesis, self-assembly property, drug release, and antitumor activity. *Bioconjugate Chemistry,* Vol. 20, No. 12, pp. 2214-2221

Westmuckett, A.D., Kakkar, V.V., Hamuro, T., Lupu, F. & Lupu, C. (2001). Bemiparin and fluid flow modulate the expression, activity and release of tissue factor pathway inhibitor in human endothelial cells in vitro. *Thrombosis and Haemostasis,* Vol. 86, No. 6, pp. 1547-1554

Williamson, J. (1957). Suramin complexes. I. Prophylactic activity against Trypanosoma congolense in small animals. *Annals of tropical medicine and parasitology,* Vol. 51, No. 4, pp. 440-456

Williamson, J. & Desowitz, R.S. (1956). Prophylactic activity of suramin complexes in animal trypanosomiasis. *Nature,* Vol. 177, No. 4519, pp. 1074-1075

Zamai, M., Caiolfa, V.R., Pines, D., Pines, E. & Parola, A.H. (1998). Nature of interaction between basic fibroblast growth factor and the antiangiogenic drug 7,7- (carbonyl-bis[imino-N-methyl-4,2- pyrrolecarbonylimino[N-methyl-4,2-pyrrole]-carbonylimino])bis- (1,3- naphthalene disulfonate). *Biophysical Journal,* Vol. 75, No. 2, pp. 672-682

Zugmaier, G., Lippman, M.E. & Wellstein, A. (1992). Inhibition by pentosan polysulfate (PPS) of heparin-binding growth factors released from tumor cells and blockage by PPS of tumor growth in animals. *Journal of the National Cancer Institute,* Vol. 84, No. 22, pp. 1716-1724

2

Regulation of Angiogenesis in Human Cancer via Vascular Endothelial Growth Factor Receptor-2 (VEGFR-2)

Shanchun Guo[1], Laronna S. Colbert[2],
Tanisha Z. McGlothen[1] and Ruben R. Gonzalez-Perez[1]
[1]*Microbiology, Biochemistry & Immunology,*
[2]*Clinical Medicine, Hematology/Oncology Section, Morehouse School of Medicine,*
Atlanta, GA,
USA

1. Introduction

Angiogenesis is the sprouting of new capillaries from pre-existing blood vessels that involves endothelial cell (EC) differentiation, proliferation, migration, cord formation and tubulogenesis (Risau 1997). This process was earlier recognized by the studies of Judah Folkman as a crucial step for tumor formation (Folkman 1971). Many endothelium-specific molecules can influence angiogenesis including members of the VEGF, angiopoietin and ephrin families. In addition, non vascular endothelium-specific factors contribute to blood vessel formation, i.e., platelet-derived growth factor, PDGF and transforming growth factor-β, TGF-β families (Yancopoulos et al. 2000). VEGF family members interact through some degree of specificity with receptor tyrosine kinases (RTK; VEGFR-1 to 3). VEGFR-1 (fms-like tyrosine kinase, Flt-1) (Shibuya et al. 1990), VEGFR-2 (fetal liver kinase, Flk-1 in mice or KDR in humans) (Matthews et al. 1991; Millauer et al. 1993; Terman et al. 1991), VEGFR-3 (Flt-4)(Pajusola et al. 1992) and a fourth receptor, Flt-3/Flk-2, belongs to the RTK family. The last receptor was identified but it does not bind to VEGF (Hannum et al. 1994). VEGF can also bind to a distinct type of high-affinity non-tyrosine kinase receptors: Neuropilin-1 and-2 (NRP-1/-2). These molecules are found in endothelial and neuronal cell surfaces (Jussila and Alitalo 2002), as well as in tumor cells (Bagri et al. 2009; Pellet-Many et al. 2008).

VEGFR-2 was discovered before the identification of its ligand, VEGF (Risau 1997; Yancopoulos et al. 2000). VEGFR-2 is a receptor-tyrosine kinase named KDR in human (Terman et al. 1992; Yancopoulos et al. 2000), Flk-1 (Matthews et al. 1991) or NYW/FLK-1 in mice (Oelrichs et al. 1993) and TKr-11 in rat (Sarzani et al. 1992) was earlier identified as a transducer of VEGF in EC (Waltenberger et al. 1994). VEGF-A is the major form that binds and signals through VEGFR-2 to develop blood vessels and to maintain the vascular network (Ferrara 1999). VEGFR-2 is thought to mediate the key effects of the endothelial-specific mitogen VEGF on cell proliferation and permeability. Therefore, the majority of VEGFR-2 actions are related to angiogenesis (Ferrara et al. 2003; Shibuya and Claesson-Welsh 2006). Homozygous deficient VEGFR-2 mice die in the second week of gestation as a consequence of insufficient development of hematopoietic and EC (Matthews et al. 1991), indicating that

VEGFR-2 is essential for life (Kabrun et al. 1997). Although, VEGF signals through VEGFR-1 (Flt-1) are required for the embryonic vasculature they are not essential for EC differentiation. Indeed, homozygous mice for targeted mutation of VEGFR-1 gene produce EC from angioblasts but develop non-functional blood vessels and die at around 10 days of gestation (Fong et al. 1995). It seems that VEGFR-1 and -2 have opposite roles in some biological contexts. VEGFR-2 mediates the major growth and permeability actions of VEGF (Shibuya 2006), whereas VEGFR-1 may have a negative role, either by acting as a decoy receptor or by suppressing signaling through VEGFR-2 (Yancopoulos et al. 2000). On the other hand, regulation of lymphatic EC is mainly dependant on VEGFR-3/VEGF-C and VEGF-D actions (Jussila and Alitalo 2002). However, VEGFR-3 is also essential for early blood vessel development and plays a role in tumor angiogenesis (Laakkonen et al. 2007; Lohela et al. 2009). Although VEGFR-1, VEGFR-2 and VEGFR-3 have similar molecular structures, the last does not bind to VEGF-A (Achen et al. 2006; Lohela et al. 2009). Flt-3/Flk-2 is expressed on CD34+ hematopoietic stem cells, myelomonocytic progenitors, primitive B cell progenitors, and thymocytes and control differentiation of hematopoietic and non-hematopoietic cells (Hannum et al. 1994; Rappold et al. 1997).

2. Structure and function of VEGFR-2

VEGFR-2 is a transmembrane receptor that plays an important role in endothelial cell development (Risau 1997; Shalaby et al. 1995). VEGFR-2 consists of 1356 and 1345 amino acids in humans and mice, respectively. VEGFR-2 consists of 4 regions: the extracellular ligand-binding domain, transmembrane domain, tyrosine kinase domain, and downstream carboxy terminal region (Matthews et al. 1991; Millauer et al. 1993; Shibuya et al. 1990; Terman et al. 1991). The presence of seven immunoglobulin (Ig)-like domains characterizes the extracellular ligand-binding domain. The ligand-binding region is localized within the second and third Ig domains (Barleon et al. 1997b; Davis-Smyth et al. 1996; Shinkai et al. 1998; Tanaka et al. 1997). Although, the third Ig-like domain is critical for ligand binding, the second and fourth domains are important for ligand association, and the fifth and sixth domains are required for retention of the ligand bound to the receptor molecule (Shinkai et al. 1998). VEGFR-2 binds VEGF-A, VEGF-C, VEGF-D and VEGF-E (Achen et al. 1998; Joukov et al. 1996b; Meyer et al. 1999; Ogawa et al. 1998; Shibuya 2003), whereas VEGFR-1 binds VEGF-A, VEGF-B and PIGF (Autiero et al. 2003; Makinen et al. 2001; Park et al. 1994). The classic interpretation of ligand-binding specificities is currently used for all aspects of vascular effects driven by VEGF-VEGFRs which have helped in elucidating their function. However, the potential formation of VEGFR heterodimers, i.e., VEGFR-2-VEGFR-1 (Huang et al. 2001) and VEGFR-2-VEGFR-3 (Dixelius et al. 2003) has generally been understated. It was noticed that substantial differences in signal transduction occur upon distinct VEGFR heterodimers complex formation because kinase domains and substrate specificities differ (Autiero et al. 2003; Dixelius et al. 2003; Huang et al. 2001; Mac Gabhann and Popel 2007; Neagoe et al. 2005). These complexes can also differentially interact with VEGF and PIGF (Autiero et al. 2003; Huang et al. 2001) resulting in unique signaling pattern and likely different feedback mechanisms (Mac Gabhann and Popel 2007).

VEGFR-2 is a type III receptor tyrosine kinase of the PDGFR family [PDGFRα/β, c-Kit, FLT3, and CSF-1 (cFMS)]. The majority of VEGFR-2 intracellular domains contain tyrosine residues (Tyr or Y) that are involved in redundant actions on vasculogenesis or angiogenesis. Major phosphorylation sites on VEGFR-2 and signaling partners have been reported as: Y^{951} (T-cell-specific adaptor, TSAd-Src); Y^{1054} and ^{1059} (kinase regulation); Y^{1175} [(PI-3K-Ras) and PI-3K-

AKT as well as phospholipase C gamma (PLCγ)-PKC-MEK)]; Y^{1214} (p38MAPK-HSP27) [(for Review see (Olsson et al. 2006; Rahimi 2006)]. pY^{951}VEGFR-2 (in the kinase insert domain) was recently found to increase angiogenesis (Tahir et al. 2009b) and seems to be also important for the interaction between VEGFR-2, PI-3K and PLCγ, which involves the adapter protein VEGF receptor-associated protein (VRAP also known as TSAd) (Wu et al. 2000). Other putatively important phosphorylated sites include Y^{996} in the kinase insert domain and Y^{1054} and Y^{1059} in the tyrosine kinase catalytic domain. These tyrosine residues, together with Y^{951}, when phosphorylated, act as docking sites to recruit molecules containing SH2, SH3 or PTB domains and to convey signals to downstream pathways (Petrova et al. 1999). Sequential activation of CDC42 and p38 MAPK by pY^{1214} (or Y^{1212} in mice) VEGFR-2 has been implicated in VEGF-induced actin remodeling (Lamalice et al. 2004). On the other hand, the upstream phosphorylation of Y^{801} within the juxtamembrane domain of VEGFR-2 seems to be required for the subsequent activation of the catalytic domain. However, the biological implications of these findings need to be further investigated (Solowiej et al. 2009). Moreover, human Y^{801} and ^{1175} VEGFR-2 (Y^{799} and ^{1173} mouse) are required for binding/activation of PI-3K and EC growth but no for migration or PLCγ1 activation (Dayanir et al. 2001). Additionally, pY^{1054} and ^{1059} in the activation loop are essential for VEGF-induced intracellular Ca^{2+} mobilization and the MAPK activation (Solowiej et al. 2009). However, the involvement of specific pY VEGFR-2 domains, activation of specific signaling pathways and driven functions is a point of controversial discussion (Guo et al. 2010). Recent data from Garonna et al., suggest that leptin (the major adipokine) treatment caused rapid phosphorylation of Y^{1175} VEGFR-2. These leptin effects positively impacted on EC cell proliferation, survival and migration. Leptin-VEGFR-2 actions in EC involved a crosstalk between p38 kinase/Akt1 and COX-2 (Garonna et al. 2011). These leptin effects were detected in absence of VEGF. Leptin induces rapid (5 min) phosphorylation of pY^{1175} VEGFR-2 in EC that was linked to proliferation, migration and tube formation in vitro (Garonna et al. 2011). We have also found leptin induces pY^{951} VEGFR-2 in 4T1 mouse breast cancer cells. However, the biological significance of this finding need to be further investigated (Guo and Gonzalez-Perez, unpublished). In addition, specific serine residues in the VEGFR-2 cytoplasmatic region are targeted by protein kinase C (PKC) and involved in regulatory mechanisms of receptor levels (ubiquitinylation and degradation) (Singh et al. 2005).

VEGF binding to VEGFR-2 triggers the specific activation of tyrosine amino acid residues within cytoplasmatic tail of the receptor inducing multiple signaling networks that result in EC survival, proliferation, migration, focal adhesion turnover, actin remodeling and vascular permeability (Kliche and Waltenberger 2001; Olsson et al. 2006; Zachary 2003). Signaling through mitogen-activated protein-kinase (MAP; including MEK-p42/p44MAPK and p38 MAPK; linked to proliferation) (Olsson et al. 2006; Takahashi and Shibuya 1997) and phosphatidylinositol 3' kinase (PI-3K)/V-akt murine thymoma viral oncogene homolog 1 (Akt1; linked to survival) (Abedi and Zachary 1997) are common receptor tyrosine kinase activation patterns. Additional signaling pathways are also triggered upon VEGFR-2 activation (i.e., PLCγ1-PKC; linked to proliferation) (Veikkola et al. 2000), focal adhesion kinase (linked to migration) (Abedi and Zachary 1997) and T Cell–Specific Adapter-Src kinase (linked to migration and vascular permeability) (Matsumoto et al. 2005) (See Fig 1). Overexpression of caveolin-1 in prostate cancer cells specifically induce pY^{951} in the VEGFR-2 cytoplasmatic tail and increases angiogenesis (Tahir et al. 2009a). On the other hand, Y^{1175} mediates both PLCγ-1 and protein kinase A (PKA)-dependent signaling pathways required for VEGF-induced release of von Willebrand factor from EC (Xiong et al. 2009). Dayanir et al, found that activation of PI-3K/S6 but not Ras/MAPK kinase pathway is responsible for

VEGFR-2-mediated cell growth (Dayanir et al. 2001). Inhibition of p38 MAPK activity enhances VEGF-induced angiogenesis *in vitro* and *in vivo* and prolonged ERK1/2 activation and increased EC survival but abrogated VEGF-induced vascular permeability (Issbrucker et al. 2003). Intriguingly, VEGF-mediated proliferation of VEGFR-2 expressing fibroblasts was slower and weaker than in EC, suggesting the cell type-specific signaling mechanism(s) (Takahashi and Shibuya 1997). These results open the possibilities for differential signaling mechanisms/responses to VEGF via VEGFR-2 in cancer compared to EC. Inconsistent reports on VEGFR-2 signaling capabilities could be due to the complex interplay of signaling and inhibiting actions of other VEGF receptors. Albeit the activation and signaling of VEGFR-2 could also be modified by the formation of VEGFR-2 heterodimers exhibiting differential signaling potential as described above.

No available data on negative regulation of VEGFR-2 by phosphorylation of specific residues are available. However, de-phosphorylation of Y residues within VEGFR-2 cytoplasmatic tail contributes to its activity regulation in EC. T-cell protein tyrosine phosphatase (TCPTP, also known as PTN2) expressed by EC and several cell types could alter VEGF signalling by controlling phosphorylation of VEGFR-2. TCPTP was reported to dephosphorylate $Y^{1054}/^{1059}$ and Y^{1214} as well as Y^{996} (this last Y dephosphorylation has not current defined functional significance). Y^{1175}, by contrast, remained phosphorylated. These actions of YCPTP inhibited VEGFR-2 kinase activity and prevented its internalization, which abrogated VEGF-mediated endothelial cell proliferation, angiogenic sprouting, chemokinesis and chemotaxis (Mattila et al. 2008).

3. The autocrine VEGF/VEGFR-2 loop: a cancer cell survival process

Intensive research has been done on VEGF/VEGFR-2 roles in vascular functions (Olsson et al. 2006). However, only a small number of reports highlight a less known function of VEGF signaling that can directly impact cancer cell survival: the autocrine loop in cancer cells. Some reports suggest that a strict molecular requirement for these autocrine actions of VEGF is the expression of VEGFR-1 as it was found in colon carcinoma (Andre et al. 2000). In line with these data, Wu et al, further reported that selective signaling through VEGFR-1 on breast cancer cells supports tumor growth through downstream activation of the p44/42 mitogen-activated protein kinase (MAPK) or Akt pathways (Wu et al. 2006). However, in breast cancer cells, VEGFR-2 isoform was not initially linked to cell survival (Andre et al. 2000; Mercurio et al. 2004).

The co-expression of NRP-1(Bachelder et al. 2001) and $\alpha6\beta4$ integrin (Mercurio et al. 2004) but not VEGFR-2 was found essential for the binding of VEGF and activation of the PI-3K survival signaling pathway in breast cancer cells. Moreover, it was suggested that breast cancer cells do not express VEGFR-2 (Bachelder et al. 2001; Mercurio et al. 2004). In contrast, VEGFR-2 overexpression and phosphorylation could be linked to drug-resistance in breast cancer. VEGF/VEGFR-2 was found essential for cell survival in either estrogen receptor (ER) positive (MCF-7) (Aesoy et al. 2008; Svensson et al. 2005) or negative cells (MDA-MB-468) (Svensson et al. 2005) after tamoxifen treatment. A signaling cascade from VEGFR-2 via ERK1/2 to Ets-2 phosphorylation was correlated to better survival of untreated patients (Svensson et al. 2005). Moreover, a VEGF/VEGFR-2/p38MAPK kinase link was involved in poor outcome for tamoxifen-treated patients (Aesoy et al. 2008). VEGF stimulation of Akt phosphorylation and activation of ERK1/2 correlated to VEGFR-2 expression and activation in various breast carcinoma cell lines and primary culture of breast carcinoma cells (Weigand et al. 2005).

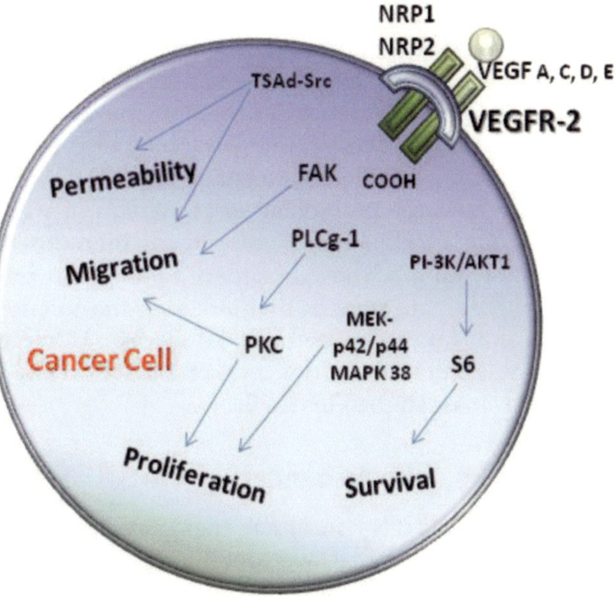

Fig. 1. VEGFR-2 signaling and biological functions.

Dimerization of VEGFR-2 occurs upon its binding to VEGF-A, -C, -D and –E. It was suggested that only mature forms of VEGF-C and VEGF-D bind with high affinity to VEGFR-2 or VEGFR-3 (Achen et al. 2005; Achen et al. 2006). NRP-1/-2 are co-receptors that stabilize the VEGFR-2 dimer. Upon ligand binding to VEGFR-2 several signaling pathways can be activated affecting diverse biological processes in endothelial and cancer cells.

Findings from our laboratory suggest that mouse (4T1, ER +) (Gonzalez et al. 2006) and human breast cancer cells (MCF-7, ER+ and MDA-MB-231, ER-) express VEGFR-2 in vitro and in vivo (Rene Gonzalez et al. 2009). Interestingly, in these cells the expression of VEGF and VEGFR-2 was linked to leptin signaling. White adipose tissue is the primary source of leptin in benign tissue but it is also expressed and secreted by cancer cells. Leptin is a known mitogenic, inflammatory and angiogenic factor for many tissues (Sierra-Honigmann et al. 1998) and increases the levels of VEGF/VEGFR-2 in cancer cells (Carino et al. 2008; Gonzalez et al. 2006; Rene Gonzalez et al. 2009). Therefore, leptin from corporal, mammary adipose tissue or cancer cells could affect cancer cells through autocrine and paracrine actions. Leptin increased the proliferation of 4T1 cells but treatment with anti-VEGFR-2 antibody resulted in a further increase in leptin-induced VEGF concentrations in the medium (Gonzalez et al 2006). This suggests a feedback loop between VEGF expression and VEGFR-2 that could be linked to cell survival/proliferation (Aesoy et al. 2008). Remarkably, inhibition of leptin signaling mediated an impressive reduction of tumor growth in mice that paralleled a significant reduction of VEGF and VEGFR-2 levels (Gonzalez et al. 2006; Rene Gonzalez et al. 2009). Moreover, leptin seems to overcome the effects of cisplatin on MCF-7 survival. A crosstalk between leptin/Notch and Wnt could be involved in the cisplatin resistance by MCF-7 (McGlothen and Gonzalez-Perez, unpublished results).

The endothelial-independent VEGF/VEGFR-2 autocrine loop was found essential for leukemia cell survival and migration in vivo (Dias et al. 2001). Results from these studies suggest that effective anti-angiogenic therapies to treat VEGF-producing and VEGFR-expressing leukemias may require blocking both paracrine and autocrine VEGF/VEGFR-2 angiogenic loops to achieve long term remission and cure (Dias et al. 2001). On the other hand, stimulation of the proliferation of prostate cancer cells by VEGF depends on the presence of VEGFR-2 through autocrine loops generated by IL-6 (H. Steiner et al. 2004a). An autocrine role for VEGF-A in chemoresistance has been demonstrated using the anti-VEGF-A antibody bevacizumab, which enhances antitumor activity of cytotoxic drugs. Moreover, combined bevacizumab and nab-paclitaxel treatment synergistically inhibited breast cancer growth, metastasis and increased the percentage of regression of well-established tumors (Volk et al. 2008). Furthermore, combination therapy using high-dosed nab-paclitaxel was found more efficient in eliminating advanced primary tumors and preexisting metastases (Volk et al. 2011). Overall these data suggest that targeting the VEGF/VEGFR-2 autocrine loop in cancer may be an innovative way to treat the disease. However, the relationships between activation of specific intracellular domains of VEGFR-2 and autocrine actions of VEGF in cancer cells remains to be studied in detail.

4. Expression of VEGFR-2 in human cancer

Because of the potential role of VEGFR-2 in tumor angiogenesis, its expression was started to investigate in malignancies soon after it was identified as a tyrosine kinase-receptor for VEGF (Waltenberger et al. 1994). VEGFR-2 was found weakly expressed in normal tissues or cells, but VEGFR-2 overexpression was reported in various cancers including lung, colon, uterus, ovarian cancer, as well as breast cancers (Giatromanolaki et al. 2007). The overexpression of VEGFR-2 not only occurs in cancer, but also the expression of VEGFR-2 relates to the disease stage, recurrence and worse outcome. Table I shows relative levels of expression of VEGFR-2 in different cancer types.

Tissue	Subtype	Positive rate	Reference
Bladder	Carcinoma	50%	(Xia et al. 2006)
Brain	Glioma	71.4%	(Steiner et al. 2004b)
Breast	Adenocarcinoma	64.5%	(Nakopoulou et al. 2002)
Cervix	Adenosquamous carcinoma	73.3%	(Longatto-Filho et al. 2009)
Colon	Carcinoma	71.4%	(Cheng et al. 2004)
Esophagus	Carcinoma	100%	(Gockel et al. 2008)
Kidney	Clear cell cancer	35%	(Badalian et al. 2007)
Lung	Non-small cell carcinoma	54.2%	(Carrillo de Santa Pau et al. 2009)
Oral	Carcinoma	↑↑	(Sato and Takeda 2009)
Ovary	Carcinoma	100%	(Chen et al. 2004)
Pancreas	Carcinoma	80%	(Itakura et al. 2000)
Prostate	Cancer*	100%	(Stadler et al. 2004)
Skin	Melanoma	↑↑	(Straume and Akslen 2003)

*Cell lines; ↑↑, overexpression of VEGFR-2

Table 1. VEGFR-2 expression in human tumors and malignant cell lines.

4.1 Breast cancer

A number of studies demonstrated that VEGFR-2 receptors are expressed in mouse and human breast cancer cell lines (Aesoy et al. 2008; Gonzalez et al. 2006; Rene Gonzalez et al. 2009; Svensson et al. 2005; Weigand et al. 2005). Upregulation of VEGFR-2 mRNA was found earlier in invasive primary and metastatic breast cancers (Brown et al. 1995). Western blot and immunohistochemical analyses of endothelium and epithelium of mammary ducts in carcinomas, fibroadenomas and fibrocystic breast disease showed positive expression of VEGFR-2 that was also found in tumor stroma (Kranz et al. 1999). VEGFR-2 expression correlated with VEGF expression that suggested these molecules were co-expressed in breast cancer but this was not significantly associated with patient survival (Ryden et al. 2003). In addition, tumor-specific expression of VEGFR-2 correlated strongly with expression of VEGF-A and progesterone receptor (PR) negativity, whereas VEGF-A was not associated with hormone receptor status (Ryden et al. 2005). Invasive and in situ breast cancers express many angiogenic factors and this process was found throughout all tumor stages (Fox et al. 2007). Nakopoulou et al, detected VEGFR-2 in 64.5% (91/141) of invasive breast carcinomas showing a widespread cytoplasmic expression in most of the neoplastic cells (Nakopoulou et al. 2002). VEGFR-2 expression was well correlated with the nuclear grade of the invasive breast carcinoma ($P = 0.003$), but demonstrated no correlation with histologic grade, stage, and patient survival (Nakopoulou et al. 2002) as was previously noticed (Ryden et al. 2003). Interestingly, in breast cancer VEGFR-2 expression was significantly correlated with two well-established proliferation indices, Ki-67 ($P = 0.037$) and topo-IIα ($P = 0.009$). This suggests VEGF may exert growth factor activities on mammary cancer cells through its receptor VEGFR-2 (Nakopoulou et al. 2002). Linderholm et al recently reported that higher VEGFR-2 levels in tumor homogenates from primary breast cancer were correlated to higher levels of VEGF ($P = 0.005$), p38 MAPK ($P = 0.018$) and absence of ER ($P = 0.008$); larger tumors ($P = 0.001$), histopathological grade III ($P = 0.018$), distant metastasis ($P = 0.044$), shorter recurrence free survival (RFS) ($P = 0.013$), and shorter breast cancer corrected survival (BCCS) ($P = 0.017$) (Linderholm et al. 2011). Their results suggest that higher intratumoral levels of VEGFR-2 would be a candidate marker of intrinsic resistance for adjuvant endocrine therapy as it was earlier reported (Aesoy et al. 2008; Svensson et al. 2005).

4.2 Cervical and endometrial cancer

Cervical cancer, the malignant neoplasm of the cervix uteri or cervical area, it is the second most frequent malignancy in women worldwide, with one-third of patients dying from pharmacoresistant disease (Legge et al. 2010). In a study, VEGFR-2 positivity was observed in 22 of 30 cases (73.3%) cervical adenosquamous carcinoma but was significantly associated with lack of metastasis ($p=0.038$) (Longatto-Filho et al. 2009). In contrast, Kuemmel et al found that VEGFR-2 levels were increased in positive lymph node patients ($p = 0.024$) and in metastatic disease ($p = 0.003$). They further determined that circulating VEGFs and their soluble receptors were present in pre-invasive, invasive and recurrent cervical cancer (Kuemmel et al. 2009).

In a recent report, VEGFR-2 was not detected in normal cervical epithelium, but was positive in cervical intraepithelial neoplasia and cervical squamous cell carcinoma. Moreover, increasing expression of VEGFR-2 and VEGF were identified in cervical carcinoma indicating a correlation between their expression and carcinoma staging (Jach et al. 2010). In other report, positive immunostaining rate was 39% for VEGF, 65% for VEGFR-1 and 68% for VEGFR-2 in endometrial carcinomas (Talvensaari-Mattila et al. 2005). These results showed a significant correlation between VEGF and its receptors, but positive immunostaining was not related to poor prognosis (Talvensaari-Mattila et al. 2005). Using a novel monoclonal antibody recognizing the activated (phosphorylated) form of VEGFR-2, Giatromanolaki et al assessed strong and consistent cytoplasmic and nuclear pVEGFR-2 staining in the normally cycling endometrium, including epithelial, stromal and endothelial cells, suggesting a role of pVEGFR-2 in the normal menstrual cycle. Moreover, approximately one-third of the 70 stage I endometrioid adenocarcinomas analyzed exhibited an intense cytoplasmic and nuclear pVEGFR-2 in both cancer cells and peritumoral vessels. These authors also observed that pVEGFR-2 reactivity in cancer cells was directly related to VEGF, VEGF/VEGFR-2 complexes and HIF1α expression. Furthermore, pVEGFR-2 levels were significantly associated with poor prognosis (Giatromanolaki et al. 2006).

4.3 Colon cancer

The American Cancer Society estimates that there will be more than 140,000 new cases of colon cancer and more than 49,000 colon cancer deaths in the United States in 2011. Colon cancer is the third most common cancer and the third leading cause of cancer death among both men and women in the U.S. Colon cancer is unique among malignancies in that it is known to arise from distinct inflammatory conditions, namely, Crohn's disease and Ulcerative colitis. The link between inflammation, hypoxia and carcinogenesis continues to be elucidated. It is known that organ and cellular adaptation to hypoxia is mediated via HIF. Stabilization of HIF occurs via hypoxia-dependent inhibition of PHDs (prolyl hydroxylases).This stabilization and subsequent activation of HIF augments tumor vascularization, an important component of carcinogenesis and metastasis (Eltzschig and Carmeliet 2011). Patients with colitis associated cancer show activated VEGFR-2 on intestinal epithelial cells (IECs). In a murine model these IECs displayed increased VEGFR-2 mediated proliferation in response to VEGF stimulation. Functional studies then demonstrated that VEGFR signaling required STAT3 to promote IECs proliferation and tumor growth in vivo. This provides additional evidence linking inflammation to the development of colon cancer (Waldner et al. 2010). Giatromanolaki et al found increased levels of pVEGFR-2 in colon cancer cells and intratumoral vasculature as compared to normal epithelium. Additionally, the highest levels of pVEGFR-2 were seen in large tumors i.e. > 6 cm, those with poor histologic differentiation and high CEF1 (the nineteen complex, a non-snRNA containing protein complex, involved in splicing of nuclear RNAs via the spliceosome alpha expression). Increased VEGFR-2 expression also correlated with high VEGF and HIF expression (Giatromanolaki et al. 2007). In addition to chronic inflammatory states obesity can also predispose patients to the development of colon cancer. Padidar et al identified leptin-regulated genes localized in the colon by in situ hybridization. The pro-inflammatory cytokines, IL-6, IL-1β, and CXCL1 were upregulated by leptin and localized to cells in the gut epithelium, lamina propria, muscularis and at the peritoneal serosal surface (Padidar et al. 2011). This further establishes the role of inflammation in the pathogenesis of colon cancer. The role of activated oncogenes and loss of tumor suppressor genes and their effect on angiogenesis and subsequent tumor survival and metastasis was further reported (Zeng et al. 2010). Among those oncogenes most prominent in colon cancer is KRAS. Mutant KRAS alleles interact with hypoxia to induce VEGF in colon cancer. In addition, an adaptive mechanism in KRAS-wild type cells was dependent upon c-Src-mediated hypoxic activation of wild type KRAS through phosphorylation of AKT and induction of VEGF expression (Zeng et al. 2010). The expression of VEGF and its receptor, VEGFR-2, and the correlation with vascularity, metastasis and proliferation was also studied by Takahashi et al. These authors conducted immunohistochemical analysis on 52 human colon carcinomas and 10 adenomas. The expression of VEGF and VEGFR-2 was higher in metastatic compared to nonmetastatic neoplasms and directly correlated with extent of neovascularization and proliferation (Takahashi et al. 1995).

4.4 Esophageal cancer

Esophageal carcinoma is one of the most common malignancies in the world. Worse prognosis is linked to lymph node metastasis. Two main types of esophageal cancer are found in humans, squamous cell carcinoma and adenocarcinoma, both of them are related to VEGFR-2. In one study of squamous cell carcinoma, twenty-four (37.5%) of the tumors showed diffuse VEGF immunoreactivity significantly correlated with tumor status ($p < 0.05$) and poor prognosis (log-rank; $p < 0.05$). VEGFR-2 immunoreactivity was detected in the cancer cell cytoplasm in 26 patients (40.6%), but did not correlate with clinicopathological factors or prognosis (Kato et al. 2002). In a recent report (Gockel et al. 2008), adenocarcinoma samples revealed different levels of expression of VEGFR-1 (97%), VEGFR-2 (94%), VEGFR-3 (77%), PDGFRα (91%), PDGFRβ (85%) and EGFR-1 (97%). Similarly, squamous cell cancers revealed VEGFR-1 (100%), VEGFR-2 (100%), VEGFR-3 (53%), PDGFRα (100%), PDGFRβ (87%) and EGFR-1 (100%) expression. In the study, 94% and 100% of the esophageal adenocarcinomas and squamous cell carcinomas, respectively, expressed at least four out of these six RTKs. These results suggest VEGFR-2 may have a high rate co-expression with other RTK in both esophageal cancer types. Therefore, the application of multi-target RTK inhibitors could be a promising and novel approach for esophageal cancer (Gockel et al. 2008).

4.5 Prostate cancer

Prostate cancer (PCa) is the most prevalent noncutaneous malignancy and the second most frequent cause of cancer-related mortality in American men. VEGFR-1 and VEGFR-2 expression was earlier reported in prostate tumors and in LNCaP, PC3, and DU145 prostate cancer cell lines (Ferrer et al. 1997; Levine et al. 1998). Further, Jackson et al., showed that VEGFR-2 induced neovascularization and proliferation of LNCaP prostate cancer cells via autocrine/paracrine mechanisms. VEGFR-1 and VEGFR-2 receptors co-localize with VEGF in prostate tumor cells, prostatic intraepithelial neoplasia, and the basal cells of normal glands. Furthermore, specific staining for both receptors was decreased in poorly differentiated cancer (Jackson et al. 2002). In view of the importance of VEGFR-2 signaling in the growth of PCa several studies have been focused on the effects of anti-angiogenic therapies for reduction of tumor growth and metastasis (Bischof et al. 2004; Stadler et al. 2004).

4.6 Ovarian cancer

Ovarian cancer is the seventh most common cancer in women. It ranks fourth as the cause of cancer deaths in women. The American Cancer Society estimated the occurrence of 21,880 new cases of ovarian cancer in the United States of America in 2010. About 13,850 women were expected to die of the disease. Human epithelial ovarian cancer (EOC) is the most lethal malignancy involving the female genital tract. EOC patients most commonly are diagnosed at an advanced stage and often present with carcinomatosis and large volume ascites. The existence of an autocrine VEGF-A/VEGFR-2 loop in EOC has been suggested in several studies. The first study of the localization of VEGFR-2 expression in nonendothelial cells was reported by Boocock et al in 1995 (Boocock et al. 1995). Their research showed that mRNAs encoding VEGF, VEGFR-1 and VEGFR-2 were detected in primary ascitic cells and in ovarian carcinoma cell lines. Elevated expression of VEGF mRNA was found in all primary tumors and metastases, especially at the margins of tumor acini. VEGFR-2 mRNA was detected not only in vascular endothelial cells but also in tumor cells at primary malignant sites (Boocock et al. 1995). Chen et al examined 42 primary EOC, 29 benign ovarian tumors and 11 normal ovarian tissue samples to determine the expression of VEGF,

VEGFR-2, P-STAT1, P-STAT3, P-STAT5 and P-STAT6. Both VEGF and VEGFR expressions were significantly higher in EOC as compared to benign tumors and normal ovarian tissues ($p < 0.001$). Additionally, the expression of VEGFR-2 was significantly correlated with STAT3 and STAT5 [correlation coefficient (r) = 0.412 and 0.481, respectively] in EOC that suggested VEGF may activate STATs pathways via VEGFR (Chen et al. 2004). Paradoxically, targeted therapy designed to inhibit both VEGFR-2 and EGFR failed to show any clinical activity when used in a phase II trial (Annunziata et al. 2010). In this study, 12 patients with recurrent, persistent or refractory EOC were administered oral vandetanib every four weeks. There was no evidence of VEGFR-2 receptor inhibition in tissues analyzed after repeated biopsies (Annunziata et al. 2010). Conversely, Koukourakis et al examined the levels of pVEGFR-2 in both EOC cells and tumor associated vessels. High pVEGFR-2 levels were noted 55% (5/9) in EOC. Additionally, high pVEGFR-2 levels was linked to higher serum VEGF levels in patients with ovarian cancer (404 +/- 214 vs. 170 +/-143, $p = 0.10$) though this association was not statistically significant (Koukourakis et al. 2011).

4.7 CNS malignancies

Tumors of the central nervous system (CNS) include both non-malignant and malignant tumors of the brain and spinal cord. Primary brain tumors encompass a diverse spectrum of malignancies which are primarily derived from glial precursors. They are the most prevalent solid tumor in children and represent the leading cause of cancer death in children younger than age fifteen. Approximately 22,000 new cases of primary malignant brain and central-nervous system-tumors were diagnosed in the United States in 2010. VEGF plays a critical role in the angiogenesis and progression of malignant brain tumors. Knizetova et al demonstrated autocrine VEGF signaling mediated via VEGFR-2 that involved the co-activation of the c-Raf/MAPK, PIK3/Akt and PLC/PKC pathways using a panel of astrocytoma (grade III and IV/GBM) derived cell lines and clinical specimens of both high and low grade astrocytomas. The VEGF-VEGFR-2 interplay affected cancer cell cycle progression and viability and radioresistance in clinical specimens. Furthermore, the use of a selective inhibitor of VEGFR-2 (SU1498) limited the VEGF-mediated proliferation and viability of astrocytoma cells in culture (Knizetova et al. 2008).

KIT, PDGFR alpha and VEGFR-2 are important clinical targets for tyrosine kinase inhibitors. Puputti et al investigated the expression and amplification of KIT, PDGFRA, VEGFR-2, and EGFR in 87 gliomas which consisted of astrocytomas, anaplastic astrocytomas, oligodendrogliomas and oligoastrocytomas. VEGFR-2 amplifications occurred in 6-17% of the gliomas at diagnosis. KIT amplification was associated with KIT protein overexpression and with the presence of PDGFRA and EGFR amplifications both at time of first glioma diagnosis and at tumor recurrence. However, KIT amplification was associated with VEGFR-2 amplification only at time of tumor recurrence (Puputti et al. 2006). In another study, Joensuu et al investigated 43 primary glioblastomas for amplification of the genes encoding tyrosine kinases. VEGFR-2 was amplified in 39% of glioblastomas and was strongly associated with amplification of KIT and PDGFRA ($p < 0.0001$). These amplified kinases may well serve as potential targets for inhibitor therapy in these CNS malignancies (Joensuu et al. 2005). Amplification and overexpression of KIT, PDGFRA, and VEGFR-2 was also studied by Blom et al. in medulloblastomas (MB) and primitive neuroectodermal tumors (PNET), the most common malignant brain tumors in children (Blom et al. 2010). Using immunohistochemistry (IHC) and chromogenic in situ hybridization (CISH) they found KIT, PDGFRA, and VEGFR-2 amplifications to be present in only 4% of MBs/PNETs.

KIT amplification was associated with concurrent PDGFRA and VEGFR-2 amplifications (p <or=0.001) but only increased copy number of PDGFRA was associated with poor overall survival ($p=0.027$) (Blom et al. 2010). A population based study conducted by Nobusawa et al of 390 glioblastomas using differential PCR demonstrated amplification of PDGFRA, KIT and VEGFR-2 genes in 33 (8.5%), 17 (4.4%) and 13 (3.3%) of glioblastomas respectively. None of these alterations were prognostic for overall survival (Nobusawa et al. 2011).

4.8 Kidney cancer

The two most common types of kidney cancer, reflecting their location within the kidney, are renal cell carcinoma (RCC) and urothelial cell carcinoma (UCC) of the renal pelvis. Tsuchiya et al investigated the expression of VEGF-related factor genes (VEGF, VEGF-B, and VEGF-C) and their receptors (VEGFR-1 and VEGFR-2) in RCC (Tsuchiya et al. 2001). They found significant differences in the expression level of VEGF, VEGFR-1 and VEGFR-2 between RCC and the corresponding normal renal tissue. Furthermore, the expression level of VEGF in the tumor tissue significantly correlated with those of VEGFR-1 and VEGFR-2. A moderate to high protein expression for VEGF, VEGFR-1, and VEGFR-2 was observed in both the tumor cells and the endothelial cells. These data suggest that VEGF and its receptors VEGFR-1 and VEGFR-2 cooperate and play a crucial role in the angiogenesis of RCC. Different RCC types may have dissimilar expression patterns of VEGF and receptor mRNA levels. In clear cell RCC, VEGFR-2 levels were higher in stage I-II than in more advanced stages, while in papillary RCC, VEGF and VEGFR-2 levels were higher in stage III than in stage I-II tumors (Ljungberg et al. 2006). In another report, the VEGFR-2 protein-positive phenotype of clear cell RCC was relatively frequent (7/20, 35%), but was lost in bone metastases (2/20, 10%) (Badalian et al. 2007). In line with the above observations in RCC, the expression of VEGF and VEGFR-2 was observed in 58% and 50%, respectively, of UCC cells (Xia et al. 2006). Moreover, VEGFR-2 expression correlated with disease stage (coefficient 0.23, $p = 0.05$). However, VEGF expression failed to correlate with clinical variables. Interestingly, VEGFR-2 expression increased with tumor invasion into the muscle ($p < 0.01$). In addition, VEGFR-2 in positive bladder cancer cell lines was also increased in response to VEGF (Xia et al. 2006). Taken together, these data suggest increased VEGFR-2 expression correlates with several features that predict progression, disease stage and invasive phenotype of UCC. In summary, VEGFR-2 is associated with tumor stage and survival of both UCC and RCC. However, diverse subtypes of these cancers may have different expression patterns of VEGFR-2 levels. Therefore, a diversity of signaling pathways might be involved in regulating angiogenesis and cancer cell survival and proliferation in the specific UCC and RCC subtypes. Detailed knowledge of tumor angiogenesis in UCC and RCC is essential when designing new treatment trials where angiogenesis inhibition will be used.

4.9 Liver cancer

The American Cancer Society reports that while still quite rare in the United States, liver cancer is more prevalent in men (17,430 new diagnoses annually) than in women (6,690 annual diagnoses). There are several types of liver cancer, including hepatoblastoma, a rare type typically affecting children, cholangiocarcinoma - a cancer that affects the cells of the bile duct, angiosarcoma- a cancer that originates in the liver blood vessels, and hepatocellular carcinoma (HCC), which is by far the most common type of liver cancer (Altekruse et al. 2009). HCC accounts for 90% of all malignant liver tumors. This typically highly vascular tumor is the fifth most common type of cancer and ranks as the third leading cause of cancer related deaths worldwide (Huang et al. 2011). It has been well established that VEGF plays a critical role in angiogenesis. If the known contributing factors to angiogenesis, namely VEGF and its receptors VEGFR-2, can be exploited, it may give rise to novel therapeutic targets for HCC (Ng et al. 2001). The hypoxic environment produced in HCC is a stimulant for the secretion of VEGF by the tumor that subsequently activates VEGFR-2 signals. Elevated expression of VEGFR-2 in HCC was correlated with worse outcome after liver transplantation. Vascular invasion was consistently associated with HCC recurrence ($p<0.01$) and overall mortality ($p<0.05$). Subjects with VEGFR-2 overexpression in tumor arterioles ($p<0.01$), venules ($p<0.05$) had worse overall survival (Kim 2008). A recent report from Huang et al showed higher expression of VEGFR-2 in HCC cells compared to normal hepatic cells ($p<0.001$). Moreover, the high expression of VEGFR-2 in HCC was related to large tumor diameter ($p=0.012$), poor differentiation ($p=0.007$), high serum α-fetoprotein ($p=0.029$), multifocal gross classification ($p=0.007$), and less than 5 years' survival ($p=0.029$). In addition, Kaplan-Meier survival and regression analyses showed that high VEGFR-2 expression ($p=0.009$) and stage grouping were independent prognostic factors (Huang et al. 2011). Anti-VEGFR-2 therapy is a promising novel potential therapy for HCC (Lang et al. 2008).

4.10 Lung cancer

Lung cancer accounts for 90% of deaths from cancer in men and approximately 80% of cancer deaths in women. Smoking increases lung cancer incidence and mortality by up to 20 times, compared to non-smokers. Additionally, lung cancer is responsible for more cancer related deaths than breast, prostate and colorectal cancer combined, as reported by the Centers for Disease Control (Tammemagi et al. 2011). Lung cancer is divided into two primary subtypes: non-small cell lung cancer (NSCLC) and small cell lung cancer (SCLC). NSCLC makes up 80% of primary lung cancers and has a 10-15% overall survival rate. While resection is an effective treatment for early stages of lung cancer, most cases of NSCLC are enough advanced that resectioning is no longer an option (Jantus-Lewintre et al. 2011). The role of VEGFR-2 as a regulator of endothelial cell migration and proliferation has been previously established (Joukov et al. 1996a; Meyer et al. 1999). It has been proposed that VEGF and its receptors contribute to the proliferation and metastasis of tumor cells. A study from Kikuchi's laboratory reported the relevance of VEGF and VEGFRs in the progression of SCLC. VEGFR-2 was detectable in five SCLC cell lines (Tanno et al. 2004). Furthermore, VEGF/VEGFR-2 autocrine loop favoring the growth of SCLC has also been suggested (Kim et al. 2010). In a study by Tanno et al, VEGFR-2 was detected in several SCLC cells lines (Tanno et al. 2004). In addition, VEGFR-2 functions were investigated in SCLC using NCI-H82 SCLC cell line that overexpresses VEGFR-2. In these cells, VEGFR-2 increased cell proliferation, thus verifying the role of VEGFR-2 in SCLC (Tanno et al. 2004). While there is currently limited information regarding the mechanism of the prolific spread of SCLC, there is evidence to support the hypothesis that VEGFR-2 plays a role in the metastasis and proliferation of this cancer type. This supports the theory that anti-cancer drugs targeting the VEGF pathway are possible therapeutic means. The VEGF pathway has also recently been identified as a viable therapeutic target in NSCLC (Nikolinakos et al. 2010).

A study utilizing a mouse model to determine if initiation and maintenance of tumor angiogenesis in NSCLC could be associated with endothelial progenitor cells (EPCs CD133+) it was found these cells express high levels of VEGFR-2. The correlation between CD133 and VEGFR-2 implicates the receptor is associated with angiogenesis and neovascularization in NSCLC (Hilbe et al. 2004). Other report using pre-clinical studies suggested that VEGF-A induced removal or shedding of VEGFR-2 in EC. VEGFR-2 shedding resulted in tumor shrinkage in NSCLC patients that was associated with expression of ADAM metalloprotease and IL-4 (Nikolinakos et al. 2010). Taken together, these results suggest that VEGFR-2 is not only a mediator of angiogenesis but a viable target. A common thread in treatment options for lung cancer seems to be the targeting of the VEGF pathway, including the VEGFR-2 receptor. Therefore, combinatorial therapies involving VEGFR-2 may prove useful in development of novel treatment options for this malignancy.

4.11 Other cancers

Some contradictory data on VEGFR-2 expression and survival of pancreatic cancer patients have been reported. A study reported that VEGFR-1 and VEGFR-2 mRNA were found in 17 and 15 of 24 pancreatic cancer samples, respectively. VEGF receptors were detected not only in blood vessels but also in pancreatic cancer cells. Remarkably, VEGFR-2 expression correlated with poor tumor differentiation and poorer survival, while VEGFR-1 expression did not correlate (Buchler et al. 2002). Accordingly, these data support the idea that VEGF/VEGFR-2 pathway regulates angiogenesis, local pancreatic tumor growth and metastasis and offers a potential new therapeutic option for this malignancy. In other report, VEGFR-2 mRNA was detected in several pancreatic cancer cell lines (Panc-1, AsPC-1, and MiaPaCa-2) (Higgins et al. 2006a). Conversely, Chung et al reported using Kaplan-Meier survival curves that VEGF and VEGFR-2 were not clearly associated with outcome in 76 tissue microarrays from pancreatic cancer. Moreover, the patients who had tumors with the lowest expression VEGFR-1 levels had the worst survival ($p = 0.0038$) (Chung et al. 2006). Causes of these opposed findings are not clearly understood.

In thyroid cancer, VEGF, VEGFR-1 and VEGFR-2 expression were analyzed on 34 papillary thyroid carcinomas (PTCs) and 18 follicular thyroid carcinomas (FTCs) and 8 poorly differentiated thyroid carcinomas (PDTCs). VEGFR-2 was found in 68% of PTCs, 56% of FTCs and 37% of PDTCs (Vieira et al. 2005). In addition, co-expression of VEGF with its receptors was observed in 50% of PTCs, 39% of FTCs and 12% of PDTCs, raising the possibility that VEGF/VEGFR-2 may signal in an autocrine loop in these neoplasias (Vieira et al. 2005). On the other hand, in metastatic medullary thyroid carcinoma (MTC) higher levels of VEGFR-2 were found in metastatic tumors as compared to primary tumors [p=2.8 x 10(-8)] (Rodriguez-Antona et al. 2010). In contrast, in a recent report, VEGFR-2 was detected in 91% (31/34) of MTC samples and had no correlation with tumor stage (tumor node metastasis) (Capp et al. 2010). Taken together these observations suggest that VEGF/VEGFR-2 expression is often found in diverse cancer types. Functions of the VEGF/VEGFR-2 appear to be expanded beyond to the development of tumor angiogenesis. Indeed, VEGF/VEGFR-2 autocrine/paracrine loop seems to play additional roles in cancer cell proliferation and survival.

5. Regulation of VEGFR-2 levels

Despite the essential role of VEGFR-2 in angiogenesis and carcinogenesis the molecular mechanisms controlling its expression are only partially known. Regulation of VEGFR-2 expression involves a series of complex mechanisms that include epigenetic changes, transcriptional regulation, cellular localization/trafficking, ligand binding, co-activator activity, adhesion molecule expression, constitutive-embryonic derived signaling pathways and cytokine-growth factor regulation. In addition, VEGFR-2 can assemble functional complexes composed of homodimers and heterodimers with other VEGFR receptors and co-receptors that can bind VEGF or other angiogenic ligands thereby affecting VEGFR-2 signaling capabilities (Fig 2).

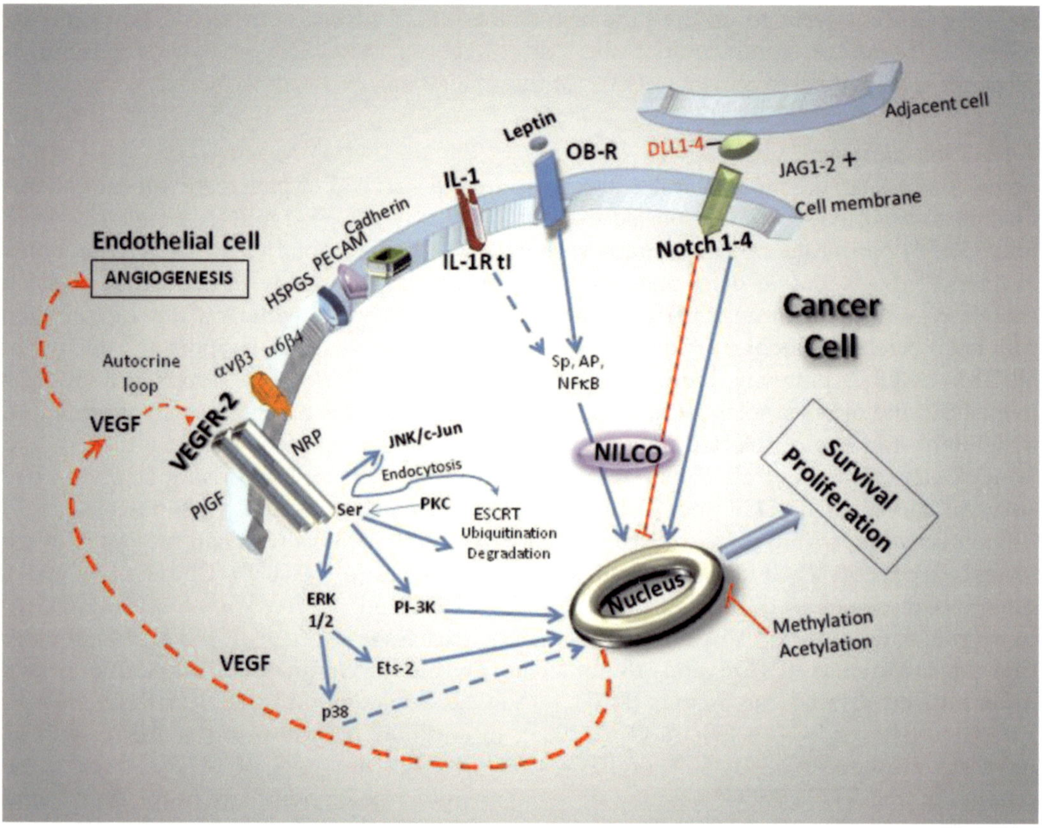

Fig. 2. Mechanisms of Regulation of VEGFR-2 levels in cancer cells

5.1 VEGFR-2 co-activators, cellular localization and trafficking

Heparin and heparan sulfates (components of proteoglycans, HSPGs) have affinity for VEGF165 (VEGF-A), the major isoform of VEGF, promoting enhanced phosphorylation of VEGFR-2. This probably occurs by enhancing ligand binding capabilities to VEGFR-2. Therefore, HSPGs affect the localization, extent and intensity of VEGFR signaling (Ashikari-Hada et al. 2005). NRP-1 can stabilize the VEGF/VEGFR-2 complex and particularly increase tumor angiogenesis (Miao et al. 2000). Blood flow could likely activate VEGFR-2 through the formation of mechanosensory complexes (Tzima et al. 2005). Adhesion molecules (PECAM-1 and VE-cadherin) (Carmeliet et al. 1999; Tzima et al. 2005) and αvβ3 integrin (Somanath et al. 2009) interplay with VEGFR-2 under diverse biological scenarios controlling VEGFR-2 expression and signaling. β3-integrin can limit the interaction of NRP-1 with VEGFR-2, thus negatively affecting VEGF-mediated angiogenesis (Robinson et al. 2009). Invasive ductal carcinoma has decreased expression of α6-integrin associated with higher tumor angiogenesis presumably linked to VEGFR-2 expression. Indeed, loss of α6-integrin correlates to overexpression of activated VEGFR-2 in murine melanoma and lung carcinoma in endothelial-specific α6-knockout mice (Germain et al. 2009). However, the specific mechanisms involved in VEGFR-2 overexpression in tumors from these mice remains to be investigated. A negative regulator of angiogenesis is thrombospondin-1. This molecule negatively modulates VEGF actions through a complex with β1-integrin and VEGFR-2 (Zhang et al. 2009a). Inverse regulation of VEGFR-1 and VEGFR-2 could play an important role in controlling the growth and differentiation of tumor-associated EC. VEGF signaling through JNK/c-Jun pathway induces endocytosis, nuclear translocation and ubiquitin-mediated downregulation of VEGFR-2 in human squamous-cell carcinomas (Zhang et al. 2009b). A model recently proposed suggests that a negative feed-back loop regulates VEGFR-2 activities through the differential segregation/localization of VEGFR-1 and VEGFR-2 (Germain et al. 2009; Robinson et al. 2009). The higher affinity of VEGFR-1 for VEGF blocks VEGFR-2 activation. In the model, Ca (2+) induces the translocation of VEGFR-1 from the trans-Golgi network to the plasma membrane allowing preferential binding of VEGF. VEGFR-2 is degraded after activation by ubiquitin-mediated proteolysis that is linked to endosomal sorting complex required for transport and to Rab GTPases (Bruns et al. 2009). This could also be stimulated by PKC pathway that requires the removal of VEGFR-2 carboxyl terminus (Bruns et al.). Differential trafficking of VEGFR-2 is potentially due to the formation of complexes with diverse angiogenic regulators. These processes occur through the endosomal pathway controlling angiogenesis (Scott and Mellor 2009).

5.2 The Notch signaling-VEGFR-2 link

Notch is a family of mammalian transmembrane proteins that function as receptors for membrane bound ligands. There are four mammalian Notch genes, Notch1–Notch4, and five ligands, Jagged1 and Jagged2 (homologs of Drosophila Serrate-like proteins) and Delta-like 1 (DLL1), DLL3 and DLL4. Notch receptors have an extracellular domain made up of multiple epidermal growth factor domains (EGF), yet, Notch intracellular domain is made up of many domain types (Kovall 2008). The Notch proteins have been proven to affect diverse cell programs (proliferation, differentiation, and apoptosis) and as result Notch influences organogenesis and morphogenesis (Artavanis-Tsakonas et al. 1999). The activation of a Notch receptor is triggered by ligands expressed on adjacent Jagged and Delta cells.

Notch signaling and its crosstalks with many signaling pathways play an important role in cancer cell growth, migration, invasion, angiogenesis and metastasis. Entangled crosstalk between Notch and other developmental signaling (Hedgehog and Wnt), and signaling triggered by growth factors, estrogens and oncogenic kinases, could impact on Notch targeted genes [for review see (Guo et al. 2011)]. This evolutionarily conserved pathway in multicellular organisms regulates embryonic and stem cell fate (Bray 2006). It is generally believed that tumor angiogenesis will not occur in absence of Notch signaling. When a Notch decoy is introduced in place of a functional Notch receptor at a tumor site in the skin during angiogenesis, cell proliferation stops and the development of the new blood vessels ceases. This suggests that the Notch protein has some significant role in angiogenesis (Phng and Gerhardt 2009; Roca and Adams 2007). Indeed, active Notch1 (Stylianou et al. 2006) or Notch4 (Imatani and Callahan 2000) signaling are involved in breast cancer angiogenesis. Soares et al, first demonstrated that a cross talk between Notch and E2 signaling occurs in breast cancer and EC. Notch gene expression was required for tubule-like structure formation in EC. Notch gene expression clustered with HIF-1α and was upregulated by E2. Thus, Notch has significant role in human breast carcinogenesis and angiogenesis (Soares et al. 2004).

Neutralization of DLL4 greatly reduced EC-mediated activation of Notch 3 signaling in T-ALL cells and blocked tumorigenesis (Indraccolo et al. 2009). Moreover, silencing Notch3 by RNA interference had marked antiproliferative and proapoptotic effects on T-ALL cells in vitro and reduced tumorigenicity in vivo (Indraccolo et al. 2009). These results elucidate Notch3 and DLL4 interaction between endothelial and tumor cells, which promotes survival and triggers tumor growth. Unlike other Notch receptors, Notch2 may possibly play a tumor-suppressive role in human cancer (Guo et al. 2011), however, the role of Notch2 in angiogenesis is not well-understood.

It has been found that DLL4 and Jagged1-Notch signaling pathways have opposing effects on angiogenesis (Benedito et al. 2009). While Jagged1-Notch signaling serves as a proangiogenic regulator (Benedito et al. 2009), DLL4-Notch signaling has been shown to significantly decrease the expression of VEGFR-2 thus inhibiting the proliferation of angiogenic cells (Williams et al. 2006). These two signals operate in equilibrium with one another, so that as the concentration of one signal increases the other will decrease proportionally. As a result of the ligand signaling competitive nature towards one another, it is plausible to speculate that the two are used as antagonistic mechanisms to help regulate the processes of angiogenesis (Benedito et al. 2009; Williams et al. 2006). In vitro, the activation of Notch1 or Notch4 in EC induces the expression of the HESR-1 transcription factor (expressed in mature vasculature but reduced in proliferating EC) that in turns downregulates VEGFR-2. Notch-mediated reduction in VEGFR-2 levels results in decreased EC proliferation. This Notch mechanism may be involved in the phenotypic changes during EC proliferation and migration to network formation (Taylor et al. 2002). Overall, one could speculate that the two types of Notch ligands operate to signal the VEGFR-2 to either continue to promote cell proliferation or move onward in the angiogenic process to EC differentiation. Activation of Notch signaling in ER-negative breast cancer cells results in direct transcriptional up-regulation of the apoptosis inhibitor and cell cycle regulator survivin (baculoviral inhibitor of apoptosis repeat-containing 5 or BIRC5). Survivin is highly expressed by cancer cells and binds and inhibits caspase-3, controlling the checkpoint in the G2/M-phase of the cell cycle. Therefore, the Notch-survivin functional gene signature is a hallmark of basal breast cancer, and may contribute to disease pathogenesis (Lee et al. 2008b; Lee et al. 2008a).

In addition, Notch signaling modulates other pathways, such as PI-3K–Akt and NFκB, also activated by VEGFR-2 signaling as discussed above. Indeed, VEGF/VEGFR-2 signals activate and regulate Notch expression in EC and cancer cells (Liu et al. 2003). VEGF or ligand-induced Notch signaling up-regulates DLL4 through a positive feed-forward mechanism. By this mechanism, DLL4 could propagate its own expression and enable synchronization of Notch expression and signaling between ECs. This signaling pathway has been suggested to serve as a negative feedback loop for endothelial sprouting. Moreover, the feedback could be bidirectional as Notch reduces VEGF responsiveness through down-regulation of VEGFR-2 in EC (Caolo et al. 2010). In addition, DLL4 expressed in tumor cells, can function as a negative regulator of tumor angiogenesis by reducing the number of blood vessels. In vitro, DLL4 did not affect the growth of cancer cells: PC3 (prostate cancer), MDA-MB-231 (breast cancer) and B16 (mouse melanoma). However, DLL4 slightly but significantly inhibited the growth of HT1080 (human fibrosarcoma) and retarded the growth of U87 (human glioblastoma). In contrast, DLL4 acted as a positive driver for tumor growth in vivo of human glioblastoma and prostate cancer xenografts (Li et al. 2007). Moreover, Notch signaling from tumor cells is able to activate EC and trigger tumor angiogenesis in vitro and in a xenograft mouse tumor model (Zeng et al. 2005). Therefore, a crosstalk between Notch and VEGFR-2 signaling may be crucial for angiogenic processes. Notch-VEGFR-2 crosstalk could also be influenced by Wnt signaling. The Notch pathway serves not only to coordinate the effects of the VEGF pathway, but its crosstalk with the Wnt pathway mediates EC function in angiogenesis (Phng and Gerhardt 2009). Furthermore, vascular remodeling in cancer is dependent upon crosstalk between the VEGF, Notch and Wnt pathways (Katoh and Katoh 2006). Deregulation of these pathways has been implicated in many tumor types, including those of the lung (Daniel et al. 2006) and liver (Martinez Arias 2003).

The Wnt pathway is made up of a family of secreted glycoproteins, ranging in size from 39-46 kDa. There are 19 known Wnt homologues that that participate in three Wnt signaling pathways: the canonical pathway, the Wnt/Ca^{2+} pathway, and the planar cell polarity pathway. The canonical pathway participates in the stabilization of β–catenin and its subsequent translocation to the nucleus where it functions as an oncogene. Abnormal activation of the canonical Wnt/β-catenin pathway is one of the most frequent signaling abnormalities known in human cancer (Brennan and Brown 2004). Interestingly, in a study conducted by Nimmagadda et al, the quail homologue to VEGFR-2 (Quek1) was found to be upregulated by Wnt1 and Wnt3a (Nimmagadda et al. 2007). Wnt1 and Wnt3a were also shown to induce proliferation in EC necessary for angiogenesis. These results are consistent with those of Wang et al that showed Wnt signaling pathway activation was vital to the development of vascular structures in embryos (Wang et al. 2006). In addition, Wnt2 was identified as an autocrine growth factor for VEGFR-2 stimulation in hepatic sinusoidal EC (HSECs) (Klein et al. 2008). Investigations from Dr. Gerhardt's laboratory showed that the Notch-regulated ankyrin repeat protein (Nrarp) acts as a molecular link between Notch and Lef1 (a chaperone for distinct factors controlling transcription of Wnt target genes)-dependent Wnt signaling in EC to control stability of new vessel connections in mouse and zebrafish. DLL4/Notch-induced expression of Nrarp limits Notch signaling and promotes Wnt/Ctnnb1 (the β–catenin gene) signaling in endothelial stalk cells through interactions with Lef1 (Phng and Gerhardt 2009). Taken together, these data suggest that multi-directional targeting of VEGFR-2, Notch and Wnt pathway components could be a worthwhile endeavor in the search for novel therapeutic targets against cancer.

In human MCF-7 BC cells over-expression of the γ-secretase (the enzyme that catalyzes intramembrane cleavage of the Notch receptor upon ligand binding required for Notch activation) liberated Notch intercellular domain and increased HIF-1α protein levels by an unknown mechanism (W. Lee et al. 2008b; Lee et al. 2008a). Notch1 signaling can promote NFκB translocation to the nucleus and DNA binding by increasing both phosphorylation of the IκB kinase α/β complex (a repressor of NFκB activation) and the expression of some NFκB family members (Monsalve et al. 2009). We have found that leptin (an adipocytokine) activated NFκB, SP1 and HIF-1α (Gonzalez-Perez et al. 2010) and increased the expression of Notch mRNA and protein in breast cancer cells under normoxic conditions (Guo and Gonzalez-Perez 2011). Remarkably, leptin induced the expression of Notch1-4, Jagged1 and VEGFR-2 in these cells. Moreover, we have recently reported that a novel and unveiled crosstalk, NILCO (Notch, IL-1 and leptin crosstalk outcome) is essential for leptin-induced proliferation, migration and VEGF/VEGFR-2 expression by breast cancer cells (Guo and Gonzalez-Perez 2011). In particular, leptin-mediated activation of NFκB increased VEGFR-2 and Notch. Furthermore, leptin increased through several signaling pathways promoter activities of VEGFR-2-Luc transfected-cells. Interestingly, leptin effects on VEGFR-2 were abrogated by a γ–secretase inhibitor. Moreover, VEGFR-2 transcription and expression was heavily depending on VEGFR-2 gene methylation and histone acetylation that could be linked to leptin and Notch effects (Guo and Gonzalez-Perez, unpublished data). However, the role of Notch-mediated regulation of VEGFR-2 and signaling crosstalk in cancer cells is so far unknown.

5.3 Estrogen-mediated regulation of VEGFR-2

Estrogens exert important regulatory functions on vessel wall components, which may contribute to the increased prevalence and severity of certain chronic inflammatory, autoimmune diseases, as well as tumor initiation, progression, particularly in tumors of the breast, endometrium, ovary and prostate (Ferreira et al. 2009; Russo and Russo 2006; Santen et al. 2009). EC have also been identified as targets for estrogens. ERs have been found in EC from various vascular beds. The regulatory functions of estrogen in EC responses are relevant to vessel inflammation, injury, and repair. In these cells estrogen affects nitric oxide production and release, modulates the expression of EC-adhesion molecules and regulates angiogenesis (Kim and Bender 2005; Rubanyi et al. 2002; Simoncini et al. 2004). The mechanisms through which estrogen regulates VEGFR-2 in angiogenesis are complex and may involve both genomic and non-genomic effects. It was earlier reported that, estrogen stimulates EC growth as well as VEGF-dependent angiogenesis by the receptor-mediated pathway, especially ERα (Suzuma et al. 1999; Tanemura et al. 2004). However, non-classical mechanisms through ERα/Sp3 and ERα/Sp4 complexes were found in some cancer cell lines, such as ZR-75 breast cancer cells. In these cells E2 activates GC-rich sites where Sp proteins but not ER-α bind to VEGFR-2 promoter to stimulate mRNA and protein expression (Higgins et al. 2006b). In contrast, in MCF-7 cells, the ERα/Sp protein-VEGFR-2 promoter interactions involve the recruitment of the co-repressors SMRT (silencing mediator of retinoid and thyroid hormone receptor) and NCoR (nuclear receptor corepressor) resulting in decreased VEGFR-2 mRNA levels (Higgins et al. 2008). Estrogens may also directly stimulate endothelial progenitor cells (EPCs). In a recently report (Baruscotti et al. 2010), physiological concentrations of E2 (10 nmol/L) was showed to increase EPC-induced capillary sprout and lumen formation in matrigel/fibrin/collagen systems. Whereas, heme oxygenase 1 (HO-1) and phosphorylation of ERK 1/2, Akt, and vVEGFR-2 were also increased, indicating that E2 via ERα promotes EPC-mediated capillary formation. The mechanism for these E2 actions probably involves non-genomic activation of RTKs and HO-1 activation.

5.4 Cytokine and growth factor regulation of VEGFR-2

VEGF-A is hypoxia-inducible showing a temporal expression pattern that generally parallels VEGFR-2 expression. Contradictory data on the direct role of hypoxia in the regulation of VEGFR-2 were reported. The differential and synergistic regulation of VEGF and VEGFR-2 by hypoxia in an organotypic cerebral slice culture system for EC was linked to a direct induction of VEGF that subsequently up-regulates VEGFR-2 in EC. VEGF-induced VEGFR-2 up-regulation was abrogated by a neutralizing anti-VEGF antibody (Kremer et al. 1997). In contrast, it was later reported that hypoxia up-regulates VEGFR-2 in cultured cells by a posttranscriptional mechanism (Gerber et al. 1997). Inflammation and angiogenesis are frequently coupled in pathological situations like breast cancer. One of the hallmarks of inflammation is an increase in vascular permeability, frequently driven by an excess of VEGF and other mediators. Inflammation induces EC activation and capillary sprouting (Arroyo and Iruela-Arispe 2010). Pathological angiogenesis is associated with the secretion of cytokines. However, the molecular and cellular mechanisms linking chronic inflammation to tumorigenesis remain largely unresolved. Many cytokines and growth factors are able to increase VEGF expression (Hicklin and Ellis 2005). However, a reduced number of these factors have been confirmed to regulate VEGFR-2 expression. Majority of inflammatory cytokines exert inflammatory effects through the induction of NFκB. a hallmark of inflammatory responses. Activation of NFκB is essential for promoting inflammation-associated cancer (Pikarsky et al. 2004). VEGF (Pikarsky et al. 2004) and VEGFR-2 (Wu and Patterson 1999) promoters have NFκB responsive cis-elements. Therefore, cytokine-activated NFκB increases angiogenesis by direct upregulation of pro-angiogenic genes. VEGFR-2 is associated to inflammatory breast cancer and is therefore a target for cancer prevention.

Cytokines have diverse effects on VEGFR-2. PIGF, erythropoietin or PDGF were unable to up-regulate VEGFR-2 (Kremer et al. 1997). Transforming growth factor-beta (TGF-β) can down-regulate VEGFR-2 (Barleon et al. 1997a) but discordant results on TNF-α mediated down-regulation (Patterson et al. 1996) and up-regulation (Giraudo et al. 1998) of VEGFR-2 have been reported. Moreover, TNF showed contradictory effects on VEGFR-2 activity. TNF induced VEGFR-2 but blocked it signals, thus delaying the VEGF-driven angiogenic response (Sainson et al. 2008). Members of the chemokine family can also regulate VEGFR-2. CCL23 (also known as MPIF-1, MIP-3, or Ckb8) is a CC chemokine initially characterized as a chemoattractant for monocytes and dendritic cells. In HUVEC, CCL23 mainly induced VEGFR-2 expression at the transcriptional level. These effects were linked to CCL23-mediated phosphorylation of SAPK/JNK (Han et al. 2009). IL-1 is a known factor in cancer development and inducer of VEGF expression in different tissues (Carmi et al. 2009; Valdivia-Silva et al. 2009). Macrophages are recruited to tumors by chemokines, cytokines and growth factors, including VEGF, produced by tumor cells and other cell types in the tumor microenvironment. In turn macrophages and tumor cells secrete IL-1 that contributes to tumor progression by facilitating angiogenesis, matrix remodeling, invasion and metastasis (Chen et al. 2009). Inhibition of IL-1 signaling by exogenous IL-1Ra negatively impacted tumor angiogenesis in nude mice (Voronov et al. 2003). We have recently demonstrated that IL-1/IL-1R tI signaling upregulates VEGFR-2 in breast cancer cells (Zhou et al. 2011).

5.4.1 Leptin regulation of VEGFR-2

Recently, leptin was added to the list of factors that upregulate VEGF-A and VEGFR-2 (Carino et al. 2008; Gonzalez et al. 2006; Rene Gonzalez et al. 2009). Leptin is a small nonglycosilated protein (16 kD) product of the ob gene. Leptin is a pleitropic adipocytokine, with mitogenic and angiogenic effects, that promotes anchorage, proliferation of breast cancer cells, microvessel and hematopoiesis and increase the levels of several factors including cell cycle regulators (Gonzalez et al. 2006; Pischon et al. 2008; Rene Gonzalez et al. 2009). Leptin actions are more often than not related to energy balance. However, leptin is also recognized for its contributions to reproduction, angiogenesis, proliferation and inflammation. Leptin's actions are now being linked to the development and pathogenesis of cancer (Hu et al. 2002; Pischon et al. 2008). Higher levels of leptin are found in female, postmenopausal women and obese individuals. The leptin levels have been related to the incidence of various types of cancer, most notably breast cancer (Cleary and Maihle 1997; Ray and Cleary). Breast carcinoma cells express higher levels of leptin and leptin receptor, OB-R, than normal mammary cells and a significant correlation between leptin/OB-R levels with metastasis and lower survival of breast cancer patients has been found (Hu et al. 2002; Laud et al. 2002; Tessitore et al. 2000). We have previously found that leptin signaling plays an important role in the growth of breast cancer that is associated with the regulation of pro-angiogenic, pro-inflammatory and pro-proliferative molecules (Rene Gonzalez et al. 2009). Leptin increases VEGFR-2 expression in endometrial cancer cells in vitro (Carino et al. 2008) and in breast cancer cells in vitro and in vivo (Gonzalez et al. 2006; Rene Gonzalez et al. 2009). Leptin upregulation of VEGF-A/VEGFR-2 was partially mediated by IL-1 system. Leptin upregulates IL-1 gene through activated SP1 and NF-κB. In addition, leptin-induced activation of PI-3K signaling pathway was related to increased levels of pmTOR, p70S6K1 and p4E-BP (Zhou et al. 2011). In human breast cancer cells ER-positive (MCF-7) or ER-negative (MDA-MB-231), leptin in a dose-response manner significantly increased the levels of VEGFR-2 protein and mRNA (Rene Gonzalez et al. 2009). However, the molecular mechanisms of how leptin signaling regulates VEGFR-2 are largely unknown (Beecken et al. 2000; Cirillo et al. 2008; Hausman and Richardson 2004). In addition, leptin induces transactivation of the HER2/*neu* proto-oncogene (*c-erbB-2*), and interacts with insulin like growth factor-1 to transactivate the EGF-receptor (EGFR) (Fiorio et al. 2008; Soma et al. 2008). Leptin stimulates aromatase expression and activation of ER (Catalano et al. 2003; Cirillo et al. 2008). A pegylated leptin peptide receptor antagonist (PEG-LPrA2) markedly reduced the growth of tumors and the expression of VEGF-A/VEGFR-2 in mouse models of syngeneic and human breast cancer xenografts (Gonzalez et al. 2006; Rene Gonzalez et al. 2009). The mice treated with PEG-LPrA2 had diminished expression of VEGF-A/VEGFR-2, OB-R, leptin, IL-1R tI, PCNA and cyclin D1 (Rene Gonzalez et al. 2009). PEG-LPrA2's effects were probably related to reduced NILCO (see Fig 2) (Guo and Gonzalez-Perez 2011). These data suggest that inhibition of leptin signaling may serve as a novel adjuvant for prevention and treatment of breast cancer. The alarming increase of incidence of obesity in the Western countries emphasizes the importance of these findings (Lee et al. 2008b; Lee et al. 2008a).

Leptin is likely linked to the growth of several cancer types and may influence the expression of VEGFR-2 in several malignancies. Results from xenografts from human ovarian cancer cells (OVCAR5 and IGROV1) subcutaneously inoculated on ovariectomized nude mice show correlations of VEGF-A/VEGFR-2 expression in all tumors. Interestingly, treatment of mice with PEG-LPrA2 induced a significant reduction of tumor growth. Moreover, incubation of ovarian cancer cells with leptin increased cell proliferation in a dose dependent fashion that was abrogated by pre-treatment with PEG-LPAr2. Furthermore, PEG-LPrA2 reduced leptin induced VEGF-A, VEGFR-2, Ki-67 as well as ERα levels. These data suggest elevated leptin would likely have pro-proliferative and pro-angiogenic effects on human ovarian cancer. Our data also suggests that leptin may be a link between obesity, estrogen and ovarian cancer (Rueda and Gonzalez-Perez, unpublished). Colon cancer development has also been linked to obesity (Frezza et al. 2006) and leptin signaling, which can orchestrate VEGF-A-driven angiogenesis and vascular development, thus providing a specific mechanism and potential target for obesity-associated cancer (Birmingham et al. 2009). A recent report stated that high levels of leptin in obese mice increased the growth of colorectal cancer induced by azoxymethane (a carcinogen) in normal mice in contrast to leptin deficient mice (*ob/ob* and *db/db*). These results suggested leptin is important for colon cancer growth in the context of obesity (Endo et al. 2011).

6. Clinical significance of targeting VEGFR-2

Solid tumor malignancies including breast, lung and prostate carcinomas are considered to be angiogenesis dependent. However, anti-angiogenic therapies have shown varying results partly because each tumor type secretes a distinct panel of angiogenic factors to sustain its own microvascular network. Additionally, recent evidence has demonstrated that tumors develop resistance to anti-angiogenic therapy by turning on alternate angiogenic pathways when one pathway is therapeutically inhibited. The redundancy of these angiogenic pathways provides a plethora of targets for intervention. It is likely that successful complete inhibition of angiogenesis will rely on the use of combination and/or sequential therapies (Hayes et al. 2007; Roy and Perez 2009).

In this section we will briefly discuss experimental therapies for angiogenesis inhibition in breast cancer. As already discussed the role of angiogenesis in carcinogenesis is complex and mediated by many different factors. The central role of the Notch receptor and its attendant Jagged and Delta cell ligands, and their role in angiogenesis have led to development of Notch signaling inhibition as a therapeutic intervention. The GSIs or small molecule inhibitors of γ-secretase have shown inhibition of tumorigenesis. The main disadvantage with the use of GSIs is their non-specificity. Many physiological processes require Notch signaling, therefore, toxicity profiles may be profound. Additionally, subsequent development of antibodies directed specifically against the Notch receptor or its ligands would offer another therapeutic alternative (Shi and Harris 2006).

Tumor hypoxia occurs as tumors grow subsequently leading to an increase in HIF-1α. Acetylation and deacetylation post-translational modifications are critical to HIF-1α signaling. As such, HDAC inhibitors can be considered as a possible therapeutic intervention in breast cancer treatment (Ellis et al. 2009). The use of HDAC inhibitors in mouse models in combination with VEGF receptor tyrosine kinase inhibitor decreases the expression of angiogenesis related genes such as angiopoietin-2 and its receptor Tie-2, and survivin in EC. HDAC inhibitors are already in clinical use in treating hematologic malignanices such as myelodisplastic syndrome (MDS) and acute myeloid leukemia (AML) (Qian et al. 2004). Regulation of VEGFR-2 expression by Sp proteins has been previously discussed in this paper. It has been suggested that VEGFR-2 can be targeted by drugs that down regulate Sp proteins or block Sp-dependent trans-activation (Higgins et al. 2006a). Activation of VEGFR-2 via binding of Sp3 and Sp4 with ERα to promoter region of VEGFR-2 is enhanced by E2. It could be hypothesized that blocking secretion of E2 would downregulate this effect and hence inhibit angiogenesis (Higgins et al. 2006b; Liang et al. 2006).

Some anti-angiogenic treatment strategies have entered the clinic to date. These agents include a humanized monoclonal antibody directed to VEGF-A (Bevacizumab; Avastin; Genentech Inc, South San Francisco, CA), a chimeric monoclonal antibody directed to the VEGFR-2 (IMC-1C11), several small molecule inhibitors of the VEGFR-2 tyrosine kinase, and a nuclease-stabilized ribozyme (Angiozyme) that specific cleaves both VEGFR-1 and VEGFR-2 mRNA (Weng and Usman 2001). Preclinical models have shown regression of solid tumor growth and angiogenesis with anti-VEGF monoclonal antibodies alone or in combination with chemotherapy (Borgstrom et al. 1999; Kim et al. 1993; Millauer et al. 1994). Clinical benefit with bevacizumab has been reported from clinically trials in metastatic colon, renal cell, and breast cancer (Hurwitz et al. 2004; Miller et al. 2005; Wedam et al. 2006; Yang et al. 2003). Bevacizumab was able to significant decrease (66.7%) phosphorylated VEGFR-2 (Y951) in tumor cells and increase in tumor apoptosis after one cycle of bevacizumab alone (Wedam et al. 2006). However, it has been reported that treatment with bevacizumab may induce alterations in human brain and tumor endothelial cells, leading to escape mechanisms from anti-VEGF-A therapy. Therefore, it is probable that VEGF-C and -D might act as alternative pro-angiogenic factors in these cirscunstances (Grau et al. 2011). Applications of bevacizumab therapy are not confined to cancer. Macular degeneration, a disorder of the retina that is enhanced by age, is the most common cause of irreversible vision loss in older people. The disease is characterized by abnormal blood vessels grow beneath the retina. Therefore, several anti-angiogenic treatments are being tested in the clinic. Among these, anti-VEGF therapies have potential successful applications. Investigations from intravitreal bevacizumab (Avastin) therapy showed promising 6-month results in patients with neovascular macular degeneration (Weigert et al. 2008).

IMC-1C11, a chimeric monoclonal antibody, binds specifically to the EC-surface extracellular domain of VEGFR-2, blocks VEGFR-VEGFR interaction and prevents VEGFR activation of the intracellular tyrosine kinase pathway (Lu et al. 2000; Zhu et al. 1998). The initial Phase I trial of IMC-1C11 was carried out in patients with metastatic colorectal carcinoma. This has provided evidence of the safety and low toxicity for an antibody blockade of VEGFR-2, as well as insight into dose and schedule requirements (Posey et al. 2003). A fully human anti-VEGFR-2 agent has been produced as a second-generation agent, which is anticipated to be nonimmunogenic for chronic administration as a single agent and in combination with chemotherapy or radiation. Semaxanib (SU5416) was the first specific synthesized potent and selective inhibitor of the VEGFR tyrosine kinase that is presently under evaluation in Phase I clinical studies for the treatment of human cancers (Fong et al. 1999). SU5416 was showed to induce growth inhibition in mouse xenotransplants of human tumors. But in several phase II trials, results were disappointing, albeit providing a good security profile (Fury et al. 2007). Other additional inhibitors of the VEGFR-2 tyrosine kinase are currently being examined in clinical trials, such as PTK 787, ZD6474, and CP547632 which have been selected on the basis of relatively selective inhibition of the VEGFR-2 ATP binding site (Ansiaux et al. 2009; Banerjee et al. 2009; Beebe et al. 2003). SCC-S2, a novel antiapoptotic molecule, has shown to decrease the proliferation and tumorigenicity of MDA-MB-435 human breast cancer cells (Kumar et al. 2004). Treatment of these cells with a cationic liposomal formulation of SCC-S2 antisense oligo correlated with decreased expression of VEGFR-2 in tumor cells as well as human lung microvascular EC and loss of cell viability (Zhang et al. 2006). Targeted therapies with the introduction of adenoviral vector expressing inducible Caspase-9, (iCaspase-9) under transcriptional regulation with EC-specific VEGFR-2 promoter induced apoptosis of proliferating human dermal microvascular EC (HDMECs) (Song et al. 2008).

Numerous studies using novel anti-angiogenic inhibitors have lent additional support to the critical role of antiangiogenesis in colon cancer pathogenesis. Sakurai et al examined the effect of a novel angiogenesis inhibitor, Ki23057, on HUVEC tube formation in colon cancer (Sakurai et al. 2007). Immunoprecipitation revealed the inhibition of tyrosine phosphorylation of VEGFR-2 in HUVECs. However, no inhibitory effect was seen on the proliferation of the colon cancer cell lines: LM-H3, LoVo and LS174T. Conversely, Ki23057 showed a significant inhibitory effect on the growth of xenografted LM-H3 tumors as well as on the spread of cancer cells to the liver. Anti-CD31 antibody staining was significantly reduced in microvessels compared to controls (Sakurai et al. 2007). Other studies demonstrated advantages of combined therapy against EGFR and VEGFR-2. Tonra et al used anti-EGFR (cetuximab) and VEGFR-2 (DC101) antibodies in pancreatic (BxPc-3) and colon cancer (GEO) cell lines. The dose response of the combined treatment revealed synergism for both cell lines (CI=0.1, $P<0.01$ for BxPC-3 and CI=0.1, $P<0.01$ for GEO) (Tonra et al. 2006). Several studies have been conducted using VEGFR-2 inhibitors for treatment highlighting the role of this pathway in the pathogenesis, proliferation and survival of PCa. The use of these agents provides another therapeutic option beyond chemotherapy for those patients who have become hormone refractory. A preclinical trial conducted by Bischof et al using a combination of irradiation, VEGFR-2 inhibition (SU5416) and chemotherapy (premetrexed) in human endothelial and tumor cells. The PCa cell line, PC3, exhibited a significant increase in antiproliferative effects ($p<0.05$) (Bischof et al. 2004). Conversely, a phase II trial employing VEGFR-2 inhibitor, SU5416, in 36 chemotherapy naive patients did not produce any significant effect on PCa growth or on in vivo PSA kinetics (Stadler et al. 2004). Additional studies are needed to fully elucidate the role of VEGFR-2 in this particular malignancy. Anti-angiogenesis treatment has been used for HCC. Combined inhibition of Raf and VEGFR-2 with the small molecule inhibitor NVP-AAL881 (Novartis, USA) was reported to efficiently disrupt oncogenic signaling and reduce tumor growth and vascularization of HCC. Hence, this strategy could prove valuable for therapy of HCC (Lang et al. 2008). New compounds/technologies are being developed to target VEGFR-2. Mice treated with VEGFR-2-based DNA vaccine showed significant reduction of renal carcinomas (Yan et al. 2009). A series of dual c-Met/VEGFR-2 kinase inhibitors were found to significantly affect growth of human xenografts (Mannion et al. 2009). Medicinal plants could be new sources for anti-VEGFR-2 drugs. Acetyl-11-keto-beta-boswellic acid (AKBA) derived from Bowawellia serrata inhibits prostate tumor growth by blocking VEGFR-2 signaling (Pang et al. 2009). Previous studies in our laboratory have demonstrated that leptin-signal inhibition resulted in decreased growth of mammary tumors derived from mouse and humans. The expression of VEGF-A and VEGFR-2 was increased under leptin signaling in cell culture and decreased by the actions of leptin peptide antagonists (PEG-LPrA2) in vitro and in vivo (Rene Gonzalez et al. 2009). Moreover, PEG-LPrA2 actions on carcinogenic (DMBA)-induced breast tumors in DIO (diet-induced-obesity) mice negatively affected VEGFR-2 and NILCO (Gonzalez-Perez, unpublished). Thus, our data strongly suggest that leptin signaling inhibition could serve as an additional preventative and/or therapeutic modality for breast cancer.

The question of which would be a more suitable target: VEGF or VEGFR-2, for tumor anti-angiogenic therapy is still unsolved. Furthermore, experimental data show inconsistent results from anti-VEGF or anti-VEGFR-2 therapies in animal models as opposed to clinical trials. Reasons for these discordant results are unknown, but most likely rely on the complexity of human cancer and redundant actions of many pro-angiogenic factors. One proposed mechanisms of tumor escape from anti-VEGF-A therapy is the upregulation of FGF2, a pleiotropic angiogenic inducer, which is expressed by several tumor types (Alessi et al. 2009). Preclinical studies investigating anti-angiogenic drug resistance by tumors show that at least 4 factors could be involved in the failure of these therapies: (1) upregulation of bFGF; (2) overexpression of MMP-9; (3) increased levels of SDF-1α (stromal-cell derived-factor 1α) and (4) HIF1α -induced recruitment of bone-marrow-derived CD45+ myeloid cells (Dempke and Heinemann 2009). In addition, results from our investigations suggest that leptin, derived either from adipose tissue or cancer cells could increase tumor angiogenesis by directly affecting EC angiogenic features by promoting proliferation, survival and secretion of VEGF-A and activating NILCO in in malignant cells (Garonna et al. 2011; Gonzalez et al. 2006; Gonzalez-Perez et al. 2010; Guo and Gonzalez-Perez 2011; Rene Gonzalez et al. 2009; Zhou et al. 2011). Probably, the more effective means to abolish VEGF-A/VEGFR-2 autocrine/paracrine effects affecting cancer cells and angiogenic features is to use combined therapies against kinase activity and crosstalk to several signaling partners, including co-receptors, adhesion molecules, developmental signaling, growth factors and cytokines (i.e., NRP-1/-2, integrins, EGF, Notch, leptin, etc). However, tumor-developed resistance to anti-angiogenic therapies would be a latent issue. Moreover, current data suggest that these combined therapies would probably show differential impact on diverse cancer/stage types.

7. Conclusions

Aberrant VEGFR-2 expression/signaling, found in majority of cancer types, are closely related to worse prognostic. Therefore, this evidence supports the idea that targeting VEGFR-2 overexpression in endothelial/malignant cells could be an effective way to treat several cancers. Many factors have been identified as potential regulators of VEGFR-2 expression and function in diverse biological scenarios. Paracrine effects of VEGF, the NILCO crosstalk and diverse cytokines/growth factors secreted by cancer cells up-regulated VEGFR-2 in EC as well as in cancer. These molecules also orchestrate autocrine/paracrine upregulation of VEGFR-2 that is essential for the survival/proliferation actions of VEGF/VEGFR-2 loop in cancer cells. Specificity of activated tyrosine amino acid residues within cytoplasmatic tail of VEGFR-2 in inducing signaling networks and biological effects in cancer require more investigation. Complexity of signals derived from activated heterodimers of VEGFR-2 and VEGFR-1 or VEGFR-3 in cancer need to be further unraveled. Additional studies are needed to advance testing and developing specific anti-VEGFR-2 therapies. Deeper understanding of VEGFR-2 regulation and signaling crosstalk mechanisms in cancer and EC cells will likely lead to the development of new therapeutic modalities. Translational studies are needed to test these agents for efficacy and toxicity in diverse cancers.

8. Acknowledgements

This work was supported in part by Grants from NIH/NCI 1SC1CA138658-01 and the Georgia Cancer Coalition Distinguished Cancer Scholar Award to R.R.G-P.; the Morehouse School of Medicine (MSM) MBRS RISE Program (NIH/NIGMS 506 GM08248) to T.Z.M., CREDO (MSCR) 2R25RR017694-06A1 to L.S.C., and facilities and support services at MSM (NIH RR03034 and 1C06 RR18386).

9. Glossary

4T1 cells: mouse mammary cancer cell line; AhR: aryl hydrocarbon receptor; Akt: protein kinase B; BAECs: bovine aortic endothelial cells; ChiPs: chromatin immunoprecipitation assays; Cyclin D1: kinase and regulator of cell cycle D1; DLL1-3: Delta-like 1-3; DMBA: 7,12 dimethylbenz[A]antracene; EC: endothelial cells; EGFR: epidermal growth factor receptor; Elf-1: Ets domain transcription factor; ER: estrogen receptor; ERK 1/2: extracellular regulated kinase 1 and 2; Ets: E-twenty six family of transcription factor; FGFR: fibroblast growth factor receptor; HAT: histone acetyltransferases; HDAC: histone deacetylases; HIF-1α: hypoxia regulated factor-1 alpha; HUVECs: human umbilical vein endothelial cells; JNK: c-Jun N-terminal kinase or SAPK (stress activated protein kinase); JunD: Transcription factor jun-D; MAPK: mitogen activated protein kinase; MCF-7: ER positive human breast cancer cell line; MDA-MB-231: ER negative human breast cancer cell line; MEK: mitogen-activated protein kinase/extracellular signal-regulated kinase; mTOR: mammalian target of rapamycin; NFκB: eukaryotic nuclear transcription factor kappa B; NILCO: Notch, IL-1 and leptin crosstalk outcome; NRP-1/-2: Neuropilin-1 and-2 receptors; OB-R: leptin receptor;

P38 kinase: extracellular regulated kinase 38; PDGF: platelet-derived growth factor; PIGF: placental growth factor or PGF; PI-3K: phosphoinositide 3-kinase; PKC: protein kinase C; RTK: receptor tyrosine kinase; SDF1α: stromal-cell derived-factor 1α; Sp1-3: Specificity protein 1-3; STAT3: signal transducer and activator of transcription 3; TGF-β: transforming growth factor beta; TNF-α: tumor necrosis factor alpha; VEGF: Vascular endothelial growth factor; VEGFR-1: Vascular endothelial growth factor receptor 1 or Flt-1; VEGFR-2: Vascular endothelial growth factor receptor 2 or KDR or Flk-1; VEGFR-3: Vascular endothelial growth factor receptor 3 or Flt-4.

10. References

Abedi, H. and Zachary, I. (1997), 'Vascular endothelial growth factor stimulates tyrosine phosphorylation and recruitment to new focal adhesions of focal adhesion kinase and paxillin in endothelial cells', *J Biol Chem,* 272 (24), 15442-51.

Achen, M. G., McColl, B. K., and Stacker, S. A. (2005), 'Focus on lymphangiogenesis in tumor metastasis', *Cancer Cell,* 7 (2), 121-7.

Achen, M. G., Mann, G. B., and Stacker, S. A. (2006), 'Targeting lymphangiogenesis to prevent tumour metastasis', *Br J Cancer,* 94 (10), 1355-60.

Achen, M. G., et al. (1998), 'Vascular endothelial growth factor D (VEGF-D) is a ligand for the tyrosine kinases VEGF receptor 2 (Flk1) and VEGF receptor 3 (Flt4)', *Proc Natl Acad Sci U S A,* 95 (2), 548-53.

Aesoy, R., et al. (2008), 'An autocrine VEGF/VEGFR2 and p38 signaling loop confers resistance to 4-hydroxytamoxifen in MCF-7 breast cancer cells', *Mol Cancer Res,* 6 (10), 1630-8.

Alessi, P., et al. (2009), 'Anti-FGF2 approaches as a strategy to compensate resistance to anti-VEGF therapy: long-pentraxin 3 as a novel antiangiogenic FGF2-antagonist', *Eur Cytokine Netw,* 20 (4), 225-34.

Altekruse, S. F., McGlynn, K. A., and Reichman, M. E. (2009), 'Hepatocellular carcinoma incidence, mortality, and survival trends in the United States from 1975 to 2005', *J Clin Oncol,* 27 (9), 1485-91.

Amino, N., et al. (2006), 'YM-359445, an orally bioavailable vascular endothelial growth factor receptor-2 tyrosine kinase inhibitor, has highly potent antitumor activity against established tumors', *Clin Cancer Res,* 12 (5), 1630-8.

Andre, T., et al. (2000), 'Vegf, Vegf-B, Vegf-C and their receptors KDR, FLT-1 and FLT-4 during the neoplastic progression of human colonic mucosa', *Int J Cancer,* 86 (2), 174-81.

Annunziata, C. M., et al. (2010), 'Vandetanib, designed to inhibit VEGFR2 and EGFR signaling, had no clinical activity as monotherapy for recurrent ovarian cancer and no detectable modulation of VEGFR2', *Clin Cancer Res,* 16 (2), 664-72.

Anonymous 'Ovarian Cancer Overview ', *http://www.cancer.org/Cancer/OvarianCancer/OverviewGuide/ovarian-cancer-overview-key-statistics.*

Anonymous 'National Cancer Institute', *http:///www.cancer.gov/cancertopics/types/brain.*

Anonymous 'Colorectal Cancer Facts & Figures 2011-2013', *American Cancer Society,* http://www.cancer.org/Research/CancerFactsFigures/ColorectalCancerFactsFigures/colorectal-cancer-facts-figures-2011-2013-page.

Ansiaux, R., et al. (2009), 'Decrease in tumor cell oxygen consumption after treatment with vandetanib (ZACTIMA; ZD6474) and its effect on response to radiotherapy', *Radiat Res,* 172 (5), 584-91.

Arroyo, A. G. and Iruela-Arispe, M. L. (2010) 'Extracellular matrix, inflammation, and the angiogenic response', *Cardiovasc Res,* 86 (2), 226-35.

Artavanis-Tsakonas, S., Rand, M. D., and Lake, R. J. (1999), 'Notch signaling: cell fate control and signal integration in development', *Science,* 284 (5415), 770-6.

Ashikari-Hada, S., et al. (2005), 'Heparin regulates vascular endothelial growth factor165-dependent mitogenic activity, tube formation, and its receptor phosphorylation of human endothelial cells. Comparison of the effects of heparin and modified heparins', *J Biol Chem,* 280 (36), 31508-15.

Autiero, M., et al. (2003), 'Role of PlGF in the intra- and intermolecular cross talk between the VEGF receptors Flt1 and Flk1', *Nat Med,* 9 (7), 936-43.

Bachelder, R. E., et al. (2001), 'Vascular endothelial growth factor is an autocrine survival factor for neuropilin-expressing breast carcinoma cells', *Cancer Res,* 61 (15), 5736-40.

Badalian, G., et al. (2007), 'EGFR and VEGFR2 protein expressions in bone metastases of clear cell renal cancer', *Anticancer Res,* 27 (2), 889-94.

Bagri, A., Tessier-Lavigne, M., and Watts, R. J. (2009), 'Neuropilins in tumor biology', *Clin Cancer Res,* 15 (6), 1860-4.

Banerjee, S., et al. (2009), 'The vascular endothelial growth factor receptor inhibitor PTK787/ZK222584 inhibits aromatase', *Cancer Res,* 69 (11), 4716-23.

Barleon, B., et al. (1997a), 'Vascular endothelial growth factor up-regulates its receptor fms-like tyrosine kinase 1 (FLT-1) and a soluble variant of FLT-1 in human vascular endothelial cells', *Cancer Res,* 57 (23), 5421-5.

--- (1997b), 'Mapping of the sites for ligand binding and receptor dimerization at the extracellular domain of the vascular endothelial growth factor receptor FLT-1', *J Biol Chem,* 272 (16), 10382-8.

Baruscotti, I., et al. (2010), 'Estradiol stimulates capillary formation by human endothelial progenitor cells: role of estrogen receptor-{alpha}/{beta}, heme oxygenase 1, and tyrosine kinase', *Hypertension,* 56 (3), 397-404.

Beebe, J. S., et al. (2003), 'Pharmacological characterization of CP-547,632, a novel vascular endothelial growth factor receptor-2 tyrosine kinase inhibitor for cancer therapy', *Cancer Res,* 63 (21), 7301-9.

Beecken, W. D., Kramer, W., and Jonas, D. (2000), 'New molecular mediators in tumor angiogenesis', *J Cell Mol Med,* 4 (4), 262-69.

Benedito, R., et al. (2009), 'The notch ligands Dll4 and Jagged1 have opposing effects on angiogenesis', *Cell,* 137 (6), 1124-35.

Birmingham, J. M., et al. (2009), 'Novel mechanism for obesity-induced colon cancer progression', *Carcinogenesis,* 30 (4), 690-7.

Biscetti, F., et al. (2009), 'Peroxisome proliferator-activated receptor alpha is crucial for iloprost-induced in vivo angiogenesis and vascular endothelial growth factor upregulation', *J Vasc Res,* 46 (2), 103-8.

Bischof, M., et al. (2004), 'Triple combination of irradiation, chemotherapy (pemetrexed), and VEGFR inhibition (SU5416) in human endothelial and tumor cells', *Int J Radiat Oncol Biol Phys,* 60 (4), 1220-32.

Blom, T., et al. (2010), 'Amplification and overexpression of KIT, PDGFRA, and VEGFR2 in medulloblastomas and primitive neuroectodermal tumors', *J Neurooncol,* 97 (2), 217-24.

Boocock, C. A., et al. (1995), 'Expression of vascular endothelial growth factor and its receptors flt and KDR in ovarian carcinoma', *J Natl Cancer Inst,* 87 (7), 506-16.

Borgstrom, P., et al. (1999), 'Importance of VEGF for breast cancer angiogenesis in vivo: implications from intravital microscopy of combination treatments with an anti-VEGF neutralizing monoclonal antibody and doxorubicin', *Anticancer Res,* 19 (5B), 4203-14.

Bray, S. J. (2006), 'Notch signalling: a simple pathway becomes complex', *Nat Rev Mol Cell Biol,* 7 (9), 678-89.

Brennan, K. R. and Brown, A. M. (2004), 'Wnt proteins in mammary development and cancer', *J Mammary Gland Biol Neoplasia,* 9 (2), 119-31.

Brown, L. F., et al. (1995), 'Expression of vascular permeability factor (vascular endothelial growth factor) and its receptors in breast cancer', *Hum Pathol,* 26 (1), 86-91.

Bruns, A. F., et al. (2009), 'VEGF-A-stimulated signalling in endothelial cells via a dual receptor tyrosine kinase system is dependent on co-ordinated trafficking and proteolysis', *Biochem Soc Trans,* 37 (Pt 6), 1193-7.

--- 'Ligand-stimulated VEGFR2 signaling is regulated by co-ordinated trafficking and proteolysis', *Traffic,* 11 (1), 161-74.

Buchler, P., et al. (2002), 'VEGF-RII influences the prognosis of pancreatic cancer', *Ann Surg,* 236 (6), 738-49; discussion 49.

Caolo, V., et al. (2010), 'Feed-forward signaling by membrane-bound ligand receptor circuit: the case of NOTCH DELTA-like 4 ligand in endothelial cells', *J Biol Chem,* 285 (52), 40681-9.

Capp, C., et al. (2010), 'Increased expression of vascular endothelial growth factor and its receptors, VEGFR-1 and VEGFR-2, in medullary thyroid carcinoma', *Thyroid,* 20 (8), 863-71.

Carino, C., et al. (2008), 'Leptin regulation of proangiogenic molecules in benign and cancerous endometrial cells', *Int J Cancer,* 123 (12), 2782-90.

Carmeliet, P., et al. (1999), 'Targeted deficiency or cytosolic truncation of the VE-cadherin gene in mice impairs VEGF-mediated endothelial survival and angiogenesis', *Cell,* 98 (2), 147-57.

Carmi, Y., et al. (2009), 'The role of macrophage-derived IL-1 in induction and maintenance of angiogenesis', *J Immunol,* 183 (7), 4705-14.

Carrillo de Santa Pau, E., et al. (2009), 'Prognostic significance of the expression of vascular endothelial growth factors A, B, C, and D and their receptors R1, R2, and R3 in patients with nonsmall cell lung cancer', *Cancer,* 115 (8), 1701-12.

Catalano, S., et al. (2003), 'Leptin enhances, via AP-1, expression of aromatase in the MCF-7 cell line', *J Biol Chem,* 278 (31), 28668-76.

Charboneau, A., et al. (2005), 'Pbx1 is required for Hox D3-mediated angiogenesis', *Angiogenesis,* 8 (4), 289-96.

Chauvet, C., et al. (2004), 'The gene encoding human retinoic acid-receptor-related orphan receptor alpha is a target for hypoxia-inducible factor 1', *Biochem J,* 384 (Pt 1), 79-85.

Chen, H., et al. (2004), 'VEGF, VEGFRs expressions and activated STATs in ovarian epithelial carcinoma', *Gynecol Oncol,* 94 (3), 630-5.

--- (2009), 'TGF-beta induces fibroblast activation protein expression; fibroblast activation protein expression increases the proliferation, adhesion, and migration of HO-8910PM [corrected]', *Exp Mol Pathol,* 87 (3), 189-94.

Chen, Z. and Han, Z. C. (2008), 'STAT3: a critical transcription activator in angiogenesis', *Med Res Rev,* 28 (2), 185-200.

Cheng, J., et al. (2004), 'Expression of vascular endothelial growth factor and receptor flk-1 in colon cancer liver metastases', *J Hepatobiliary Pancreat Surg,* 11 (3), 164-70.

Chung, G. G., et al. (2006), 'Vascular endothelial growth factor, FLT-1, and FLK-1 analysis in a pancreatic cancer tissue microarray', *Cancer,* 106 (8), 1677-84.

Cirillo, D., et al. (2008), 'Leptin signaling in breast cancer: an overview', *J Cell Biochem,* 105 (4), 956-64.

Cleary, M. P. and Maihle, N. J. (1997), 'The role of body mass index in the relative risk of developing premenopausal versus postmenopausal breast cancer', *Proc Soc Exp Biol Med,* 216 (1), 28-43.

Daniel, V. C., Peacock, C. D., and Watkins, D. N. (2006), 'Developmental signalling pathways in lung cancer', *Respirology,* 11 (3), 234-40.

Davis-Smyth, T., et al. (1996), 'The second immunoglobulin-like domain of the VEGF tyrosine kinase receptor Flt-1 determines ligand binding and may initiate a signal transduction cascade', *EMBO J,* 15 (18), 4919-27.

Davis, R., et al. (2009), 'Sulforaphane inhibits angiogenesis through activation of FOXO transcription factors', *Oncol Rep,* 22 (6), 1473-8.

Dayanir, V., et al. (2001), 'Identification of tyrosine residues in vascular endothelial growth factor receptor-2/FLK-1 involved in activation of phosphatidylinositol 3-kinase and cell proliferation', *J Biol Chem,* 276 (21), 17686-92.

Dempke, W. C. and Heinemann, V. (2009), 'Resistance to EGF-R (erbB-1) and VEGF-R modulating agents', *Eur J Cancer,* 45 (7), 1117-28.

Dias, S., et al. (2001), 'Inhibition of both paracrine and autocrine VEGF/ VEGFR-2 signaling pathways is essential to induce long-term remission of xenotransplanted human leukemias', *Proc Natl Acad Sci U S A,* 98 (19), 10857-62.

Dineen, S. P., et al. (2008), 'The Adnectin CT-322 is a novel VEGF receptor 2 inhibitor that decreases tumor burden in an orthotopic mouse model of pancreatic cancer', *BMC Cancer,* 8, 352.

Dixelius, J., et al. (2003), 'Ligand-induced vascular endothelial growth factor receptor-3 (VEGFR-3) heterodimerization with VEGFR-2 in primary lymphatic endothelial cells regulates tyrosine phosphorylation sites', *J Biol Chem,* 278 (42), 40973-9.

Drevs, J., et al. (2007), 'Phase I clinical study of AZD2171, an oral vascular endothelial growth factor signaling inhibitor, in patients with advanced solid tumors', *J Clin Oncol,* 25 (21), 3045-54.

Ellis, L., Hammers, H., and Pili, R. (2009), 'Targeting tumor angiogenesis with histone deacetylase inhibitors', *Cancer Lett,* 280 (2), 145-53.

Eltzschig, H. K. and Carmeliet, P. (2011), 'Hypoxia and inflammation', *N Engl J Med,* 364 (7), 656-65.

Endo, H., et al. (2011), 'Leptin acts as a growth factor for colorectal tumours at stages subsequent to tumour initiation in murine colon carcinogenesis', *Gut.*

Ferrara, N. (1999), 'Vascular endothelial growth factor: molecular and biological aspects', *Curr Top Microbiol Immunol,* 237, 1-30.

Ferrara, N., Gerber, H. P., and LeCouter, J. (2003), 'The biology of VEGF and its receptors', *Nat Med,* 9 (6), 669-76.

Ferreira, A. M., et al. (2009), 'Estrogens, MSI and Lynch syndrome-associated tumors', *Biochim Biophys Acta,* 1796 (2), 194-200.

Ferrer, F. A., et al. (1997), 'Vascular endothelial growth factor (VEGF) expression in human prostate cancer: in situ and in vitro expression of VEGF by human prostate cancer cells', *J Urol,* 157 (6), 2329-33.

Fiorio, E., et al. (2008), 'Leptin/HER2 crosstalk in breast cancer: in vitro study and preliminary in vivo analysis', *BMC Cancer,* 8, 305.

Folkman, J. (1971), 'Tumor angiogenesis: therapeutic implications', *N Engl J Med,* 285 (21), 1182-6.

Fong, G. H., et al. (1995), 'Role of the Flt-1 receptor tyrosine kinase in regulating the assembly of vascular endothelium', *Nature,* 376 (6535), 66-70.

Fong, T. A., et al. (1999), 'SU5416 is a potent and selective inhibitor of the vascular endothelial growth factor receptor (Flk-1/KDR) that inhibits tyrosine kinase catalysis, tumor vascularization, and growth of multiple tumor types', *Cancer Res,* 59 (1), 99-106.

Fox, S. B., Generali, D. G., and Harris, A. L. (2007), 'Breast tumour angiogenesis', *Breast Cancer Res,* 9 (6), 216.

Frezza, E. E., Wachtel, M. S., and Chiriva-Internati, M. (2006), 'Influence of obesity on the risk of developing colon cancer', *Gut,* 55 (2), 285-91.

Fritz, W. A., Lin, T. M., and Peterson, R. E. (2008), 'The aryl hydrocarbon receptor (AhR) inhibits vanadate-induced vascular endothelial growth factor (VEGF) production in TRAMP prostates', *Carcinogenesis,* 29 (5), 1077-82.

Fury, M. G., et al. (2007), 'A Phase II study of SU5416 in patients with advanced or recurrent head and neck cancers', *Invest New Drugs,* 25 (2), 165-72.

Gaetano, C., et al. (2001), 'Retinoids induce fibroblast growth factor-2 production in endothelial cells via retinoic acid receptor alpha activation and stimulate angiogenesis in vitro and in vivo', *Circ Res,* 88 (4), E38-47.

Garonna, E., et al. (2011), 'Vascular endothelial growth factor receptor-2 couples cyclo-oxygenase-2 with pro-angiogenic actions of leptin on human endothelial cells', *Plos one,* 6 (4), e18823.

Gerald, D., et al. (2004), 'JunD reduces tumor angiogenesis by protecting cells from oxidative stress', *Cell,* 118 (6), 781-94.

Gerber, H. P., et al. (1997), 'Differential transcriptional regulation of the two vascular endothelial growth factor receptor genes. Flt-1, but not Flk-1/KDR, is up-regulated by hypoxia', *J Biol Chem,* 272 (38), 23659-67.

Germain, M., et al. (2009), 'Genetic ablation of the alpha 6-integrin subunit in Tie1Cre mice enhances tumour angiogenesis', *J Pathol.*

Giatromanolaki, A., et al. (2006), 'Phosphorylated KDR expression in endometrial cancer cells relates to HIF1alpha/VEGF pathway and unfavourable prognosis', *Mod Pathol,* 19 (5), 701-7.

--- (2007), 'Activated VEGFR2/KDR pathway in tumour cells and tumour associated vessels of colorectal cancer', *Eur J Clin Invest,* 37 (11), 878-86.

Giraudo, E., et al. (1998), 'Tumor necrosis factor-alpha regulates expression of vascular endothelial growth factor receptor-2 and of its co-receptor neuropilin-1 in human vascular endothelial cells', *J Biol Chem,* 273 (34), 22128-35.

Gockel, I., et al. (2008), 'Co-expression of receptor tyrosine kinases in esophageal adenocarcinoma and squamous cell cancer', *Oncol Rep,* 20 (4), 845-50.

Gonzalez-Perez, R. R., et al. (2010), 'Leptin upregulates VEGF in breast cancer via canonic and non-canonical signalling pathways and NFkappaB/HIF-1alpha activation', *Cell Signal,* 22 (9), 1350-62.

Gonzalez, R. R., et al. (2006), 'Leptin signaling promotes the growth of mammary tumors and increases the expression of vascular endothelial growth factor (VEGF) and its receptor type two (VEGF-R2)', *J Biol Chem,* 281 (36), 26320-8.

Grau, S., et al. (2011), 'Bevacizumab can induce reactivity to VEGF-C and -D in human brain and tumour derived endothelial cells', *J Neurooncol.*

Guo, S. and Gonzalez-Perez, R. R. (2011), 'Notch, IL-1 and leptin crosstalk outcome (NILCO) is critical for leptin-induced proliferation, migration and VEGF/VEGFR-2 expression in breast cancer', *PLoS One,* 6(6): e21467 (doi:10.1371/journal.pone.0021467).

Guo, S., Liu, M., and Gonzalez-Perez, R. R. (2011), 'Role of Notch and its oncogenic signaling crosstalk in breast cancer', *Biochim Biophys Acta,* 1815 (2), 197-213.

Guo, S., et al. (2010), 'Vascular endothelial growth factor receptor-2 in breast cancer', *Biochim Biophys Acta,* 1806 (1), 108-21.

Han, K. Y., et al. (2009), 'CCL23 up-regulates expression of KDR/Flk-1 and potentiates VEGF-induced proliferation and migration of human endothelial cells', *Biochem Biophys Res Commun,* 382 (1), 124-8.

Hannum, C., et al. (1994), 'Ligand for FLT3/FLK2 receptor tyrosine kinase regulates growth of haematopoietic stem cells and is encoded by variant RNAs', *Nature,* 368 (6472), 643-8.

Hata, Y., et al. (1998), 'Transcription factors Sp1 and Sp3 alter vascular endothelial growth factor receptor expression through a novel recognition sequence', *J Biol Chem,* 273 (30), 19294-303.

Hausman, G. J. and Richardson, R. L. (2004), 'Adipose tissue angiogenesis', *J Anim Sci,* 82 (3), 925-34.

Hayes, D. F., Miller, K., and Sledge, G. (2007), 'Angiogenesis as targeted breast cancer therapy', *Breast,* 16 Suppl 2, S17-9.

Hicklin, D. J. and Ellis, L. M. (2005), 'Role of the vascular endothelial growth factor pathway in tumor growth and angiogenesis', *J Clin Oncol,* 23 (5), 1011-27.

Higgins, K. J., et al. (2006a), 'Regulation of vascular endothelial growth factor receptor-2 expression in pancreatic cancer cells by Sp proteins', *Biochem Biophys Res Commun,* 345 (1), 292-301.

--- (2006b), 'Vascular endothelial growth factor receptor-2 expression is induced by 17beta-estradiol in ZR-75 breast cancer cells by estrogen receptor alpha/Sp proteins', *Endocrinology,* 147 (7), 3285-95.

--- (2008), 'Vascular endothelial growth factor receptor-2 expression is down-regulated by 17beta-estradiol in MCF-7 breast cancer cells by estrogen receptor alpha/Sp proteins', *Mol Endocrinol,* 22 (2), 388-402.

Hilbe, W., et al. (2004), 'CD133 positive endothelial progenitor cells contribute to the tumour vasculature in non-small cell lung cancer', *J Clin Pathol,* 57 (9), 965-9.

Hu, X., et al. (2002), 'Leptin--a growth factor in normal and malignant breast cells and for normal mammary gland development', *J Natl Cancer Inst,* 94 (22), 1704-11.

Huang, J., et al. (2011), 'Prognostic significance and potential therapeutic target of VEGFR2 in hepatocellular carcinoma', *J Clin Pathol,* 64 (4), 343-8.

Huang, K., et al. (2001), 'Signaling properties of VEGF receptor-1 and -2 homo- and heterodimers', *Int J Biochem Cell Biol,* 33 (4), 315-24.

Huang, X., et al. (2006), 'Critical role for the Ets transcription factor ELF-1 in the development of tumor angiogenesis', *Blood,* 107 (8), 3153-60.

Hurwitz, H., et al. (2004), 'Bevacizumab plus irinotecan, fluorouracil, and leucovorin for metastatic colorectal cancer', *N Engl J Med,* 350 (23), 2335-42.

Imatani, A. and Callahan, R. (2000), 'Identification of a novel NOTCH-4/INT-3 RNA species encoding an activated gene product in certain human tumor cell lines', *Oncogene,* 19 (2), 223-31.

Indraccolo, S., et al. (2009), 'Cross-talk between tumor and endothelial cells involving the Notch3-Dll4 interaction marks escape from tumor dormancy', *Cancer Res,* 69 (4), 1314-23.

Issbrucker, K., et al. (2003), 'p38 MAP kinase--a molecular switch between VEGF-induced angiogenesis and vascular hyperpermeability', *FASEB J,* 17 (2), 262-4.

Itakura, J., et al. (2000), 'Concomitant over-expression of vascular endothelial growth factor and its receptors in pancreatic cancer', *Int J Cancer,* 85 (1), 27-34.

Jach, R., et al. (2010), 'Expression of VEGF, VEGF-C and VEGFR-2 in in situ and invasive SCC of cervix', *Front Biosci (Elite Ed),* 2, 411-23.

Jackson, M. W., et al. (2002), 'A potential autocrine role for vascular endothelial growth factor in prostate cancer', *Cancer Res,* 62 (3), 854-9.

Jantus-Lewintre, E., et al. (2011), 'Combined VEGF-A and VEGFR-2 concentrations in plasma: Diagnostic and prognostic implications in patients with advanced NSCLC', *Lung Cancer.*

Jenuwein, T. (2001), 'Re-SET-ting heterochromatin by histone methyltransferases', *Trends Cell Biol,* 11 (6), 266-73.

Jenuwein, T. and Allis, C. D. (2001), 'Translating the histone code', *Science,* 293 (5532), 1074-80.

Joensuu, H., et al. (2005), 'Amplification of genes encoding KIT, PDGFRalpha and VEGFR2 receptor tyrosine kinases is frequent in glioblastoma multiforme', *J Pathol,* 207 (2), 224-31.

Jones-Bolin, S., et al. (2006), 'The effects of the oral, pan-VEGF-R kinase inhibitor CEP-7055 and chemotherapy in orthotopic models of glioblastoma and colon carcinoma in mice', *Mol Cancer Ther,* 5 (7), 1744-53.

Jones, P. A. and Baylin, S. B. (2002), 'The fundamental role of epigenetic events in cancer', *Nat Rev Genet,* 3 (6), 415-28.

Joukov, V., et al. (1996a), 'A novel vascular endothelial growth factor, VEGF-C, is a ligand for the Flt4 (VEGFR-3) and KDR (VEGFR-2) receptor tyrosine kinases', *EMBO J,* 15 (2), 290-98.

--- (1996b), 'A novel vascular endothelial growth factor, VEGF-C, is a ligand for the Flt4 (VEGFR-3) and KDR (VEGFR-2) receptor tyrosine kinases', *EMBO J,* 15 (7), 1751.

Joung, Y. H., et al. (2005), 'Hypoxia activates the cyclin D1 promoter via the Jak2/STAT5b pathway in breast cancer cells', *Exp Mol Med,* 37 (4), 353-64.

Jussila, L. and Alitalo, K. (2002), 'Vascular growth factors and lymphangiogenesis', *Physiol Rev,* 82 (3), 673-700.

Kabrun, N., et al. (1997), 'Flk-1 expression defines a population of early embryonic hematopoietic precursors', *Development,* 124 (10), 2039-48.

Kato, H., et al. (2002), 'Expression of vascular endothelial growth factor (VEGF) and its receptors (Flt-1 and Flk-1) in esophageal squamous cell carcinoma', *Anticancer Res,* 22 (6C), 3977-84.

Katoh, Y. and Katoh, M. (2006), 'Comparative integromics on VEGF family members', *Int J Oncol,* 28 (6), 1585-9.

Kim ES, et al. (2010), 'The BATTLE trial (Bio- marker-integrated Approaches of Targeted Therapy for Lung Cancer Elimination): personalizing therapy for lung cancer. ', *101st Annual Meeting of the American Association for Cancer Research,* April 17-21, (Washington, DC.).

Kim, J. Y., et al. (2009), 'The expression of VEGF receptor genes is concurrently influenced by epigenetic gene silencing of the genes and VEGF activation', *Epigenetics,* 4 (5), 313-21.

Kim, K. H. and Bender, J. R. (2005), 'Rapid, estrogen receptor-mediated signaling: why is the endothelium so special?', *Sci STKE,* 2005 (288), pe28.

Kim, K. J., et al. (1993), 'Inhibition of vascular endothelial growth factor-induced angiogenesis suppresses tumour growth in vivo', *Nature,* 362 (6423), 841-4.

Klein, D., et al. (2008), 'Wnt2 acts as a cell type-specific, autocrine growth factor in rat hepatic sinusoidal endothelial cells cross-stimulating the VEGF pathway', *Hepatology,* 47 (3), 1018-31.

Kliche, S. and Waltenberger, J. (2001), 'VEGF receptor signaling and endothelial function', *IUBMB Life,* 52 (1-2), 61-6.

Knizetova, P., et al. (2008), 'Autocrine regulation of glioblastoma cell cycle progression, viability and radioresistance through the VEGF-VEGFR2 (KDR) interplay', *Cell Cycle,* 7 (16), 2553-61.

Koukourakis, M. I., et al. (2011), 'Serum VEGF levels and tissue activation of VEGFR2/KDR receptors in patients with breast and gynecologic cancer', *Cytokine,* 53 (3), 370-5.

Kouzarides, T. (2007), 'Chromatin modifications and their function', *Cell,* 128 (4), 693-705.

Kovall, R. A. (2008), 'More complicated than it looks: assembly of Notch pathway transcription complexes', *Oncogene,* 27 (38), 5099-109.

Kranz, A., Mattfeldt, T., and Waltenberger, J. (1999), 'Molecular mediators of tumor angiogenesis: enhanced expression and activation of vascular endothelial growth factor receptor KDR in primary breast cancer', *Int J Cancer,* 84 (3), 293-8.

Kremer, C., et al. (1997), 'Up-regulation of flk-1/vascular endothelial growth factor receptor 2 by its ligand in a cerebral slice culture system', *Cancer Res,* 57 (17), 3852-9.

Kuemmel, S., et al. (2009), 'Circulating vascular endothelial growth factors and their soluble receptors in pre-invasive, invasive and recurrent cervical cancer', *Anticancer Res,* 29 (2), 641-5.

Kuenen, B. C., et al. (2005), 'Dose-finding study of the multitargeted tyrosine kinase inhibitor SU6668 in patients with advanced malignancies', *Clin Cancer Res,* 11 (17), 6240-6.

Kumar, D., et al. (2004), 'Expression of SCC-S2, an antiapoptotic molecule, correlates with enhanced proliferation and tumorigenicity of MDA-MB 435 cells', *Oncogene,* 23 (2), 612-6.

Kunizaki, M., et al. (2007), 'The lysine 831 of vascular endothelial growth factor receptor 1 is a novel target of methylation by SMYD3', *Cancer Res,* 67 (22), 10759-65.

Kuo, M. H. and Allis, C. D. (1998), 'Roles of histone acetyltransferases and deacetylases in gene regulation', *Bioessays,* 20 (8), 615-26.

Laakkonen, P., et al. (2007), 'Vascular endothelial growth factor receptor 3 is involved in tumor angiogenesis and growth', *Cancer Res,* 67 (2), 593-9.

Lamalice, L., et al. (2004), 'Phosphorylation of tyrosine 1214 on VEGFR2 is required for VEGF-induced activation of Cdc42 upstream of SAPK2/p38', *Oncogene,* 23 (2), 434-45.

Lang, S. A., et al. (2008), 'Dual inhibition of Raf and VEGFR2 reduces growth and vascularization of hepatocellular carcinoma in an experimental model', *Langenbecks Arch Surg,* 393 (3), 333-41.

Laud, K., et al. (2002), 'Identification of leptin receptors in human breast cancer: functional activity in the T47-D breast cancer cell line', *Mol Cell Endocrinol,* 188 (1-2), 219-26.

Laurie, S. A., et al. (2008), 'Phase I and pharmacokinetic study of daily oral AZD2171, an inhibitor of vascular endothelial growth factor tyrosine kinases, in combination with carboplatin and paclitaxel in patients with advanced non-small-cell lung cancer: the National Cancer Institute of Canada clinical trials group', *J Clin Oncol,* 26 (11), 1871-8.

Lee, C. W., et al. (2008a), 'Molecular dependence of estrogen receptor-negative breast cancer on a notch-survivin signaling axis', *Cancer Res,* 68 (13), 5273-81.

--- (2008b), 'A functional Notch-survivin gene signature in basal breast cancer', *Breast Cancer Res,* 10 (6), R97.

Lee, J. H., et al. (2008c), 'Interferon regulatory factor-1 (IRF-1) regulates VEGF-induced angiogenesis in HUVECs', *Biochim Biophys Acta,* 1783 (9), 1654-62.

Legge, F., et al. (2010), 'Pharmacotherapy of cervical cancer', *Expert Opin Pharmacother,* 11 (12), 2059-75.

Levine, A. C., et al. (1998), 'Androgens induce the expression of vascular endothelial growth factor in human fetal prostatic fibroblasts', *Endocrinology,* 139 (11), 4672-8.

Li, J. L., et al. (2007), 'Delta-like 4 Notch ligand regulates tumor angiogenesis, improves tumor vascular function, and promotes tumor growth in vivo', *Cancer Res,* 67 (23), 11244-53.

Liang, Y., Brekken, R. A., and Hyder, S. M. (2006), 'Vascular endothelial growth factor induces proliferation of breast cancer cells and inhibits the anti-proliferative activity of anti-hormones', *Endocr Relat Cancer,* 13 (3), 905-19.

Linderholm, B. K., et al. (2011), 'Vascular endothelial growth factor receptor 2 and downstream p38 mitogen-activated protein kinase are possible candidate markers of intrinsic resistance to adjuvant endocrine treatment in steroid receptor positive breast cancer', *Breast Cancer Res Treat,* 125 (2), 457-65.

Liu, Z. J., et al. (2003), 'Regulation of Notch1 and Dll4 by vascular endothelial growth factor in arterial endothelial cells: implications for modulating arteriogenesis and angiogenesis', *Mol Cell Biol,* 23 (1), 14-25.

Ljungberg, B. J., et al. (2006), 'Different vascular endothelial growth factor (VEGF), VEGF-receptor 1 and -2 mRNA expression profiles between clear cell and papillary renal cell carcinoma', *BJU Int,* 98 (3), 661-7.

Lohela, M., et al. (2009), 'VEGFs and receptors involved in angiogenesis versus lymphangiogenesis', *Curr Opin Cell Biol,* 21 (2), 154-65.

Longatto-Filho, A., et al. (2009), 'Molecular characterization of EGFR, PDGFRA and VEGFR2 in cervical adenosquamous carcinoma', *BMC Cancer,* 9, 212.

Lu, D., et al. (2000), 'Identification of the residues in the extracellular region of KDR important for interaction with vascular endothelial growth factor and neutralizing anti-KDR antibodies', *J Biol Chem,* 275 (19), 14321-30.

M. Barr, Gray, K. Gately, N. Al-Sarraf, G.P. Pidgeon and K.J. O'Byrne (2009), 'VEGF and the epigenetic regulation of its receptors in non-small cell lung cancer ', *Lung Cancer,* Volume 63, Supplement 1, , S1, S1–S38.

Mac Gabhann, F. and Popel, A. S. (2007), 'Dimerization of VEGF receptors and implications for signal transduction: a computational study', *Biophys Chem,* 128 (2-3), 125-39.

Makinen, T., et al. (2001), 'Inhibition of lymphangiogenesis with resulting lymphedema in transgenic mice expressing soluble VEGF receptor-3', *Nat Med,* 7 (2), 199-205.

Mannion, M., et al. (2009), 'N-(4-(6,7-Disubstituted-quinolin-4-yloxy)-3-fluorophenyl)-2-oxo-3-phenylimidazoli dine-1-carboxamides: a novel series of dual c-Met/VEGFR2 receptor tyrosine kinase inhibitors', *Bioorg Med Chem Lett,* 19 (23), 6552-6.

Martin, D., Galisteo, R., and Gutkind, J. S. (2009), 'CXCL8/IL8 stimulates vascular endothelial growth factor (VEGF) expression and the autocrine activation of

VEGFR2 in endothelial cells by activating NFkappaB through the CBM (Carma3/Bcl10/Malt1) complex', *J Biol Chem,* 284 (10), 6038-42.

Martinez Arias, A. (2003), 'Wnts as morphogens? The view from the wing of Drosophila', *Nat Rev Mol Cell Biol,* 4 (4), 321-5.

Matsumoto, T., et al. (2005), 'VEGF receptor-2 Y951 signaling and a role for the adapter molecule TSAd in tumor angiogenesis', *EMBO J,* 24 (13), 2342-53.

Matthews, W., et al. (1991), 'A receptor tyrosine kinase cDNA isolated from a population of enriched primitive hematopoietic cells and exhibiting close genetic linkage to c-kit', *Proc Natl Acad Sci U S A,* 88 (20), 9026-30.

Mattila, E., et al. (2008), 'The protein tyrosine phosphatase TCPTP controls VEGFR2 signalling', *J Cell Sci,* 121 (Pt 21), 3570-80.

Meissner, M., et al. (2009), 'Inhibition of Rac1 GTPase downregulates vascular endothelial growth factor receptor-2 expression by suppressing Sp1-dependent DNA binding in human endothelial cells', *Exp Dermatol,* 18 (10), 863-9.

Mercurio, A. M., et al. (2004), 'Autocrine signaling in carcinoma: VEGF and the alpha6beta4 integrin', *Semin Cancer Biol,* 14 (2), 115-22.

Meyer, M., et al. (1999), 'A novel vascular endothelial growth factor encoded by Orf virus, VEGF-E, mediates angiogenesis via signalling through VEGFR-2 (KDR) but not VEGFR-1 (Flt-1) receptor tyrosine kinases', *EMBO J,* 18 (2), 363-74.

Miao, H. Q., et al. (2000), 'Neuropilin-1 expression by tumor cells promotes tumor angiogenesis and progression', *FASEB J,* 14 (15), 2532-9.

Millauer, B., et al. (1994), 'Glioblastoma growth inhibited in vivo by a dominant-negative Flk-1 mutant', *Nature,* 367 (6463), 576-9.

--- (1993), 'High affinity VEGF binding and developmental expression suggest Flk-1 as a major regulator of vasculogenesis and angiogenesis', *Cell,* 72 (6), 835-46.

Miller, K. D., et al. (2005), 'Randomized phase III trial of capecitabine compared with bevacizumab plus capecitabine in patients with previously treated metastatic breast cancer', *J Clin Oncol,* 23 (4), 792-9.

Monsalve, E., et al. (2009), 'Notch1 upregulates LPS-induced macrophage activation by increasing NF-kappaB activity', *Eur J Immunol,* 39 (9), 2556-70.

Nakopoulou, L., et al. (2002), 'Expression of the vascular endothelial growth factor receptor-2/Flk-1 in breast carcinomas: correlation with proliferation', *Hum Pathol,* 33 (9), 863-70.

Neagoe, P. E., Lemieux, C., and Sirois, M. G. (2005), 'Vascular endothelial growth factor (VEGF)-A165-induced prostacyclin synthesis requires the activation of VEGF receptor-1 and -2 heterodimer', *J Biol Chem,* 280 (11), 9904-12.

Ng, I. O., et al. (2001), 'Microvessel density, vascular endothelial growth factor and its receptors Flt-1 and Flk-1/KDR in hepatocellular carcinoma', *Am J Clin Pathol,* 116 (6), 838-45.

Nikolinakos, P. G., et al. (2010), 'Plasma cytokine and angiogenic factor profiling identifies markers associated with tumor shrinkage in early-stage non-small cell lung cancer patients treated with pazopanib', *Cancer Res,* 70 (6), 2171-9.

Nimmagadda, S., et al. (2007), 'FGFs, Wnts and BMPs mediate induction of VEGFR-2 (Quek-1) expression during avian somite development', *Dev Biol,* 305 (2), 421-9.

Nobusawa, S., et al. (2011), 'Amplification of the PDGFRA, KIT and KDR genes in glioblastoma: a population-based study', *Neuropathology.*

Oelrichs, R. B., et al. (1993), 'NYK/FLK-1: a putative receptor protein tyrosine kinase isolated from E10 embryonic neuroepithelium is expressed in endothelial cells of the developing embryo', *Oncogene,* 8 (1), 11-8.

Ogawa, S., et al. (1998), 'A novel type of vascular endothelial growth factor, VEGF-E (NZ-7 VEGF), preferentially utilizes KDR/Flk-1 receptor and carries a potent mitotic activity without heparin-binding domain', *J Biol Chem,* 273 (47), 31273-82.

Olsson, A. K., et al. (2006), 'VEGF receptor signalling - in control of vascular function', *Nat Rev Mol Cell Biol,* 7 (5), 359-71.

Padidar, S., et al. (2011), 'Leptin up-regulates pro-inflammatory cytokines in discrete cells within mouse colon', *J Cell Physiol,* 226 (8), 2123-30.

Pajusola, K., et al. (1992), 'FLT4 receptor tyrosine kinase contains seven immunoglobulin-like loops and is expressed in multiple human tissues and cell lines', *Cancer Res,* 52 (20), 5738-43.

Pang, X., et al. (2009), 'Acetyl-11-keto-beta-boswellic acid inhibits prostate tumor growth by suppressing vascular endothelial growth factor receptor 2-mediated angiogenesis', *Cancer Res,* 69 (14), 5893-900.

Park, J. E., et al. (1994), 'Placenta growth factor. Potentiation of vascular endothelial growth factor bioactivity, in vitro and in vivo, and high affinity binding to Flt-1 but not to Flk-1/KDR', *J Biol Chem,* 269 (41), 25646-54.

Patterson, C., et al. (1995), 'Cloning and functional analysis of the promoter for KDR/flk-1, a receptor for vascular endothelial growth factor', *J Biol Chem,* 270 (39), 23111-8.

--- (1996), 'Downregulation of vascular endothelial growth factor receptors by tumor necrosis factor-alpha in cultured human vascular endothelial cells', *J Clin Invest,* 98 (2), 490-6.

--- (1997), 'Nuclear protein interactions with the human KDR/flk-1 promoter in vivo. Regulation of Sp1 binding is associated with cell type-specific expression', *J Biol Chem,* 272 (13), 8410-6.

Pellet-Many, C., et al. (2008), 'Neuropilins: structure, function and role in disease', *Biochem J,* 411 (2), 211-26.

Petrova, T. V., Makinen, T., and Alitalo, K. (1999), 'Signaling via vascular endothelial growth factor receptors', *Exp Cell Res,* 253 (1), 117-30.

Phng, L. K. and Gerhardt, H. (2009), 'Angiogenesis: a team effort coordinated by notch', *Dev Cell,* 16 (2), 196-208.

Pikarsky, E., et al. (2004), 'NF-kappaB functions as a tumour promoter in inflammation-associated cancer', *Nature,* 431 (7007), 461-6.

Pischon, T., Nothlings, U., and Boeing, H. (2008), 'Obesity and cancer', *Proc Nutr Soc,* 67 (2), 128-45.

Polyzos, A. (2008), 'Activity of SU11248, a multitargeted inhibitor of vascular endothelial growth factor receptor and platelet-derived growth factor receptor, in patients with metastatic renal cell carcinoma and various other solid tumors', *J Steroid Biochem Mol Biol,* 108 (3-5), 261-6.

Posey, J. A., et al. (2003), 'A phase I study of anti-kinase insert domain-containing receptor antibody, IMC-1C11, in patients with liver metastases from colorectal carcinoma', *Clin Cancer Res,* 9 (4), 1323-32.

Puputti, M., et al. (2006), 'Amplification of KIT, PDGFRA, VEGFR2, and EGFR in gliomas', *Mol Cancer Res,* 4 (12), 927-34.

Qian, D. Z., et al. (2004), 'The histone deacetylase inhibitor NVP-LAQ824 inhibits angiogenesis and has a greater antitumor effect in combination with the vascular endothelial growth factor receptor tyrosine kinase inhibitor PTK787/ZK222584', *Cancer Res,* 64 (18), 6626-34.

R. D. Kim, A. Lazaryan, F. Aucejo et al (2008), 'Vascular endothelial growth factor receptor 2 (VEGFr2) expression and recurrence of hepatocellular carcinoma following liver transplantation: The Cleveland Clinic experience. ', *J Clin Oncol* abstr 4594.

Rahimi, N. (2006), 'VEGFR-1 and VEGFR-2: two non-identical twins with a unique physiognomy', *Front Biosci,* 11, 818-29.

Rappold, I., et al. (1997), 'Functional and phenotypic characterization of cord blood and bone marrow subsets expressing FLT3 (CD135) receptor tyrosine kinase', *Blood,* 90 (1), 111-25.

Ray, A. and Cleary, M. P. 'Leptin as a potential therapeutic target for breast cancer prevention and treatment', *Expert Opin Ther Targets,* 14 (4), 443-51.

Razny, U., et al. (2009), 'Hepatocyte RXR alpha deletion in mice leads to inhibition of angiogenesis', *Genes Nutr,* 4 (1), 69-72.

Rene Gonzalez, R., et al. (2009), 'Leptin-signaling inhibition results in efficient anti-tumor activity in estrogen receptor positive or negative breast cancer', *Breast Cancer Res,* 11 (3), R36.

Risau, W. (1997), 'Mechanisms of angiogenesis', *Nature,* 386 (6626), 671-4.

Robertson, J. D., et al. (2009), 'Phase III trial of FOLFOX plus bevacizumab or cediranib (AZD2171) as first-line treatment of patients with metastatic colorectal cancer: HORIZON III', *Clin Colorectal Cancer,* 8 (1), 59-60.

Robinson, S. D., et al. (2009), 'Alphav beta3 integrin limits the contribution of neuropilin-1 to vascular endothelial growth factor-induced angiogenesis', *J Biol Chem,* 284 (49), 33966-81.

Roca, C. and Adams, R. H. (2007), 'Regulation of vascular morphogenesis by Notch signaling', *Genes Dev,* 21 (20), 2511-24.

Rodriguez-Antona, C., et al. (2010), 'Overexpression and activation of EGFR and VEGFR2 in medullary thyroid carcinomas is related to metastasis', *Endocr Relat Cancer,* 17 (1), 7-16.

Ronicke, V., Risau, W., and Breier, G. (1996), 'Characterization of the endothelium-specific murine vascular endothelial growth factor receptor-2 (Flk-1) promoter', *Circ Res,* 79 (2), 277-85.

Roy, V. and Perez, E. A. (2009), 'Biologic therapy of breast cancer: focus on co-inhibition of endocrine and angiogenesis pathways', *Breast Cancer Res Treat,* 116 (1), 31-8.

Rubanyi, G. M., Johns, A., and Kauser, K. (2002), 'Effect of estrogen on endothelial function and angiogenesis', *Vascul Pharmacol,* 38 (2), 89-98.

Ruggeri, B., et al. (2003), 'CEP-7055: a novel, orally active pan inhibitor of vascular endothelial growth factor receptor tyrosine kinases with potent antiangiogenic activity and antitumor efficacy in preclinical models', *Cancer Res,* 63 (18), 5978-91.

Russo, J. and Russo, I. H. (2006), 'The role of estrogen in the initiation of breast cancer', *J Steroid Biochem Mol Biol,* 102 (1-5), 89-96.

Ryden, L., et al. (2003), 'Tumor specific VEGF-A and VEGFR2/KDR protein are co-expressed in breast cancer', *Breast Cancer Res Treat,* 82 (3), 147-54.

--- (2005), 'Tumor-specific VEGF-A and VEGFR2 in postmenopausal breast cancer patients with long-term follow-up. Implication of a link between VEGF pathway and tamoxifen response', *Breast Cancer Res Treat,* 89 (2), 135-43.

Sainson, R. C., et al. (2008), 'TNF primes endothelial cells for angiogenic sprouting by inducing a tip cell phenotype', *Blood,* 111 (10), 4997-5007.

Sakurai, K., et al. (2007), 'A novel angiogenesis inhibitor, Ki23057, is useful for preventing the progression of colon cancer and the spreading of cancer cells to the liver', *Eur J Cancer,* 43 (17), 2612-20.

Santen, R., et al. (2009), 'Estrogen mediation of breast tumor formation involves estrogen receptor-dependent, as well as independent, genotoxic effects', *Ann N Y Acad Sci,* 1155, 132-40.

Sarzani, R., et al. (1992), 'A novel endothelial tyrosine kinase cDNA homologous to platelet-derived growth factor receptor cDNA', *Biochem Biophys Res Commun,* 186 (2), 706-14.

Sato, H. and Takeda, Y. (2009), 'VEGFR2 expression and relationship between tumor neovascularization and histologic characteristics in oral squamous cell carcinoma', *J Oral Sci,* 51 (4), 551-7.

Scott, A. and Mellor, H. (2009), 'VEGF receptor trafficking in angiogenesis', *Biochem Soc Trans,* 37 (Pt 6), 1184-8.

Shalaby, F., et al. (1995), 'Failure of blood-island formation and vasculogenesis in Flk-1-deficient mice', *Nature,* 376 (6535), 62-6.

Shi, W. and Harris, A. L. (2006), 'Notch signaling in breast cancer and tumor angiogenesis: cross-talk and therapeutic potentials', *J Mammary Gland Biol Neoplasia,* 11 (1), 41-52.

Shibuya, M. (2003), 'Vascular endothelial growth factor receptor-2: its unique signaling and specific ligand, VEGF-E', *Cancer Sci,* 94 (9), 751-6.

--- (2006), 'Differential roles of vascular endothelial growth factor receptor-1 and receptor-2 in angiogenesis', *J Biochem Mol Biol,* 39 (5), 469-78.

Shibuya, M. and Claesson-Welsh, L. (2006), 'Signal transduction by VEGF receptors in regulation of angiogenesis and lymphangiogenesis', *Exp Cell Res,* 312 (5), 549-60.

Shibuya, M., et al. (1990), 'Nucleotide sequence and expression of a novel human receptor-type tyrosine kinase gene (flt) closely related to the fms family', *Oncogene,* 5 (4), 519-24.

Shinkai, A., et al. (1998), 'Mapping of the sites involved in ligand association and dissociation at the extracellular domain of the kinase insert domain-containing receptor for vascular endothelial growth factor', *J Biol Chem,* 273 (47), 31283-8.

Sierra-Honigmann, M. R., et al. (1998), 'Biological action of leptin as an angiogenic factor', *Science,* 281 (5383), 1683-6.

Simoncini, T., et al. (2004), 'Genomic and non-genomic effects of estrogens on endothelial cells', *Steroids,* 69 (8-9), 537-42.

Singh, A. J., et al. (2005), 'The carboxyl terminus of VEGFR-2 is required for PKC-mediated down-regulation', *Mol Biol Cell,* 16 (4), 2106-18.

Soares, R., et al. (2004), 'Evidence for the notch signaling pathway on the role of estrogen in angiogenesis', *Mol Endocrinol,* 18 (9), 2333-43.

Solowiej, J., et al. (2009), 'Characterizing the effects of the juxtamembrane domain on vascular endothelial growth factor receptor-2 enzymatic activity, autophosphorylation, and inhibition by axitinib', *Biochemistry,* 48 (29), 7019-31.

Soma, D., et al. (2008), 'Leptin augments proliferation of breast cancer cells via transactivation of HER2', *J Surg Res,* 149 (1), 9-14.

Somanath, P. R., Malinin, N. L., and Byzova, T. V. (2009), 'Cooperation between integrin alphavbeta3 and VEGFR2 in angiogenesis', *Angiogenesis,* 12 (2), 177-85.

Song, W., et al. (2008), 'Cancer gene therapy with iCaspase-9 transcriptionally targeted to tumor endothelial cells', *Cancer Gene Ther,* 15 (10), 667-75.

Stadler, W. M., et al. (2004), 'A randomized Phase II trial of the antiangiogenic agent SU5416 in hormone-refractory prostate cancer', *Clin Cancer Res,* 10 (10), 3365-70.

Steiner, H., et al. (2004a), 'An autocrine loop for vascular endothelial growth factor is established in prostate cancer cells generated after prolonged treatment with interleukin 6', *Eur J Cancer,* 40 (7), 1066-72.

Steiner, H. H., et al. (2004b), 'Autocrine pathways of the vascular endothelial growth factor (VEGF) in glioblastoma multiforme: clinical relevance of radiation-induced increase of VEGF levels', *J Neurooncol,* 66 (1-2), 129-38.

Strahl, B. D. and Allis, C. D. (2000), 'The language of covalent histone modifications', *Nature,* 403 (6765), 41-5.

Straume, O. and Akslen, L. A. (2003), 'Increased expression of VEGF-receptors (FLT-1, KDR, NRP-1) and thrombospondin-1 is associated with glomeruloid microvascular proliferation, an aggressive angiogenic phenotype, in malignant melanoma', *Angiogenesis,* 6 (4), 295-301.

Stylianou, S., Clarke, R. B., and Brennan, K. (2006), 'Aberrant activation of notch signaling in human breast cancer', *Cancer Res,* 66 (3), 1517-25.

Suzuma, I., et al. (1999), '17 Beta-estradiol increases VEGF receptor-2 and promotes DNA synthesis in retinal microvascular endothelial cells', *Invest Ophthalmol Vis Sci,* 40 (9), 2122-9.

Svensson, S., et al. (2005), 'ERK phosphorylation is linked to VEGFR2 expression and Ets-2 phosphorylation in breast cancer and is associated with tamoxifen treatment resistance and small tumours with good prognosis', *Oncogene,* 24 (27), 4370-9.

Tahir, S. A., Park, S., and Thompson, T. C. (2009a), 'Caveolin-1 regulates VEGF-stimulated angiogenic activities in prostate cancer and endothelial cells', *Cancer Biol Ther,* 8 (23).

--- (2009b), 'Caveolin-1 regulates VEGF-stimulated angiogenic activities in prostate cancer and endothelial cells', *Cancer Biol Ther,* 8 (23), 2286-96.

Takahashi, T. and Shibuya, M. (1997), 'The 230 kDa mature form of KDR/Flk-1 (VEGF receptor-2) activates the PLC-gamma pathway and partially induces mitotic signals in NIH3T3 fibroblasts', *Oncogene,* 14 (17), 2079-89.

Takahashi, Y., et al. (1995), 'Expression of vascular endothelial growth factor and its receptor, KDR, correlates with vascularity, metastasis, and proliferation of human colon cancer', *Cancer Res,* 55 (18), 3964-8.

Talvensaari-Mattila, A., Soini, Y., and Santala, M. (2005), 'VEGF and its receptors (flt-1 and KDR/flk-1) as prognostic indicators in endometrial carcinoma', *Tumour Biol,* 26 (2), 81-7.

Tammemagi, C. M., et al. (2011), 'Lung Cancer Risk Prediction: Prostate, Lung, Colorectal and Ovarian Cancer Screening Trial Models and Validation', *J Natl Cancer Inst.*

Tanaka, K., et al. (1997), 'Characterization of the extracellular domain in vascular endothelial growth factor receptor-1 (Flt-1 tyrosine kinase)', *Jpn J Cancer Res,* 88 (9), 867-76.

Tanemura, M., et al. (2004), 'The role of estrogen and estrogen receptorbeta in choroidal neovascularization', *Mol Vis,* 10, 923-32.

Tanno, S., et al. (2004), 'Human small cell lung cancer cells express functional VEGF receptors, VEGFR-2 and VEGFR-3', *Lung Cancer,* 46 (1), 11-9.

Taylor, K. L., Henderson, A. M., and Hughes, C. C. (2002), 'Notch activation during endothelial cell network formation in vitro targets the basic HLH transcription factor HESR-1 and downregulates VEGFR-2/KDR expression', *Microvasc Res,* 64 (3), 372-83.

Teodoro, J. G., Evans, S. K., and Green, M. R. (2007), 'Inhibition of tumor angiogenesis by p53: a new role for the guardian of the genome', *J Mol Med,* 85 (11), 1175-86.

Terman, B. I., et al. (1991), 'Identification of a new endothelial cell growth factor receptor tyrosine kinase', *Oncogene,* 6 (9), 1677-83.
--- (1992), 'Identification of the KDR tyrosine kinase as a receptor for vascular endothelial cell growth factor', *Biochem Biophys Res Commun,* 187 (3), 1579-86.
Tessitore, L., et al. (2000), 'Leptin expression in colorectal and breast cancer patients', *Int J Mol Med,* 5 (4), 421-6.
Tonra, J. R., et al. (2006), 'Synergistic antitumor effects of combined epidermal growth factor receptor and vascular endothelial growth factor receptor-2 targeted therapy', *Clin Cancer Res,* 12 (7 Pt 1), 2197-207.
Tsuchiya, N., et al. (2001), 'Quantitative analysis of gene expressions of vascular endothelial growth factor-related factors and their receptors in renal cell carcinoma', *Tohoku J Exp Med,* 195 (2), 101-13.
Tzima, E., et al. (2005), 'A mechanosensory complex that mediates the endothelial cell response to fluid shear stress', *Nature,* 437 (7057), 426-31.
Urbich, C., et al. (2003), 'Fluid shear stress-induced transcriptional activation of the vascular endothelial growth factor receptor-2 gene requires Sp1-dependent DNA binding', *FEBS Lett,* 535 (1-3), 87-93.
Valdivia-Silva, J. E., et al. (2009), 'Effect of pro-inflammatory cytokine stimulation on human breast cancer: implications of chemokine receptor expression in cancer metastasis', *Cancer Lett,* 283 (2), 176-85.
Veikkola, T., et al. (2000), 'Regulation of angiogenesis via vascular endothelial growth factor receptors', *Cancer Res,* 60 (2), 203-12.
Vieira, J. M., et al. (2005), 'Expression of vascular endothelial growth factor (VEGF) and its receptors in thyroid carcinomas of follicular origin: a potential autocrine loop', *Eur J Endocrinol,* 153 (5), 701-9.
Volk, L. D., et al. (2011), 'Synergy of nab-paclitaxel and bevacizumab in eradicating large orthotopic breast tumors and preexisting metastases', *Neoplasia,* 13 (4), 327-38.
--- (2008), 'Nab-paclitaxel efficacy in the orthotopic model of human breast cancer is significantly enhanced by concurrent anti-vascular endothelial growth factor A therapy', *Neoplasia,* 10 (6), 613-23.
Voronov, E., et al. (2003), 'IL-1 is required for tumor invasiveness and angiogenesis', *Proc Natl Acad Sci U S A,* 100 (5), 2645-50.
Wade, P. A. and Wolffe, A. P. (1997), 'Histone acetyltransferases in control', *Curr Biol,* 7 (2), R82-4.
Waldner, M. J., et al. (2010), 'VEGF receptor signaling links inflammation and tumorigenesis in colitis-associated cancer', *J Exp Med,* 207 (13), 2855-68.
Waltenberger, J., et al. (1994), 'Different signal transduction properties of KDR and Flt1, two receptors for vascular endothelial growth factor', *J Biol Chem,* 269 (43), 26988-95.
Wang, H., et al. (2006), 'Gene expression profile signatures indicate a role for Wnt signaling in endothelial commitment from embryonic stem cells', *Circ Res,* 98 (10), 1331-9.
Wedam, S. B., et al. (2006), 'Antiangiogenic and antitumor effects of bevacizumab in patients with inflammatory and locally advanced breast cancer', *J Clin Oncol,* 24 (5), 769-77.
Weigand, M., et al. (2005), 'Autocrine vascular endothelial growth factor signalling in breast cancer. Evidence from cell lines and primary breast cancer cultures in vitro', *Angiogenesis,* 8 (3), 197-204.
Weigert, G., et al. (2008), 'Intravitreal bevacizumab (Avastin) therapy versus photodynamic therapy plus intravitreal triamcinolone for neovascular age-related macular

degeneration: 6-month results of a prospective, randomised, controlled clinical study', *Br J Ophthalmol,* 92 (3), 356-60.
Weng, D. E. and Usman, N. (2001), 'Angiozyme: a novel angiogenesis inhibitor', *Curr Oncol Rep,* 3 (2), 141-6.
Williams, C. K., et al. (2006), 'Up-regulation of the Notch ligand Delta-like 4 inhibits VEGF-induced endothelial cell function', *Blood,* 107 (3), 931-9.
Wu, L. W., et al. (2000), 'VRAP is an adaptor protein that binds KDR, a receptor for vascular endothelial cell growth factor', *J Biol Chem,* 275 (9), 6059-62.
Wu, Y. and Patterson, C. (1999), 'The human KDR/flk-1 gene contains a functional initiator element that is bound and transactivated by TFII-I', *J Biol Chem,* 274 (5), 3207-14.
Wu, Y., et al. (2006), 'The vascular endothelial growth factor receptor (VEGFR-1) supports growth and survival of human breast carcinoma', *Int J Cancer,* 119 (7), 1519-29.
Xia, G., et al. (2006), 'Expression and significance of vascular endothelial growth factor receptor 2 in bladder cancer', *J Urol,* 175 (4), 1245-52.
Xiong, H. Q., et al. (2004), 'A phase I surrogate endpoint study of SU6668 in patients with solid tumors', *Invest New Drugs,* 22 (4), 459-66.
Xiong, Y., et al. (2009), 'Vascular endothelial growth factor (VEGF) receptor-2 tyrosine 1175 signaling controls VEGF-induced von Willebrand factor release from endothelial cells via phospholipase C-gamma 1- and protein kinase A-dependent pathways', *J Biol Chem,* 284 (35), 23217-24.
Yamada, Y., et al. (2003), 'Aberrant methylation of the vascular endothelial growth factor receptor-1 gene in prostate cancer', *Cancer Sci,* 94 (6), 536-9.
Yan, J., et al. (2009), 'A promising new approach of VEGFR2-based DNA vaccine for tumor immunotherapy', *Immunol Lett,* 126 (1-2), 60-6.
Yancopoulos, G. D., et al. (2000), 'Vascular-specific growth factors and blood vessel formation', *Nature,* 407 (6801), 242-8.
Yang, J. C., et al. (2003), 'A randomized trial of bevacizumab, an anti-vascular endothelial growth factor antibody, for metastatic renal cancer', *N Engl J Med,* 349 (5), 427-34.
Zachary, I. (2003), 'VEGF signalling: integration and multi-tasking in endothelial cell biology', *Biochem Soc Trans,* 31 (Pt 6), 1171-7.
Zeng, M., et al. (2010), 'Hypoxia activates the K-ras proto-oncogene to stimulate angiogenesis and inhibit apoptosis in colon cancer cells', *Plos one,* 5 (6), e10966.
Zeng, Q., et al. (2005), 'Crosstalk between tumor and endothelial cells promotes tumor angiogenesis by MAPK activation of Notch signaling', *Cancer Cell,* 8 (1), 13-23.
Zhang, C., et al. (2006), 'Role of SCC-S2 in experimental metastasis and modulation of VEGFR-2, MMP-1, and MMP-9 expression', *Mol Ther,* 13 (5), 947-55.
Zhang, X., et al. (2009a), 'Thrombospondin-1 modulates vascular endothelial growth factor activity at the receptor level', *FASEB J,* 23 (10), 3368-76.
Zhang, Z., et al. (2009b), 'VEGF-dependent tumor angiogenesis requires inverse and reciprocal regulation of VEGFR1 and VEGFR2', *Cell Death Differ.*
Zhou, W., Guo, S., and Gonzalez-Perez, R. R. (2011), 'Leptin pro-angiogenic signature in breast cancer is linked to IL-1 signalling', *Br J Cancer,* 104 (1), 128-37.
Zhu, Z., et al. (1998), 'Inhibition of vascular endothelial growth factor-induced receptor activation with anti-kinase insert domain-containing receptor single-chain antibodies from a phage display library', *Cancer Res,* 58 (15), 3209-14.

3

The Effect of Chinese Herb on Tumor Angiogenesis by Inhibiting Vessel Endothelial Cells

Jian Jin, Li-Ying Qiu, Hui Hua and Lei Feng
The School of Medicine and Pharmaceutics, Jiang Nan University, China

1. Introduction

Currently, anti-angiogenesis drugs are the popular treatment for cancer, which, however, are not without serious drawbacks. Virtually all such drugs are recombinant peptides/proteins or therapeutic antibodies and thus can only be administered via intravenous injection. In addition, these drugs tend to have low stability and short half life in vivo, which demands long treatment at high doses, which in turn renders the therapy expansive and could lead to high occurrences of side effects. Furthermore, these drugs usually target only one, out of many, step or pathway of angiogenesis and are not very effective. Even Avastin, the top-selling anti-tumor angiogenesis drug on the market, can only extend patients' life span by 4~6 months without a cure. Therefore, it is necessary to develop efficacious, affordable, and orally available angiogenesis-inhibiting drugs.
We report here the high-throughput screening (HTS) of over 500 Chinese medicinal herbs and plants in human vessel endothelial cell (HMEC-1) proliferation inhibition assay, which leads to the discovery of several candidate drugs with neovascularization inhibition property. Study on seropharmacology of several medicinal herbs/plants including albizia bark and *Semen Vaccariae* demonstrated their specific inhibition on HMEC-1 growth, suggesting their potential use as oral drugs for neovascularization inhibition. (seropharmacology as a new screen method to study Chinese medical effects *in vitro*, which cultive cells by medium containing a serum from animals of oral adminstrated a medicine. It is to be proved that the medicine has the effect after oral the medicine. And it paves a highway for investigation of traditional Chinese medicine. The standardized methodology of seropharmacology was initiaed to help to the exensive application of this technology.) Our study aims to investigate the efficacy and mechanism of such inhibition of albizia bark extracts, its effective moiety and effective monomer in multiple angiogenesis models.

2. Reagents and methods

2.1 Reagents

MEM culture media was obtained from Gibco (City, Country). Sulforhodamine B (SRB) and bFGF were obtained from Sigma (St. Louis, MO, USA). FCS, trypsin, L-glutamine were purchased from Huamei Biological Company (Bejing, China). Anti- CD31 monoclonal antibody and immunohistochemisty kit were purchased from Zhongshan Jinqiao

Biotechnology Technical Service Co. Ltd. (Beijing, China). DAPI kit, TUNEL apoptosis kit, JC-1, Caspase-3, 9 spectrophotometry kit, mitotic cycle kit, and Annexin V-FITC apoptosis kit were obtained from Kaiji Biological Company (Nanjing, China). Cortex albiziae and licorice root were purchased from Shanhe Pharmaceutical Co. Ltd (Wuxi, China).

2.2 Cell lines

CPAE was kindly provided by Dr. J. Badet (Créteil University, Paris, France). **Human microvascular endothelial cell line** (HMEC-1) and human lung embryonic fibrocyte (MRC-5) were generous gifts from Dr. He Lu (INSERM U553, National Institute for Health and Medicine Research, France). B_{16} melanoma, breast cancer cell (MCF-7) and Hepatocellular carcinoma ($HepG_{2)}$ were purchased from Institute, Chinese Academy of Sciences (Beijing, China). Cells are routinely maintained in MCDB complete culture medium in a 37^0C incubator with a humidified atmosphere containing 5% CO_2.

2.3 Animals

Swiss nude mice and BALB/c mice were purchased from Shanghai Laboratory Animal Center, Chinese Academy of Sciences (Shanghai, China). Nude and C57bl/6 mice were used for human C51 colon cancer and mouse Lewis lung carcinoma ,respecctively,which were obtained from Tumor Research Center, Chinese Academy of Sciences (Beijing, China). Fertilized eggs were purchased from Mashan Poultry Center (Wuxi, China).

2.4 Herbal extracts

Albizia bark and licorice root were soaked in 5-volume of cold water for 2h, boiled for 30 min, and strained. The remaining herbal material was returned to boil for 30 min in 3-volume of water and strained. Both filtrates were combined and condensed in a waterbath to a concentrate of 1g of starting herbal material per mL. It totally get finished for 2 or 3 days

2.5 Purification of active monomer

Albizia bark extracts was loaded onto a D-101 resin column. About 70% of the ethanol elutes containing active ingredient were collected, as monitored by an in vitro activity assay. Further purification was carried out using standard silica gel column chromatography with a solvent system of chloroform–methanol–water for elution, antiphase styrene column chromatography, and antiphase C18 column chromatography to obtain the active ingredient at a purity of more than 90%. It is named *julibroside J_8, its* constituents identified as 3-o-[β-D-xylopyranosyl-(1→2)-β-D-fucopyranosyl-(1→6)-β-D-gluCopyranosyl]-21-o-{(6s)-2-trans-2-hydroxymethyl-6-methyl-6-o-[4-o-((6R)-2-trans-2,6-dimethyl-6-o-β-D-quinovopyranosyl)-2,7-octadienoyl)-β-D-quinovopyranosyl]-2,7-octadienoyl}-acacicacid-28-o-β-D-glucopyranosyl-(1→3)-[α-L-arabinofuranosyl-(1→4)]-α-L-rhamnopyranosyl-(1→2)-β-D-glucopyranosyl ester (structure shown in Fig. 1).

2.6 HMEC-1 cell proliferation inhibition assay

HMEC-1 cells were seeded in 96-well plates at 7000 ~ 8000 cells per well and cultured for 24h and the volume of cell suspension in each plate is 150μL. Following the addition of herbal extract with 150μL in each plate, cells were cultured for another 48h. Wells containing culture medium alone and those with untreated cells were served as blank and negative control, respectively. The experiment was carried out in quadruplicate and analyzed by SRB method.

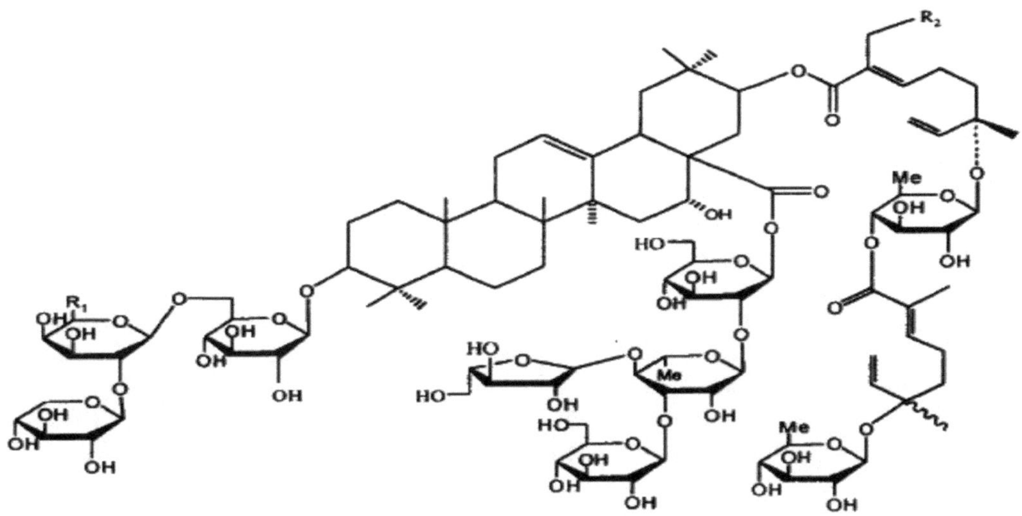

Fig. 1. Chemical structure of compound j8.

SRB assay was used to get the result of drug sensitivity assay of carcinoma. The effect of compound on proliferation inhibition was calculated according to the formula listed below:

$$\text{percentage inhibition } (\%) = \frac{(\text{negative control signal} - \text{test well signal})}{(\text{negative control signal} - \text{blank well signal})} \times 100$$

2.7 Chick chorioallantoic membrane (CAM) assay

Fresh fertilized eggs (50 ± 5 g each) with intact shell were selected for the experiment. They were soaked in 0.1% benzalkonium bromide for 3 min, and then placed in an incubator maintained at 37.8 ± 0.5 0C with a relative humidity of 65% ~ 70%. The eggs were turned daily once in the morning and once in the evening and sorted into groups of 10, based on their embryonic age. Three treatment groups were dosed with albizia bark extract at 100, 500 and 1000 μg/mL, whereas the negative control group were given normal saline only. Compounds were spotted onto sterile filter paper discs (4 mm x 4 mm) and air dried. The discs were subsequently placed onto the CAM between two vitelline veins through a window made in the eggshell and the window was sealed with sterile clear tape. Following an additional incubation for 2~3 days, seals were removed to expose the CAM; the blood vessels surround the disc (within a radius of 8mm) was counted and sorted into 3 categories based on their size; their vascular branching pattern and density were also noted.

2.8 Matrigel plug assay [1-2]

Eight-week-old female Swiss nude mice (18-22 g) were randomized into four groups (N=5 per group) injected with 0.3ml Martrigel subcutaneously at ventral lateral side; an oral dosing regimen was followed and started on the same day. One group received albizia bark extract at 8mg/kg per day, while the other were given normal saline and served as control. Mice were sacrificed after seven consecutive days of daily dosing; Matrigel plugs were removed, fixed in ethanol, and embedded in paraffin. Immunohistochemistry was performed on the sections for PECAM-1, a vessel endothelial cell marker, and blood vessels were counted on BX-40 optical microscope (Olympus, Japan).

2.9 Pharmacodynamic analysis of Albizia bark extract in C_{51} nude mice model of colon cancer

Fifteen nude mice (about 20g) were randomly assigned to three groups (N=5 per group) and inoculated subcutaneously with $5x10^7$ of C51 colon cancer cells under right armpit. Daily oral dosing started 10 days after inoculation, when the size of tumor reached 8-10 mm^3, and lasted for 4 weeks. The blank group received normal saline, control group licorice extract (8 mg/kg), and treatment group albizia bark extract (8mg/kg). Mice were sacrificed by cervical dislocation on Day 28. A portion of tumor tissue was fixed in 4% formaldehyde, embedded in paraffin and sectioned, sectioned into a thickness of 5μ m, and then stained with. Immunohistochemistry was performed on the sections for PECAM-1, blood vessels counted on BX-40 optical microscope (Olympus, Japan) with an overall magnification of 200x, and microvascular density (MVD) determined as previously described. It has been done for two weeks.

2.10 Pharmacodynamic analysis of albizia bark extract in nude mice model of lung cancer metastasis

Seven-week-old female C57BL/6 mice (18-20g) were randomized into three groups (N = 8~10 per group) and inoculated with 0.2ml of Lewis lung cancer (LLC) cell suspension ($5x10^6$/L) by ventral subcutaneous injection. Seven days later, treatment group were administered albizia bark ingredients or licorice by gavage daily, whereas control group received normal saline. Mice were sacrificed after 15 days. Lungs were fixed , in 4% formaldehyde and embedded in paraffin and sectioned for H&E staining. Three nonconsecutive sections from each sample were analyzed to determine the mean numbleof lung metastases.

2.11 Cell migration assay using scratch wound healing[3]

HMEC-1 cells were seeded in 24-well plate at $8x10^4$ cells per well, respectively, and incubated for 24h to allow attachment. A scratch of 1mm in width was introduced at the center of each well by drawing a plastic pipette tip across the surface of cell monolayer and detached cells were washed off with PBS. Media containing drugs at various concentrations were then added to each well and cells were photographed immediately with a 100x magnification and the resulting image was defined as the migration map at 0h. Subsequently, cells were photographed in the same visual field at 6h, 12h, 24h, and 48h respectively. Images obtained were processed with software IPWin60C and the distance between two opposing wound margins was measured. Cell mobility was calculated based on 6 measurements taken at randomly selected sites per image.

2.12 Tube formation assay[4]

Matrigel was thawed at 4^0C O/N and added to 24-well plates that had been pre-chilled on ice at 150 μl per well. The plates were placed in a 37^0C / 5% CO_2 incubator for 30 min. 3B11 cell suspension ($4x10^5$ cells/ml) was mixed with equal volume of cell culture media containing different concentrations of drugs and a total volume of 200 μl was plated in each well of a Matrigel plate. Cells were incubated in a 37^0C / 5% CO_2 incubator for 12h and photographed periodically.

2.13 H&E staining

HMEC-1 single cell suspension was add to a 6-well plate at 10^4 or 10^5 per well and cultured on glass coverslips for 24h, followed by further culture of 48h in the presence of drugs at various concentration. After decanting culture media, coverslips were washed three times with PBS, fixed with formalin for 10 min, and stained with hematoxylin and eosin. 10 Kunming mice (20-22g) were administered J8 for 10 days, mice were sacrificed. Lungs liver, and kidney were fixed, embedded in paraffin and sectioned for H&E staining. The change in cell morphology was observed under the microscope.

2.14 DAPI staining

HMEC-1 cells in logarithmic phase were plated in tissue culture dish and cultured on glass coverslip for 24h to allow adhesion. *Julibroside J_8* was added to a final concentration of 0.5, 1.0, and 2.5 μg / mL, while the control received no compound, and cells were cultured for another 24h. Coverslips were washed in PBS followed by DAPI staining buffer, stained in DAPI working solution at 37^0C for 15 min, rinsed in methanol and mounted in glycerol. The nuclear staining was examined on a fluorescence microscope with an oil-immersion lens.

2.15 TUNEL assay

HMEC-1 cells in logarithmic phase were plated in tissue culture dish and cultured on glass coverslips for 24h. *Julibroside J_8* was added to a final concentration of 0.5, 1.0, and 2.5 μg / mL, while the control received no compound, and cells were cultured for another 24h. Coverslips were fixed in freshly prepared 4% paraformaldehyde (PFA) at RT for 15 min ~1h. blocked in 3% H_2O_2 /MeOH at RT for 10 min, and permeabilized in freshly prepared 0.1% Triton X-100 / 0.1% sodium citrate on ice for 2 minutes. Washed samples were incubated with 50 μL fresh TdT reaction mix in the dark for 60 minutes at 37^0C in a humidified chamber. Negative controls were incubated with TdT reaction mix without TdT enzyme. Samples were washed in PBS three times and incubated with 50 μL Streptavidin-HRP solution in the dark for 30 minutes at 37^0C in a humidified chamber. Fresh DAB solution was applied to washed coverslips for 10 minutes at RT, which were subsequently rinsed, counterstained with hematoxylin and mounted.

2.16 Detection of cell death and apoptosis by flow cytometry (FCM)

HMEC-1 cells in logarithmic growth phase were inoculated into cell culture flask at 5×10^5 cell/ml in MCDB complete medium for 24h. *Julibroside J_8* was added to a final concentration of 0.5~2.5 μg/ml and cells were cultured for another 48h. The blank control received no compound. Cells were trypsinized, washed three times with PBS, and resuspended in 200μL binding buffer. 10 μL Annexin V-FITC was added into the cell suspension and incubated at RT protected from light for 30 min, followed by the addition of 5μL propidium iodide (PI) and continued incubation for another 5 min. With the addition of 400μL Binding buffer working solution, cells were ready for FCM.

2.17 Analysis of cell cycle and DNA content by FCM

HMEC-1 cells in logarithmic growth phase were inoculated into cell culture flask at 5×10^5 cell/ml in MCDB complete medium for 24h. *Julibroside J_8* was added to a final concentration of 0.5~2.5 μg/ml and cells were further cultured for 48h. The blank control received no compound. Cells were trypsinized, washed twice with PBS, and resuspended in 500 μL PBS. While gently mixing, 1.5 mL of cold 70% EtOH in PBS (pre-chilled at -20^{0}C) were added into cell suspension dropwise and the mixture was placed in the refrigerator for at least 24h. Prior to FCM analysis, cells were washed twice with PBS, resuspended in 1ml PI staining solution (PI at 100 μg/ml in PBS with 100 μg /ml DNase-free RNase A) and incubated at 4^{0}C for 30 min protected from light. The stained cells were washed in PBS, then resuspended in up to 1 ml of PBS, and strained through a 200 mesh screen. The cells were put through FCM; data from 5,000-10,000 cells per sample were analyzed using software Cellfit (BD Biosciences, USA).

2.18 Analysis of mitochondrial membrane potential by FCM

HMEC-1 cells in logarithmic growth phase were inoculated into cell culture flask at 5 x 10^5 cell/ml in MCDB complete medium for 24h. *Julibroside* J_8 was added to a final concentration of 0.5~2.5 μg/ml and cells were cultured for another 24h. The blank control received no compound. Cells were trypsinized and washed twice with PBS. No more than 10^6 cells were collected and resuspended in 500 ul lipophilic cation 5,5',6,6'-tetrachloro-1,1',3,3'-tetraethylbenzimidazolcarbocyanine iodide (JC-1) staining solution. JC-1 is more advantageous over rhodamines and other carbocyanines, capable of entering selectively into mitochondria, since it changes reversibly its color from green to orange as membrane potentials increase (over values of about 80-100 mV). This property is due to the reversible formation of JC-1 aggregates upon membrane polarization that causes shifts in emitted light from 530 nm (i.e., emission of JC-1 monomeric form) to 590 nm (i.e., emission of J-aggregate) when excited at 490 nm; the color of the dye changes reversibly from green to greenish orange as the mitochondrial membrane becomes more polarized. Both colors can be detected using the filters commonly mounted in all flow cytometers, so that green emission can be analyzed in fluorescence channel 1 (FL1) and greenish orange emission in channel 2 (FL2), subsequently incubated in a CO2 incubator at 37^{0}C for 15 ~ 20 min. Cells were then pelleted at RT (2000 rpm, 5 min) and washed twice with incubation buffer. Finally, cells were resuspended in 500 ul of incubation buffer and ready for FCM.

2.19 Determination of Caspase-3, 9 content in endothelial cells by spectrophotometer

HMEC-1 cells of logarithmic growth phase were seeded in cell culture flasks at 5×10^5 cell/mL. After 24h, *julibroside* J_8 was added to a final concentration of 1.5 μg /mL. Cells were harvested at 4, 8 and 12 hours after drug treatment and 5×10^6 cells were collected at each time point. Cells were washed twice with PBS. After the 2nd wash, cells were centrifuged at 2000 rpm for 5 min and the supernatant was discarded. 150 μL of ice-cold Lysis Buffer was used to resuspend the cell pellet; the resulting cell extraction was placed on ice for 20 ~ 60 min, with 3 ~ 4 short vortexes (10 sec each time) in between. The extraction was centrifuged at 4°C (10,000 rpm, 1min) and the supernatant, or the lysate, was carefully transferred to a fresh eppendorf (EP)tube and stored on ice. 50 μL of cell lysate was used for caspase-3 and caspase-9 enzyme activity measurement with caspase-3 and caspase-9 activity assay kits by spectrophotometry. Meanwhile, the protein concentration was determined by Bradford assay to normalize caspase activity by mg of protein. All assays were performed according to manufactures' instructions.

3. Results

3.1 Albizia bark extracts on neovascularization

3.1.1 Albizia bark extracts inhibit neovascularization in CAM assay

CAM assay is one of several classical in vivo models for studying angiogenesis. We found here that CAM treated with normal saline showed prominent angiogenesis. A large number of vessels radiated from underneath the control disc and were highly branched, which led to abundant capillaries that are responsible for the vibrant color of the CAM (Fig. 2, left panels). However, the number of vessels radiating from disc treated with albizia at 500 ug/mL was greatly reduced, and the vessels were sparse, disorganized, with a light yellow appearance (Fig. 2, right panels). The effect was dose-dependent and the phenotype was more pronounced with increased albiziae at 1000 ug/mL (Table 1), suggesting that albizia extract is an inhibitor of neovascularization.

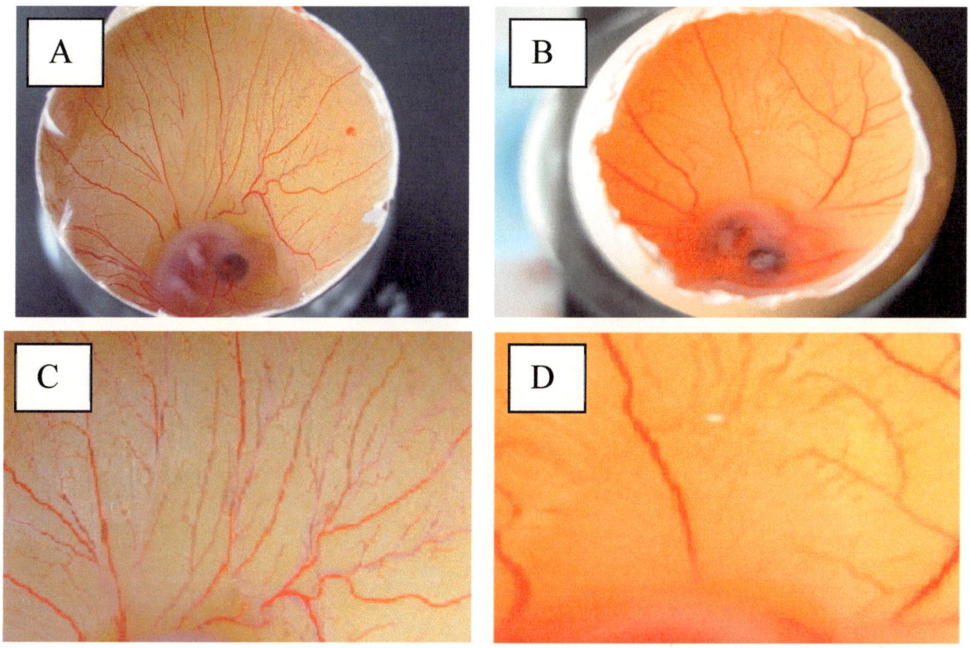

A and C: control with normal saline, B and D: albiziae treatment.

Fig. 2. Effect of *Albizia julibrissin* extracts on neovascularization in CAM (top, 10x; bottom, 20x).

albiziae extract	No. of blood vessel		
(μg/mL)	Large	Medium	Small
0 (control)	2.5±0.20	3.5±0.67	19.7±0.47
100	2.1±0.34	3.9±0.53	15.6±0.29
500	2.6±0.54	2.8±0.97	10.7±0.19*
1000	2.5±0.67	2.5±0.27	6.8±0.48 **

* $P<0.05$, ** $P<0.01$ vs Control

Table 1. Effect of *Albizia julibrissin* extracts on neovascularization in CAM ($\bar{x} \pm s$, n =10)

3.1.2 Albizia bark extracts inhibit vascularization in bFGF-induced Matrigel plugs

Paraffin sections were obtained from implanted Matrigel plugs and stained for endothelial marker CD31 (Fig. 3A, as shown in brown). bFGF to induce substantial microvasculature formation in Matrigel plugs, as evidenced by the presence of abundant endothelial cells which were positively stained for CD31. Treatment with albizia extract decreased the amount of endothelial cells in bFGF-induced Matrigel plugs, suggesting an inhibition of microvasculature formation, while treatment with licorice extract had no discernable effect on angiogenesis. Plugs from uninduced Matrigel were rarely populated by endothelial cells.

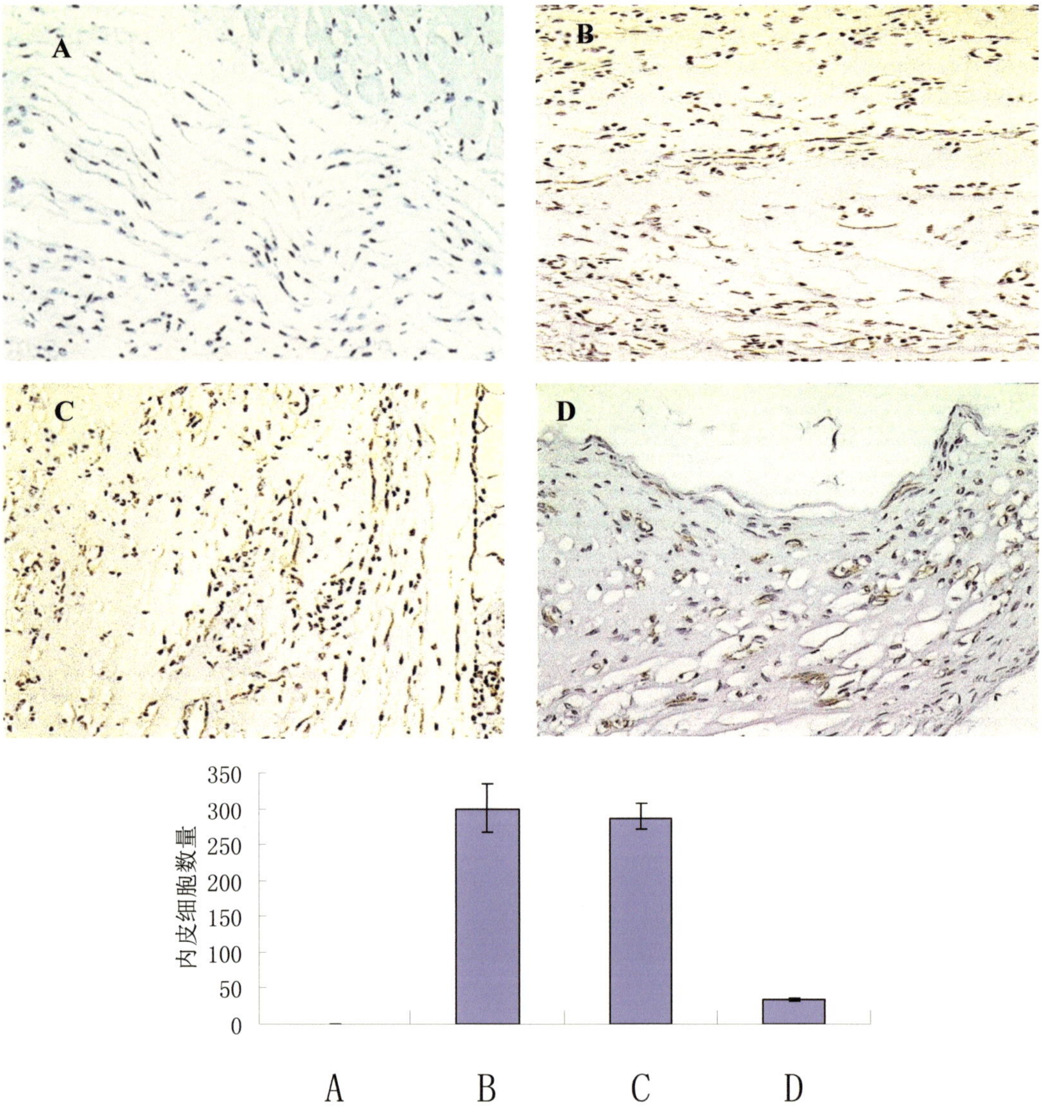

A: -bFGF (Blank) B: +bFGF
C: +bFGF / licorice D: +bFGF/ albizia

Fig. 3. Effect of *Albizia julibrissin* extracts on angiogenesis in matrigel plug (100x).

3.1.3 Albizia bark extracts inhibit neovascularization in C51 colon cancer mouse model

Nude mice inoculated with C51 colon cancer cells developed tumor, which contained in blood vessels. Compared to control group that were administered with saline, albiziae treatment caused a 67.5% reduction in tumor growth, while licorice extract showed only a slight inhibition rate (IR)f 10% (Table 2). IHC of endothelial marker CD31 on tumor tissue sections revealed extensive vessel formation in control group (Fig. 4). Microvessel density (MVD) was measured with a light microscope in a single area of invasive tumor (200x field or 0.74 mm^2) representative of the highest microvessel density (neovascular "hot spot"). This was done after endothelial cells, lining the microvessels, had been highlighted with anti-factor VIII-related antigen/von Willebrand's factor (F8RA/vWF). Subsequent studies by other investigators, using either anti-F8RA/vWF or other relatively vessel-specific reagents such as anti-CD31. MVD was drastically reduced in albiziae-treated tumors, demonstrating that albiziae is a potent inhibitor of tumor neovascularization. Despite of its mild inhibition on tumor growth, licorice extract did not seem to have much effect on neovascularization, and there were no statistically significant differences between the control and licorice-treated groups.

$$\text{The rate of inhibition (IR) (\%)} = \frac{(\text{negative control volume} - \text{test well volume})}{(\text{negative control volume})} \times 100$$

CD3

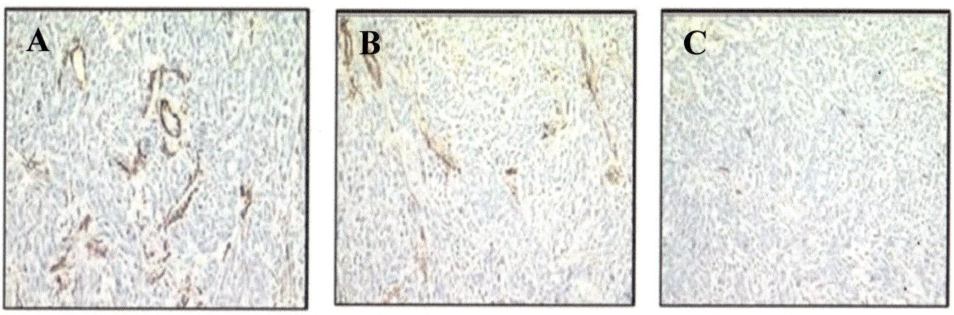

A: control B: licorice extract C: alzabiae extract

Fig. 4. *Albizia julibrissin* extracts reduced microvessel density in tumor.

Group	No. of mice	IR (%)	MVD
Blank	5	0	31.6±2.89
Licorice	5	10	29.1±1.78
albiziae	5	67.5	10.5±0.98 *

* P <0.05. vs Control

Table 2. The rate of inhibition (IR) of tumor growth and microvessel density (MVD) of different groups.

3.1.4 Albiziae extract inhibits metastasis in mouse LLC model

Nude mice were inoculated with LLC cells and their lungs harvested and examined for the appearance of tumor as sign of metastasis. Five out of 10 mice in saline control group developed lung cancer with large nodules, the average size of tumor at 4.5±6.6 mm^3; the tumor cells were variable in size, sometimes with giant cancer cells. The nodules appeared highly invasive and with abundant interstitial vessels (Fig. 5A). Normal lung tissues were compressed and damaged, and infiltrated by large number of inflammatory cells. The histopathology of tumor in licorice extract group showed no marked difference from saline group (Fig. 5B). Albiziae bark extracts, on the other hand, significantly improved and stabilized the cancer. Compared to the 50% metastasis rate in control group, only 1 in 8 mice from albiziae extracts group developed lung cancer, with an average size of 0.5±1.4 mm^3. The nodule showed much reduced cell nuclear division and interstitial vasculature. No substantial infiltration by inflammatory cells was discovered. The combined results showed clear inhibition of LCC metastasis by albiziae extracts.

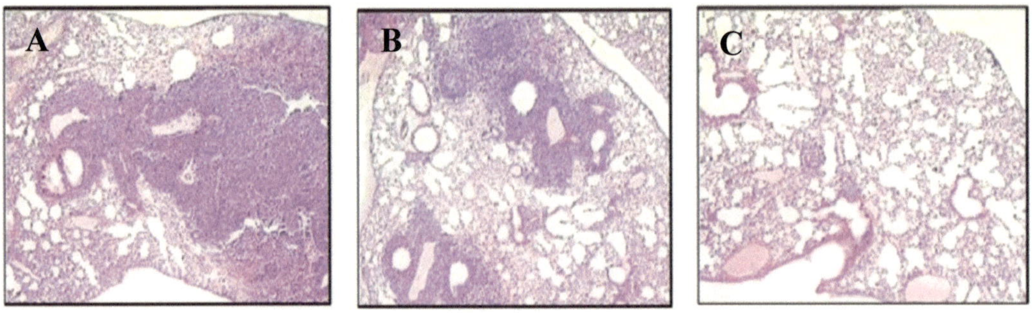

A: negative control B: licorice extracts C: albizia extracts

Fig. 5. Antitumor effect of *Albizia julibrissin* extracts in mice implanted with LLC.

3.2 The effect of albiziae effective monomer *julibroside J_8* on neovascularization

3.2.1 *Julibroside J_8* readily inhibits HMEC-1 cell proliferation

In order to identify the specificity of anti-angiogenic of *Julibroside J_8 in vitro*, We first investigated the effect of *Julibroside J_8* (1μg/ml,2μg/ml,5μg/ml,10μg/ml,20μg/ml) on proliferation of B16, MCF-7, hepG2, MRC-5 and HMEC-1. The results indicated that *Julibroside J_8* caused a decrease in proliferation of B16, MCF-7, hepG2 and HMEC-1. The IC_{50} was estimated to be 10μg/ml, 9.5μg/ml, 8.8μg/ml and 1.2μg/ml, respectively. But it did not significantly inhibit proliferation of normal cell (MRC-5) at the concentration of 20μg/ml. Another experiment in mice proved that *julibroside J_8* had little effects on the quiescent vessels of kidney, lung, and liver.(Fig 6). The results show that *J_8* has specific action on anti-angiogenic *in vitro* and *in vivo*.

A (lung)

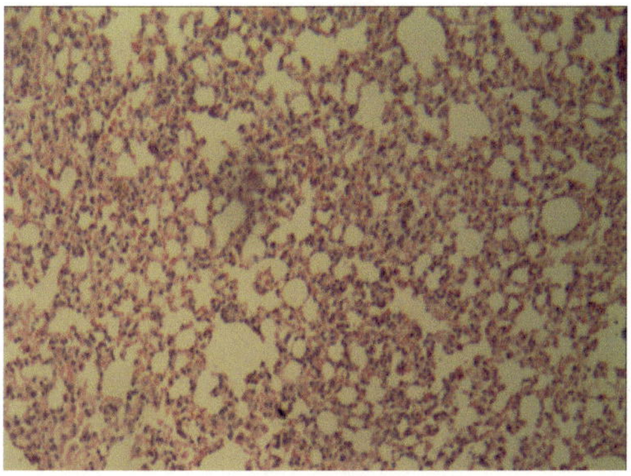

B (liver)

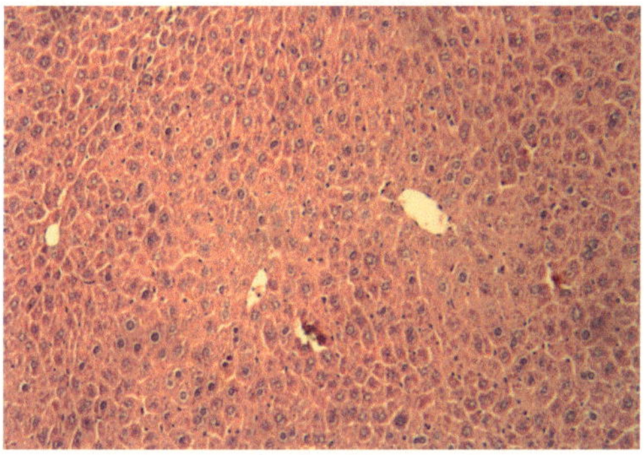

C (kidney)

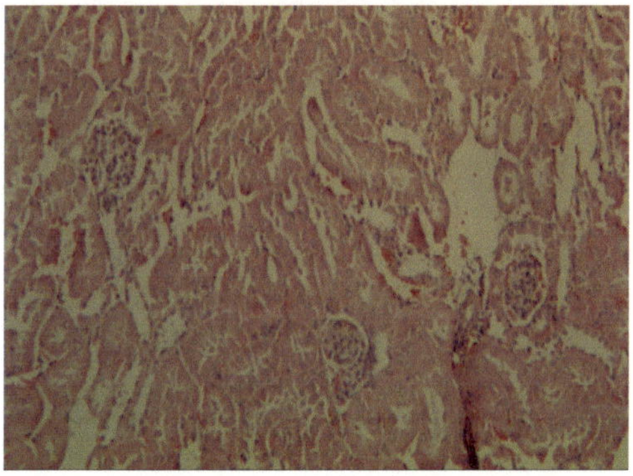

Fig. 6. No significant effect of *julibroside* J_8 on the quiescent vessels. 10×

3.2.2 *julibroside* J_8 inhibits Matrigel tube formation in vitro

As shown in Fig. 6, *julibroside* J_8 Demonstrated dose-dependent inhibition in Matrigel tube formation assay (Fig. 7). At 1 µg/mL of *julibroside* J_8, the number of tube formed was reduced. At 2.0 µg/mL, HMEC-1 cells showed limited mobility and formed few tubes. At 4.0 µg/mL, HMEC-1 cells had difficulty attaching.

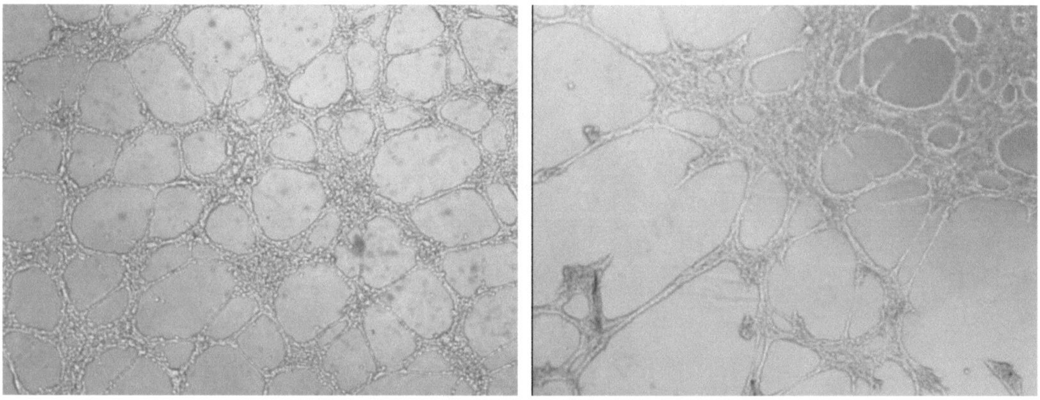

A (control) B (*J8* treatment)

Fig. 7. Effect of *julibroside* J_8 on tube formation of HMEC-1.

3.2.3 *julibroside* J_8 inhibits microvessel formation in CAM assay

Compared to the microvessels formed in saline control group, the ones in *julibroside* J_8 treatment group were abnormal in appearance and sparsely distributed (Fig. 7) and the number of blood vessel in all three size categories (L, M, S) were reduced (Table 3) in a dose-dependent manner, demonstrating a clear inhibition of neovascularization by *julibroside* J_8.

julibroside J_8 (μg/mL)	No. of blood vessels		
	Large	Medium	Small
0 (control)	2.8±0.20	4.5±0.87	21.8±1.89
10	2.1±0.34	3.8±0.36	16.6±0.65
50	2.6±0.54	2.8±0.97	9.9±0.30 *
100	2.3±0.67	2.5±0.27	4.9±0.57 **

* $P<0.05$, **$P<0.01$ vs Control

Table 3. Effect of *julibroside* J_8 on neovascularization in CAM ($\bar{x} \pm s$, n =10).

3.2.4 *julibroside* J_8 arrests cell cycle at G2/M phase

FCM cell cycle analysis of HMEC-1 cells treated with *julibroside* J_8 at various concentrations for 48 hrs showed a dose-dependent reduction of dividing cells (Table 4 and Fig. 8). At 0.5, 1.5 and 2.5 μg/mL of *julibroside* J_8, the percentage of cells in S phase was decreased to 30.20%, 14.43% and 11.25%, respectively, compared to 38.92% in the control group. In the mean time, increased number of cells was found in G_2/M and sub G1 phases, while the number of cells in G_1 phase remained constant.

Cell Cycle	*julibroside J_8* (μg/mL)			
	0	0.5	1.5	2.5
S	38.92%	30.20%	14.43%	11.25%
G_2/M	8.66%	21.35%	29.15%	30.25%
G_1	52.42%	48.43%	56.47%	54.2%
Sub G_1	0%	7.11%	15.85%	16.49%

Table 4. Cell cycle analysis of HMEC-1 cells treated with *julibroside J_8*.

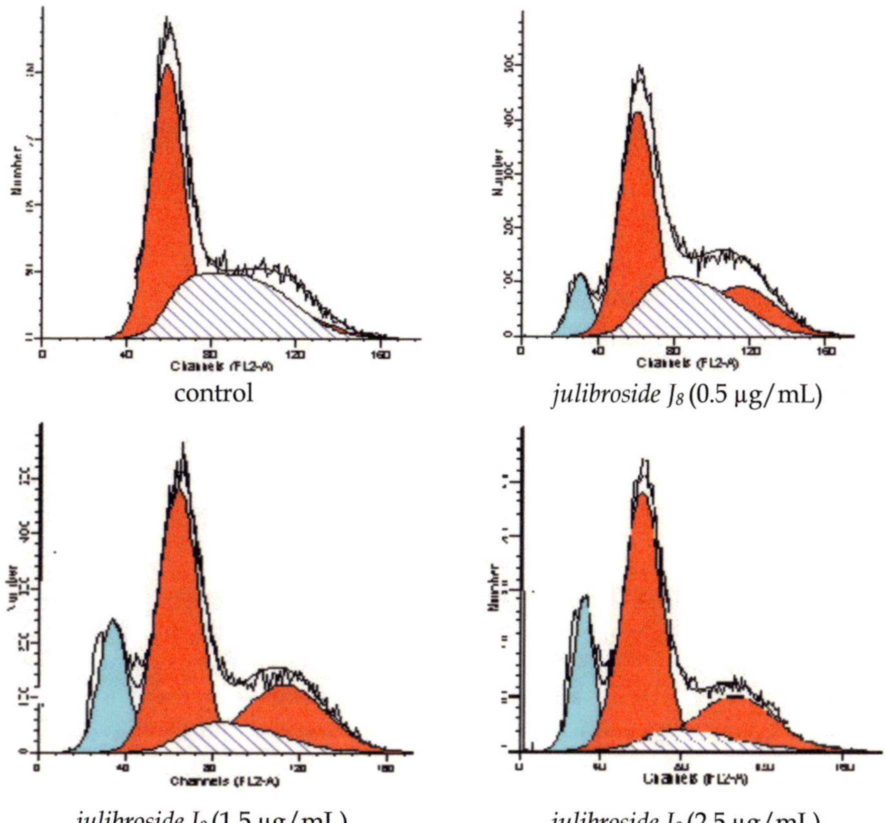

Fig. 8. Effects on cell cycle and apoptosis of HMEC-1 after treated with different concentration *julibroside J_8*.for 48h.

3.3 Effect of *julibroside J_8* on apoptosis and its mechanism

3.3.1 Observation of nuclear structure by DAPI staining

HMCE-1 cells cultured on coverslips were stained with DAPI and their nuclear morphology was observed by fluorescent microscopy (Fig. 9). Control group in general showed weaker fluorescence, which was enhanced upon fixation. The nuclei appeared round, clear-edged, and uniformly stained. HMCE-1 cells treated with *julibroside J_8* exhibited a stronger blue stain and displayed many characteristics associated with apoptotic cells, such as irregular edges around the nucleus, chromosome concentration in the nucleus, heavier coloring, and, with nuclear pyknosis, an increased number of nuclear body fragments.

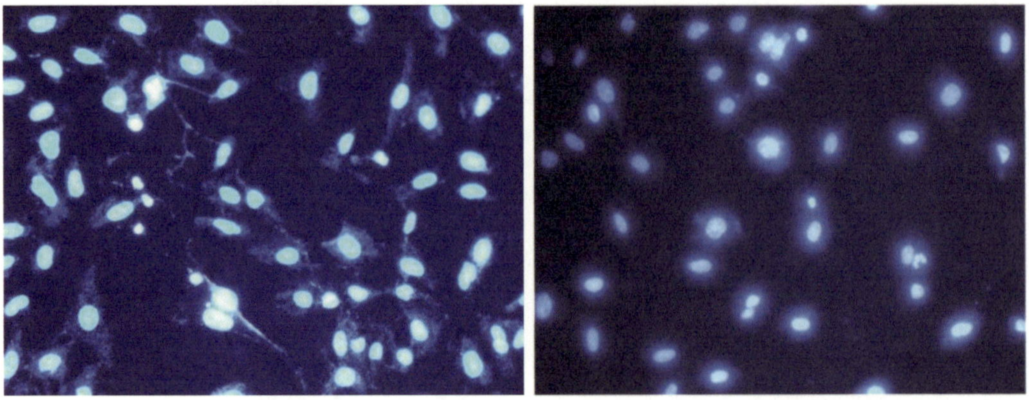

control (×40) *julibroside* J_8 (2.0 ug/ml) (×40)

Fig. 9. The morphological change of HMEC-1 cells by DAPI.

3.3.2 Determination of DNA fragmentation by TUNEL assay

HMEC-1 cells grown on coverslips were stained for terminal deoxynucleotidyl transferase activity, an indication of DNA fragmentation and hallmark of late stage apoptosis. The reaction was developed with DAB chromogen and images examined by light microscopy (Fig. 10). Few nuclei were stained dark brown in untreated cells, whereas an increase of stained nuclei was detected in *julibroside* J_8-treated HMEC-1 cells in a dose-dependent manner, indicating *julibroside* J_8 is able to induce apoptosis.

3.3.3 FCM analysis of Annexin V/ PI double labeling

Annexin V/PI double staining coupled with FAM analysis allows the distinguishing of live cells (Annexin V ^{neg}, PI ^{neg}), early apoptotic cells (Annexin V ^{pos}, PI ^{neg}), and late apoptotic cells (Annexin V ^{pos}, PI ^{pos}). It was discovered that under treatment of increasing concentration of *julibroside* J_8 for 48 hr, increased cell number appeared in the two right quadrants of the histogram which was indicative of early and late apoptotic events. Compared to the combined apoptotic rate of 8.34% in the control group, *julibroside* J_8 treatment at 0.5, 1.5 and 2.5 μg/mL resulted in an significantly higher apoptotic rate of 13.63%, 19.55% and 32.32%, respectively (Table 5).

Julibroside J_8 (μg/mL)	HMEC-1(%)			
	Live cells	Early apoptotic cells	Late apoptotic cells	Dead cells
0	90.81	5.15	3.19	0.86
0.5	82.91	8.14	7.79	1.16
1.5	78.15	7.65	11.90	2.28
2.5	67.96	8.94	21.38	1.72

Table 5. Effects of *julibroside* J_8 on necrosis and apoptosis rate in HMEC-1 cells.

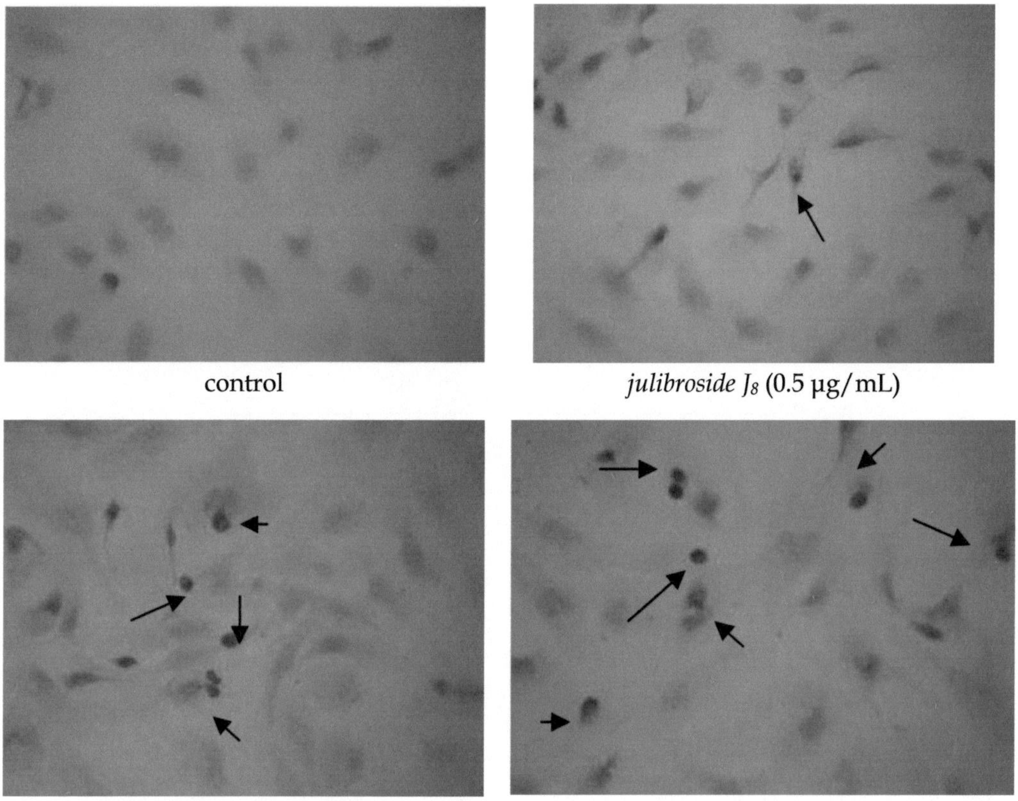

control | *julibroside J_8* (0.5 μg/mL)

julibroside J_8 (1.5 μg/mL) | *julibroside J_8* (2.5 μg/mL)

Fig. 10. Effect of *julibroside J_8* on DNA fragmentation in HMEC-1 cells (400x).

3.3.4 *julibroside J_8* does not affect mitochondrial membrane potential (ΔΨm)

As shown in Fig. 12, treatment with increasing dose of *julibroside J_8* did not result in change in HMEC-1 ΔΨm accordingly, and there were no statistically significant differences between treated groups and control group, indicating that ΔΨm is not involved in HMEC-1 cell apoptosis induced by *julibroside J_8*.

3.3.5 Effect of *julibroside J_8* on Caspase-3, 9 of HMEC-1

As demonstrated in Table 6, treatment with *julibroside J_8* did not change the activities of Caspase-3, 9, suggesting *julibroside J_8*-induced apoptosis is unrelated to Caspase-3, 9.

	lysis+reaction buffer	blank	negative control	4 h	10 h	24 h
Caspase-3	0.053	0.063	0.231	0.258	0.234	0.214
Caspase-9	0.053	0.060	0.219	0.229	0.203	0.199

Table 6. The effect of *julibroside J_8* (2 μg/mL) on Caspase-3, 9 activities in HMEC-1 cell.

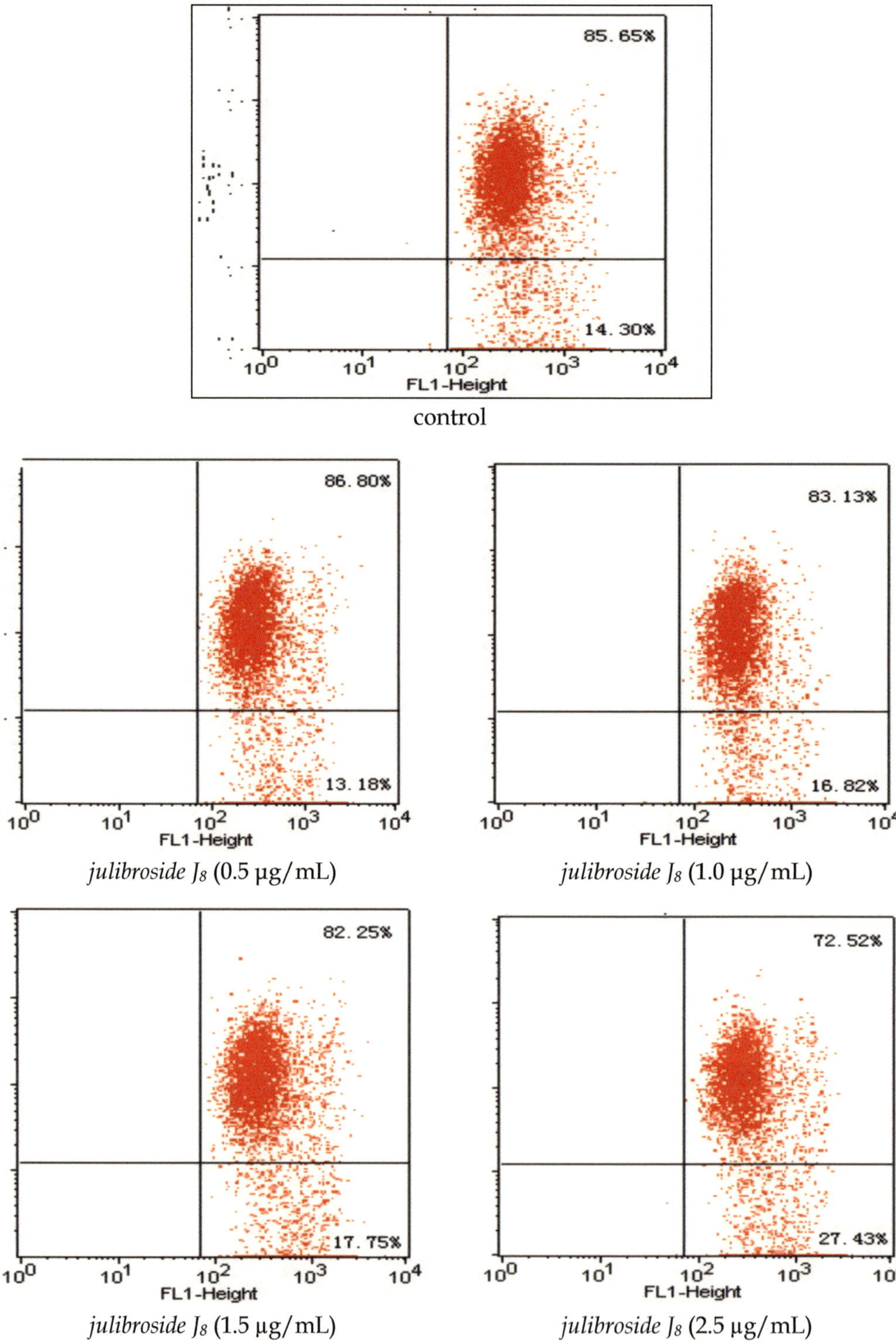

control

julibroside J8 (0.5 µg/mL)

julibroside J8 (1.0 µg/mL)

julibroside J8 (1.5 µg/mL)

julibroside J8 (2.5 µg/mL)

Fig. 11. Effect of *julibroside J8* on ΔΨm in HMEC-1 cells after incubation for 24 h.

4. Discussion

Invasiveness, metastasis and hyperproliferation are the key issues in tumor cell biology. Since Folkman proposed the concept of angiogeneis in 1972, tumor neovascularization has attracted much interest from the field of biological medicine and pharmaceutical industry, and been applied to the research and development of novel anticancer drugs, namely angiogenesis inhibitors targeting vessel endothelial cells to block the blood and nutrient supply to tumor and thus its growth and metastasis[5-6]. Using HMEC-1 cell proliferation inhibition assay as HTS read-out, our study identified 4, out of 500, medicinal herbs that function as neovascularization inhibitors, and among which albizia bark extract was shown to be able to inhibit tumor neovascularization and metastasis by *in vitro* and *in vivo* assays.

Monitored by HMEC-1 proliferation inhibition assay, we obtained effective monomer *julibroside* J_8 through a series of separation and purification steps. *In vitro* cell-based assay determined the IC_{50} of *julibroside* J_8 on HMEC-1 proliferation as 1.2 μg/mL. *Julibroside* J_8 can also inhibit Matrigel tube formation in vitro and neovascularization in CAM assay.

Our results showed that *julibroside* J_8 treatment changed cell cycle distribution, resulting in more cells at G_2/M phase and less at S phase, and the appearance of sub-G_1 peak of apoptosis, which demonstrate that *julibroside* J_8 is capable of cell proliferation inhibition and induction of apoptosis. Similarly, apoptosis was detected by Annexin V-FITC/PI double labeling.

Apoptosis is a cellular response to certain environmental messages and thus regulated by various endogenous and exogenous factors. Mitochondria are a vital cell organelle whose main function is energy conversion. In addition, mitochondria are involved in a range of other processes, such as signaling, cellular differentiation, cell death, as well as the control of the cell cycle and cell growth. A large body of work has established the involvement of mitochondria in apoptosis, and alterations in $\Delta\Psi m$ has been regarded as one of the earliest events in cell death, prior to the appearance of such hallmarks as chromatin condensation and DNA fragmentation. Once $\Delta\Psi m$ collapses, apoptosis becomes irreversible. Our study showed that *julibroside* J_8 treatment leads to the decrease in HMEC-1 cell number. DAPI stain illustrated cell shrinkage, membrane blebbing and increasing cellular debris when cells were treated with high concentration of *julibroside* J_8. In addition, DNA fragmentation was identified by TUNEL Apoptosis assay. FCM analysis revealed that cells were arrested at G_2/M phase of the cell cycle following *julibroside* J_8, accompanied by a sizable peak of apoptosis. Further analysis by Annexin-V/PI double labeling proved the dose-dependent effect of *julibroside* J_8 on apoptosis. However, $\Delta\Psi m$ did not seem to be affected.

Members of caspase family play a vital role in mitochondria-mediated apoptosis; the key players among them are caspase-3 and 9. Both are present in cytosol under normal physiological conditions as inactive precursors. When cellular stress (eg. DNA damage) occurs, procaspase-9 is activated by cytochrome c released from mitochondria; the resulting caspase-9 in turn activates the downstream procaspase-3. The activated caspase-3, a key factor in apoptosis execution, cleaves a host of downstream substrate and cell undergoes apoptosis. However, our study did not detect the change in caspase-3/9 acitivity as a function of time, suggesting *julibroside* J_8 induces apoptosis in HMCE-1 cells in mechanism independent of mitochondria pathway.

In all, we conclude that *julibroside* J_8, a novel molecule purified from albizia bark extracts, is able to inhibit HMEC-1 cell proliferation by cell cycle arrest at G_2/M phase. In addition, we proved by multiple means that *julibroside* J_8 can induce apoptosis. However, *julibroside* J_8 does not seem to affect $\Delta\Psi_M$ nor caspase-3/9 activity, suggesting a mitochondria-independent apoptosis pathway.

5. References

[1] Akhtar, N., Dickerson, E.B., Auerbach, R. The sponge/matrigel angiogenesis assay. Angiogenesis 2002, 5, 75–80.

[2] Ley, C.D., Olsen, M.W.B., Lund, E.L., et al. Angiogenic synergy of bFGF and VEGF is antagonized by angiopoietin-2 in a modified in vivo matrigel assay. Microvascular Research2004, 68, 161–168.

[3] Valster, A., Tran, N.L., Nakada, M., et al. Cell migration and invasionassays. Methods 2005, 37, 208–215.

[4] Soeda, S., Kozako, T., Iwata, K., et al. Oversulfated fucoidan inhibits the basic fibroblast growth factor-induced tube formation by human umbilical vein endothelial cells: its possible mechanism of action. Biochim.Biophys. Acta 2000,1497, 127–134.

[5] Kowanetz M, Ferrara N: Vascular endothelial growth factor signaling pathways: therapeutic perspective. Clin Cancer Res 2006, 12:5018-5022.

[6] Goodwin AM. In vitro assays of angiogenesis for assessment of angiogenic and anti-angiogenic agents. Microvasc Res 2007, 74:172–183

4

Beyond VEGF: The NOTCH and ALK1 Signaling Pathways as Tumor Angiogenesis Targets

Olivier Nolan-Stevaux and H. Toni Jun
Amgen, Inc.
USA

1. Introduction

The clinical validation of several anti-angiogenic agents targeting the VEGF pathway for the treatment of metastatic colorectal cancer (Hurwitz et al., 2004), non-small cell lung cancer (Sandler et al., 2006), hepatocellular carcinoma (Llovet et al., 2008) and metastatic renal cell carcinoma (mRCC) (Motzer et al., 2009) has provided evidence that angiogenesis inhibition can lead to increased overall patient survival. Although these treatments achieve sustained tumor regression in isolated cases, the average clinical gains from individual therapeutics are measured in only weeks to months. In most patients, cancer progression resumes following initial disease stabilization as tumors acquire resistance to anti-angiogenic agents (Ellis and Hicklin, 2008; Rini and Atkins, 2009). In some disease, such as metastatic breast cancer (Miller et al., 2007), the clinical benefits from VEGF-targeted therapies appear marginal from the outset, while still other cancer types, such as melanoma (Hauschild et al., 2009) and pancreatic ductal adenocarcinoma (Kindler et al., 2007), appear to be refractory to anti-angiogenic drugs from the outset and are deemed "intrinsically" resistant (Bergers and Hanahan, 2008).

Acquired and intrinsic resistance to VEGF-targeted therapies stem from multiple pro-angiogenic mechanisms: VEGF signaling upregulation (Rini and Atkins, 2009); secretion of alternative angiogenic factors (Casanovas, 2011; Kopetz et al., 2010; Loges et al., 2010); acquisition of new blood vessels in an angiogenesis-independent manner via vasculogenesis, vessel co-option or vascular mimicry (Kerbel, 2008; Loges et al., 2010); and activation of stromal components such as myeloid cells and cancer associated fibroblasts, which can cooperate to rescue or expand the tumor vasculature (Bergers and Hanahan, 2008; Crawford and Ferrara, 2009). To overcome acquired resistance mechanisms, some clinicians currently shift patients from one VEGF-targeted therapy to another and are able to achieve lasting clinical benefit at least in the case of metastatic renal cell carcinoma (mRCC), suggesting that upregulation of the VEGF signaling pathway itself is one of the major initial routes of resistance in this cancer type (Rini and Atkins, 2009). However, all cancers eventually acquire resistance to even the most potent VEGF receptor inhibitors, underscoring the need for additional anti-angiogenic therapies targeted at alternative signaling pathways to overcome these resistance mechanisms.

In this chapter, we will review two signaling pathways that play critical functions at distinct phases of angiogenesis and against which experimental drugs are currently in development: the NOTCH and BMP9-ALK1 signaling axes. In each case, we will present the genetic and experimental evidence demonstrating the function of these signaling axes in angiogenesis, the signal transduction events they mediate during angiogenesis and the pre-clinical evidence indicating that targeted inhibition of these pathways leads to the disruption of tumor angiogenesis and decreased tumor growth.

2. Function of NOTCH signaling in angiogenesis

Named after the notched wing appearance of its Drosophila phenotype (Mohr, 1919; Morgan and Bridges, 1916), the NOTCH pathway is a highly conserved signaling system that plays a role in multiple critical processes, including stem cell maintenance, pattern formation, and cell fate determination. In vertebrates, this signaling system is comprised of four NOTCH receptors, and five trans-membrane ligands. This section will summarize the data that demonstrate the role of individual members of this signaling pathway in vascular development and discuss the evidence that suggests that NOTCH signaling may represent an attractive point of therapeutic intervention for angiogenic therapy.

2.1 Expression of NOTCH receptors and ligands in endothelial cells and in tumors

Expression analysis of the NOTCH signaling pathway in human cancer samples provides encouraging evidence of a role for NOTCH signaling in human disease. Expression of the NOTCH ligand Delta-like 4 (DLL4) is upregulated in human breast cancer and not found in normal breast tissue (Li et al 2007). Similar studies have also demonstrated an upregulation of DLL4 expression in the tumor endothelium of clear cell renal cell carcinoma (CC-RCC) patients compared to normal kidney vasculature (Figure 1; Patel 2005) as well as in bladder carcinoma compared to normal bladder tissue (Patel et al., 2006). Mouse studies corroborate a role for DLL4 in the tumor vasculature. In a mouse reporter line where LacZ expression is driven by the DLL4 promoter, there is preferential expression in the tumor vasculature of implanted Lewis lung carcinoma tumors compared to the adjacent normal vasculature. Interestingly, a VEGF-Trap molecule that induces a VEGF signaling blockade effectively blocks the upregulation of DLL4 in the tumor vasculature of C6 glioma xenograft tumors, suggesting that DLL4 upregulation may be VEGF dependent (Gale et al., 2004; Noguera-Troise et al., 2006).

The NOTCH ligands may also signal from the tumor itself to the vasculature. Jagged1 (JAG1) expression in head and neck squamous cell carcinoma (HNSCC) cell lines is upregulated in response to multiple growth factors, such as HGF, EGF, and TGF-alpha, pathways that are commonly altered in human cancer. In an HNSCC xenograft model, tumor expressed JAG1 enhanced neovascularization and tumor growth in vivo, and correlated with vessel content and disease progression, suggesting JAG1 may signal from the tumor to the tumor vasculature via murine NOTCH expressed on ECs (Zeng et al., 2005). There have also been reports of tumor expression of DLL4 in colorectal cancer (Jubb et al., 2009), although it has been hypothesized to play a direct role in cancer stem cell survival rather than tumor signaling to the endothelium (Hoey et al., 2009).

2.2 Functional role of NOTCH receptors in developmental angiogenesis

The phenotypes associated with genetic alteration of individual components of the NOTCH signaling pathway validate a role for multiple pathway members in embryonic vascular development. Each of the NOTCH receptors is expressed in the mouse vasculature and deletion of some individual NOTCH receptors show embryonic lethality, demonstrating non-overlapping functions during development. For example, NOTCH1 null mice are

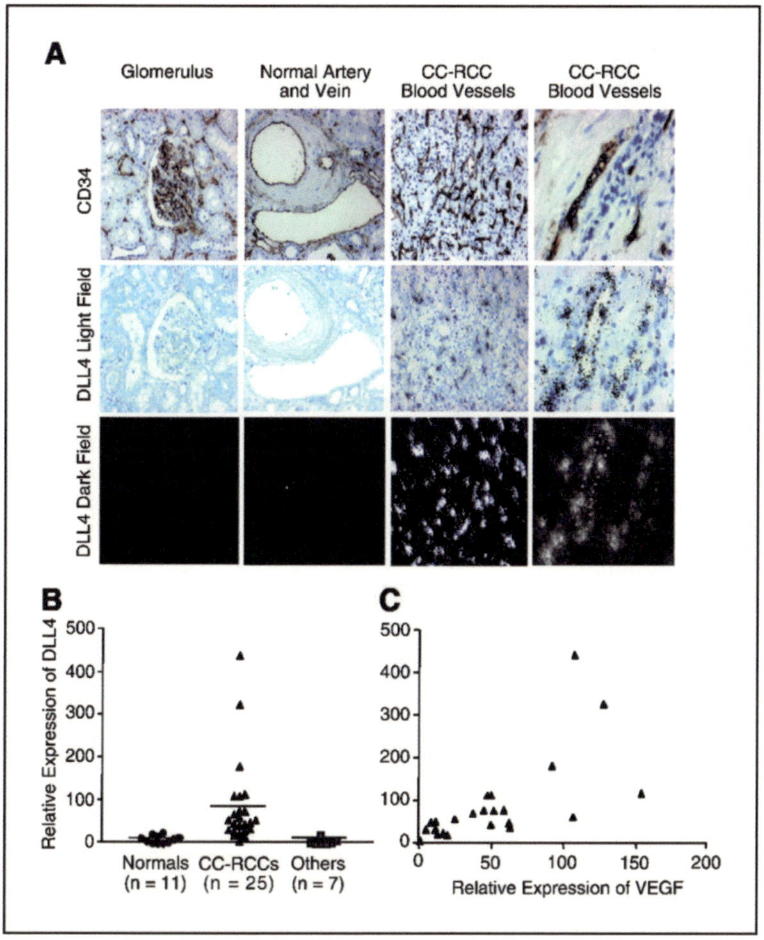

Fig. 1. Differential expression of DLL4 in renal cancer.
In situ analysis (A) or RT-PCR (B) demonstrates higher relative expression (up to nine-fold) of human DLL4 in CC-RCC samples compared to normal kidney tissue. (C) DLL4 expression correlates with elevated VEGF-A expression. ©Adapted and reprinted by permission from the American Association for Cancer Research: Patel et al, Up-regulation of delta-like 4 ligand in human tumor vasculature and the role of basal expression in endothelial cell function, Cancer Res, 2005, (19) 65: 8692.

non-viable due to severe vascular defects and impaired somitogenesis with extensive cell death resulting in lethality by embryonic day 9.5 (Conlon et al., 1995) -10.5 with complete resorption by d11.5 (Swiatek et al., 1994). Endothelial cell specific deletion of NOTCH1 has a similar phenotype, demonstrating the critical endothelial compartment function of NOTCH1 in early vascular development (Limbourg et al., 2005). While the NOTCH4 knockout mouse is viable, compound loss of NOTCH1 and NOTCH4 shows a more profound vascular phenotype than deletion of either single gene alone (Krebs et al., 2000), suggesting a possible NOTCH1 redundancy for NOTCH4 in development.

NOTCH2 is also expressed in the mouse vasculature, most notably in the developing heart (Loomes et al., 2002). However, mice expressing a NOTCH2 deletion mutant that lacks all but one of the ankyrin repeats in the N2ICD die prior to NOTCH2 heart expression at d11.5 with abnormalities observed in the neuroepithelium and cranial ganglia cells, as well as the optic and otic vesicles (Hamada et al., 1999). A NOTCH2 hypomorph allele causes perinatal lethality due to defects in the glomerular development in the kidney (McCright et al., 2001). Taken together, these data suggest that NOTCH2 may have non-vascular roles in development.

Despite expression of NOTCH3 in the mouse heart (Loomes et al., 2002), NOTCH3 null mice are viable, fertile and show no overt phenotype either alone, and unlike NOTCH4, does not show increased vascular defects on a NOTCH1 null background (Krebs et al., 2003). A detailed analysis of the NOTCH3 phenotype indicates that this receptor may play a role in arterial identity of vascular smooth muscle cells, as distal arteries exhibit structural lesions and defective arterial myogenic responses (Domenga et al., 2004). In humans, NOTCH3 mutations are associated with Cerebral Autosomal Dominant Arteriopathy with Subcortical Infarcts and Leukoencephalopathy (CADASIL), an adult onset vascular disorder caused by systemic vascular lesions that result in a myriad of symptoms, including recurrent ischemic strokes (Joutel et al., 1996). These mutations do not seem to affect ligand/receptor interaction nor do they disrupt subsequent signaling (Haritunians et al., 2002). The mutations allow accumulation of a soluble NOTCH3 ECD (Joutel et al., 2000), and this could locally interfere with signaling of multiple intact NOTCH receptors and their ligands as there is substantial binding promiscuity among NOTCH receptors and ligands.

2.3 Functional role of NOTCH ligands in developmental angiogenesis

Knockout of JAG1 in the mouse results in embryonic lethality by E10 -10.5 and can be identified by hemorrhage and the lack of large blood vessels in the yolk sac, reminiscent of the NOTCH1 null phenotype. Additional vascular defects and hemorrhage are also present in the cranial area and there is an overall loss of vessel branching and reduced vessel diameter (Xue et al., 1999). Like the NOTCH1 deletion, the phenotype is similar when the knockout is restricted to the endothelial cell compartment suggesting that the early lethality is due to JAG1 expression in the vasculature (High et al., 2008). Detailed examination shows that vascular smooth muscle cell (VSMC) markers are severely diminished despite intact NOTCH signaling in the endothelial cells themselves. The primary role of JAG1 may therefore be to signal to the VSMC, and other ligands may be able to compensate for the loss of JAG1-triggered signaling in the endothelial cells. Other studies using conditional loss or overexpression of JAG1 suggest that JAG1 plays a proangiogenic role in the presence of other ligands in the developing retina and can act as a partial antagonist to DLL4 to modulate NOTCH pathway signaling (Benedito et al., 2009). In humans, JAG1 mutations have been associated with Allagille syndrome (AGS), which has a variety of symptoms including reduced numbers of intrahepatic bile ducts, cardiac defects (including pulmonary artery stenosis and hypoplasia, pulmonic valve stenosis and tetralogy of Fallot), skeletal defects, ophthalmological abnormalities, renal and pancreatic abnormalities, and intracranial bleeding. Although mutations in NOTCH2 have not been associated with AGS, combined mutations of both NOTCH2 and JAG1 best recapitulate the human pathology of AGS in the mouse (McCright et al., 2002).

DLL4 is expressed throughout the vascular endothelium, most notably in the endothelial cells of actively growing capillaries at the leading front of the superficial vascular plexus, while mature capillaries have lower levels of DLL4 expression as analyzed in situ (Shutter et al., 2000) or by reporter construct (Lobov et al., 2007). Over time, DLL4 expression decreases in mature veins but increases in the arteries. DLL4 inactivation results in an early lethality and haploinsufficiency by E9.5 in some mouse strains. DLL4 knockout embryos exhibit an avascular yolk sac, arterio-venous malformations (AVMs), growth retardation, and an overall lack of major arteries and vascular remodeling (Krebs et al., 2004) In rare cases of heterozygote survival, defects are also observed in the developing retina characterized by enhanced angiogenic sprouting and endothelial cell proliferation, which is a hallmark of a DLL4 blockade (Lobov et al., 2007).

Delta-like 1(DLL1) has been reported to be expressed in the endothelium of the developing embryo in both arteries and veins (Beckers et al., 1999). DLL1 is detectable in fetal arterial endothelial cells beginning at embryonic day 13.5, and is a critical regulator of arterial identity. Disruption of DLL1 leads to lethality by E12 with aberrant somite compartmentalization and hemorrhagic events (Hrabe de Angelis et al., 1997). Loss of DLL1 in the mouse also leads to a downregulation of VEGF receptor 2 (VEGFR2) and neuropilin (NRP) expression as well as a reduction in the levels of activated NOTCH1 receptor, despite the expression of DLL4 and JAG1 in the endothelium (Sorensen et al., 2009). The role of DLL1 is not restricted to the developing embryo, as heterozygous adult mice display impaired arteriogenesis after induction by ischemia (Limbourg et al., 2007).

Knockout of the Jagged2 (JAG2) gene in mouse die at birth due to cleft palate and lack observable defects in the vascualture. Future studies using a conditional allele may illuminate a role of JAG2 in the vasculature of the adult mouse (Xu et al., 2010). A targeted Delta-like 3 (DLL3) knockout mouse is viable, but homozygous mutants have growth defects with disorganized vertebrae and costal defects resulting from defective segmentation in the embryo and delayed and irregular somite formation. Similarly, two viable spontaneous mutations of DLL3, *pudgy* and *omagari*, have abnormal formation and patterning of somites. Although clearly important for normal development, neither the JAG2 nor the DLL3 null mice have apparent signs of an angiogenic defect. However, this does not exclude a vascular role beyond their essential functions in development.

2.4 Overview of NOTCH signaling

The four NOTCH receptors are single pass transmembrane proteins with a large number (25-29) of epidermal growth factor-like (EGF-like) motifs that are repeated throughout their extracellular domains (ECD) (see Kopan and Ilagan, 2009 for a recent comprehensive review). They are each synthesized as a proreceptor before cleavage by a furin-like protease during their transport to the surface (Blaumueller et al., 1997; Logeat et al., 1998). The ECDs of NOTCH receptors also contain 3 LIN12/NOTCH repeat (LNR) domains that are noncovalently linked to the rest of the receptor through a heterodimerization (HD) domain. The HD and LNR domains collectively make up the negative regulatory region (NRR), which overall prevents activation of the receptor in its non-ligand bound state (Sanchez-Irizarry et al., 2004).

The classical NOTCH ligands are also single pass transmembrane proteins. (Figure 2) The ligands have multiple EGF repeats as well as a Delta, Serrate, and Lag-z (DSL) domain that is essential for interaction with the NOTCH receptors. Jagged ligands distinguish themselves from the Delta-like ligands by an additional cysteine rich domain (reviewed by Kopan, 2009). There are also non-classical ligands that can activate NOTCH receptors in specific contexts, such as the Delta/NOTCH-like EGF-related receptor (DNER), which acts as a NOTCH ligand in neurons for glial cell differentiation (Eiraku et al., 2005) or F3/cortactin, which is involved in NOTCH activation during oligodendrocyte maturation (Hu et al., 2003). Ligands and receptors are proposed to be expressed on opposing cells and

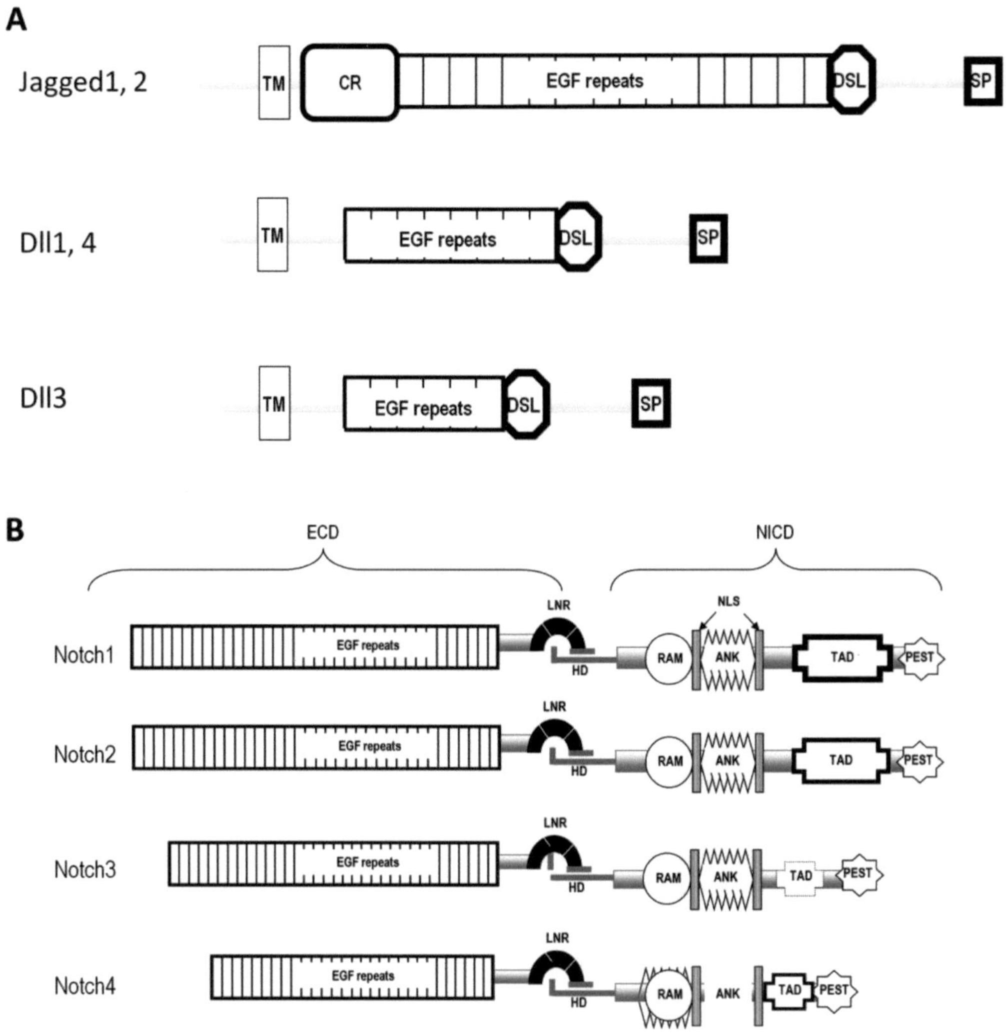

Fig. 2. Diagram of the NOTCH ligands and receptors.
A. The NOTCH ligand family has five distinct transmembrane ligands, each encoded by its own gene. The extracellular domains of all the receptors contain a signal peptide (SP), multiple EGF repeats, and a Delta/Serrate/Lag-2 (DSL) as well as a transmembrane (TM) domain. The Jagged ligands also have a cysteine rich domain. All ligands have a small intracellular domain as well. B. The NOTCH receptor family has four distinct transmembrane receptors, each encoded by its own gene. The extracellular domains of all the receptors contain multiple EGF repeats as well as an LNR domain which protects the receptors from cleavage and thereby preventing activation. Ligand binding is thought to be mediated by EGF repeats 11-13. The intracellular domains contain a RAM domain, six ANK repeats, two NLS sequences, and a PEST domain to regulate the stability of the protein. NOTCH3 has a weak transcriptional activation domain (TAD) compared to other receptor family members.

operate as a short-range signaling system. When a NOTCH ligand binds to a NOTCH receptor, the interaction induces a conformational change in the NRR region allowing exposure of additional cleavage sites (reviewed in Gordon et al., 2008). The first cleavage is mediated by ADAM-type metalloproteases on the ECD side of the protein (Gordon et al., 2007). Nicastrin, a transmembrane glycoprotein protein in the presenilin/γ-secretase protease complex, helps mediate the second cleavage by docking NOTCH into the protease (Chen et al., 2001), resulting in the release of the NOTCH intracellular domain (NICD) (Struhl and Greenwald, 1999). The NICD contains a nuclear localization signal (NLS) that regulates translocation into the nucleus (Figure 3) (Schroeter et al., 1998).

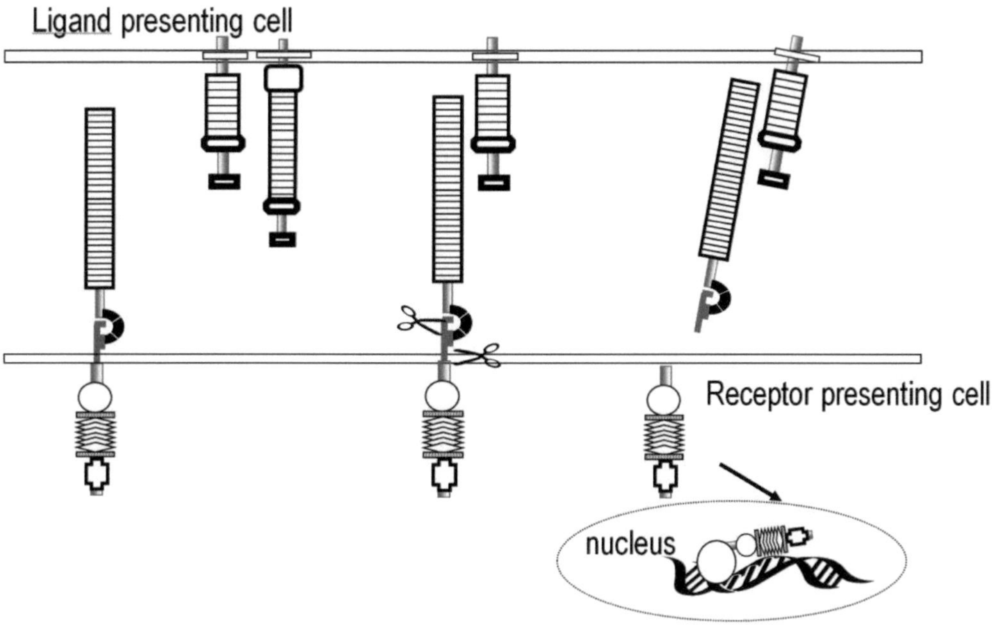

Fig. 3. Canonical NOTCH receptor signaling.
Ligand presentation by an adjacent cell can activate the receptor by promoting two sequential cleavages (denoted by scissors) by the TACE family of proteases and γ-secretase. These cleavages liberate the NOTCH receptor intracellular domain and allow it to translocate to the nucleus. NICD then interacts with the CSL family of transcription factors and induces expression of NOTCH target genes.

The NICD of all four NOTCH receptors contains a regulation of amino acid (RAM) domain, ankyrin (ANK) repeats, a nuclear localization signal (NLS) (Lieber et al., 1993), and a proline, glutamate, serine, threonine (PEST) domain (Figure 2). Cdk8 directly phosphorylates the PEST domain in all NICDs, which then become substrates for the nuclear ubiquitin ligase Sel10, regulating NICD turnover. (Fryer et al., 2002; Fryer et al., 2004; Oberg et al., 2001). Prior to destruction, the NICD interacts via its ANK repeats with the DNA binding protein CBF1/Drosophila Su(H)/C.Elegans LAG-1 (CSL), which, in the absence of NOTCH, associates with co-repressors and histone deacetylases to prevent transcription of key gene targets (Jarriault et al., 1995). Once NICD is present and binds to CSL, the co-repressors are displaced allowing recruitment of mastermind (MAML) and conversion into a transcriptional activation complex. The co-regulator SKIP and histone

deacetylase p300 are also recruited to the same promoters (Wallberg et al., 2002; Zhou et al., 2000). This allows the transcription of members of the Hes and Hey family of transcriptional repressors (Ohtsuka et al., 1999), reviewed in (Iso et al., 2003). The strength of the transcriptional signal varies among family members and seems to depend upon cofactor association as well as binding site orientation (Ong et al., 2006).
NOTCH signaling between receptors and ligands can be further regulated by post-translational glycosylation of the receptors and ligands which contain multiple potential sites for N- and O- linked glycosylation. The Fringe family of glycosyltransferases can mediate O-fucose elongation on the NOTCH ECD (Moloney et al., 2000) thereby changing affinity of NOTCH receptors for their ligands. For example Fringe modification of NOTCH1 increases activation by Delta1 but decreases activation by JAG1 (Yang et al., 2005). Dynamic fringe family expression can thereby substantially modify NOTCH signaling (reviewed by (Haines and Irvine, 2003). Rumi has also been identified in Drosophilla as an enzyme that can add O-glucose to the NOTCH ECD and may affect NOTCH signaling by enhancing cleavage and activation of NOTCH by its ligands (Acar et al., 2008).

2.5 Preclinical data using pharmacological inhibitors targeting NOTCH signaling

The genetic data ascribing a key role for NOTCH signaling in angiogenesis has encouraged multiple groups to create molecules to specifically inhibit NOTCH signaling and evaluate their subsequent effects on the tumor vasculature. Such agents include soluble DLL4 (SolDLL4) fused to Fc and neutralizing antibodies specific to DLL4 or NOTCH1 that inhibit the receptor/ligand interaction (Funahashi et al., 2008; Noguera-Troise et al., 2006; Ridgway et al., 2006; Wu et al., 2010). These agents have demonstrated an anti-tumor effect in a broad spectrum of xenograft models, including those with intrinsic or acquired resistance to VEGF therapy. Examination of the tumor vasculature with all agents revealed an increase in sprouting leading to an overall expansion of non-productive vasculature, as evidenced by greater hypoxia in the tumor itself and decreased perfusion of these new vessels. Subsequent studies using live-cell imaging suggest that the aberrant sprouting is due to the fact that tip cell positioning is dynamic and migration of vessel stalk cells creates competition for the tip position among ECs. Regulation and organization of the vessel is determined by DLL4 expression, via modulation by VEGF receptor 1 and 2 (VEGFR1 and VEGFR2) levels, to allow tip formation only towards the highest concentrations of VEGF-A. Disruption of DLL4/NOTCH signaling using pharmacological inhibitors subsequently disrupts the ability of the vessel to organize (Jakobsson et al., 2010).
Blockade of DLL4 signaling has been reported to be enhanced with blockade of other angiogenic signaling pathways. Notably, the efficacy of anti-DLL4 treatment was increased upon the addition of agents designed to inhibit VEGF signaling, either with an anti-VEGF-A antibody (Ridgway et al., 2006), or a soluble VEGFR2-Fc fusion protein (Noguera-Troise et al., 2006). As bevacizumab is already an approved agent for human use, there is clear potential for use as a clinical combination. A recent study has also demonstrated that inhibition of EphrinB4 signaling by a soluble EphB4 albumin fusion protein in combination with either allelic deletion or a soluble DLL4-Fc fusion construct could also enhance efficacy in the RipTag model, a highly angiogenic model of pancreatic islet carcinogenesis (Djokovic et al., 2010).

2.6 Potential preclinical toxicities associated with chronic NOTCH signaling inhibition

Although these data suggest that NOTCH signaling is an attractive target for therapeutic intervention in tumor angiogenesis, there may be substantial side effects associated with short and long term blockade of NOTCH signaling. Several studies suggest that NOTCH signaling acts as a tumor suppressor in specific tissues. For example, skin specific ablation of NOTCH1 results in hyperproliferation of the basal epidermal layer in young mice and epidermal and corneal hyperplasia in older mice (Nicolas et al., 2003). A recent study has also demonstrated that NOTCH1 can act as a tumor suppressor in a K-Ras driven model of pancreatic cancer. Pancreas specific K-Ras^{G12D} expression causes early stage lesions of pancreatic cancer, reminiscent of ADM/Tc, PanIN1A or PanIN1B stages in human disease (Hingorani et al., 2003). Pancreas specific NOTCH loss in this background significantly accelerates pancreatic lesions and produced a more advanced grade (PanIN1B to PanIN2), suggesting that loss of NOTCH results in increased tumor incidence and progression (Hanlon et al., 2010). In both cases, increased proliferation was observed as assessed by Ki67 staining of affected tissue. NOTCH signaling may also have a tumor suppression role in myeloid leukemia due to altered fate specification. Deletion of NOTCH1 and NOTCH2 or Nicastrin results in a murine form of chronic myelomonocytic leukemia (CMML) due to accumulation of granulocyte/monocyte progenitors. Loss of NOTCH dependent inhibition of genes that specify myelomonocytic fate for the blood cells causes resultant pathology. Interestingly, mutations in NOTCH signaling were found in 5/42 patient samples with CMML (Klinakis et al., 2011) suggesting that this may be relevant to the development of human disease.

Another intriguing genetic study that demonstrated the effects of long term NOTCH loss used a model in which the endogenous NOTCH1 gene was replaced with NOTCH1-Cre fusion protein (Vooijs et al., 2007). When crossed with a mouse containing a floxed NOTCH1 allele, it allows progressive inactivation of NOTCH1 dependent signaling in its physiologic context, i.e. as NOTCH1 is activated, it is lost. Beyond a broad effect on overall survival due to hemorrhage and vascular tumors, 11 out of 13 mice in this system demonstrated aberrations in multiple organs, including the liver, ovary, testis, skin, lymph nodes, uterus, and colon. The liver in particular, was the organ most affected by NOTCH1 activated loss and had evidence of hemangiomas and proliferation specifically associated with NOTCH1 loss (Liu et al., 2011).

In other preclinical studies, pharmacological agents causing long term blockade, such as an anti-DLL4 antibody, also caused unexpected proliferative effects in select tissues (Yan et al., 2010). Dose dependent ulcerating subcutaneous tumors (mouse) as well as sinusoidal dilation and centrilobular hepatocyte atrophy in the liver (mouse, rat, monkey) was observed. It was also noted that similar liver effects were seen with both an anti-NOTCH1 antibody and a γ-secretase inhibitor, which would inhibit processing or activation of all NOTCH recetpors, suggesting that the effects were likely pathway associated. However, impact on overall survival was not observed as was seen in the genetic study, possibly due to shorter exposure as compared to genetic loss. It is unknown if the other vascular beds that were described to be affected in the genetic study were affected by antibody inhibition as they were not discussed. Interestingly, there may be mechanisms to counteract NOTCH signaling induced proliferation. For example, hepatic lesions caused by DLL4 inhibition were prevented when combined with systemic Ephrin B2/EphB4 inhibition, (Djokovic et al., 2010). As mentioned earlier, this combination enhanced anti-DLL4 efficacy, and that combination therapy may be a possible approach to mitigate NOTCH pathway associated toxicities while preserving anti-tumor effects.

2.7 Clinical perspectives

Despite the possible toxicities described above, the compelling preclinical efficacy data generated with neutralizing agents to DLL4 and NOTCH1 have encouraged efforts to evaluate these agents in the clinic. Currently two companies have active clinical trials that target DLL4 (www.clinicaltrials.gov). OMP-21M18 (Oncomed Pharmaceuticals) is a neutralizing anti-DLL4 mAb that is currently in Phase 1 and 1b clinical trials in combination with chemotherapy. OMP-21M18 is specific for human DLL4, and preclinical data with this antibody demonstrates a direct anti-tumor effect for primary human xenografts that express huDLL4. However, OMP-21M18 combined with an antibody that recognizes muDLL4 demonstrated increased efficacy, suggesting that DLL4 signaling has a role in both tumor and stroma in primary human xenograft growth (Hoey, 2009). A second human anti-DLL4 mAb, REGN-421, created by Regeneron pharmaceuticals, is also in Phase 1 clinical trials. Given the preclinical data, there may be benefit to combination of an agent targeting DLL4 with bevacizumab. A recent retrospective analysis demonstrates that DLL4 expression, along with VEGF-C and neuropilin-1, indicated a poor response to bevacizumab treatment and may be a path of resistance in human disease (Jubb et al., 2011).

3. Function of ALK1 / Endoglin signaling in angiogenesis

A second angiogenic signaling axis with potential for therapeutic intervention is the ALK1/Endoglin pathway. In recent years, therapeutics directed at the ALK1/Endoglin signaling axis have entered phase 1 and 2 clinical trials, marking a clinical transition for a field of research dating back more than 20 years with the cloning of Endoglin (ENG or CD105) and ALK1 (Attisano et al., 1993; Gougos and Letarte, 1990). ENG, a homo-dimeric membrane glycoprotein highly expressed in endothelial cells (Gougos and Letarte, 1988), has homology to betaglycan and is capable of binding several cytokines of the TGFβ-super family, leading to its classification as a Type III TGFβ co-receptor. ALK1, the product of the *Activin receptor-like kinase 1* gene (*ACVRL1*), is an endothelial-specific serine/threonine kinase belonging to the Type I TGFβ receptor family (Attisano et al., 1993). Together, ENG and ALK1 define a signaling receptor complex for the BMP9 and BMP10 cytokines at the surface of endothelial cells. ENG and ALK1 are required for angiogenesis and vascular morphogenesis and anti-ENG and anti-ALK1 targeted agents have the potential to disrupt tumor angiogenesis independently or cooperatively with anti-VEGF treatment.

3.1 Normal and tumor endothelial expression of ENG and ALK1

ENG and ALK1 are both preferentially expressed in endothelial cells. During development, *ENG* and *ALK1* present very similar expression patterns in areas of vasculogenesis (yolk sac, early embryonic vasculature) and angiogenesis (throughout the late embryonic vascular endothelium) (Jonker and Arthur, 2002; Roelen et al., 1997; Seki et al., 2003). *ENG* is detected in veins, liver sinusoidal endothelial cells and arteries, while *ALK1* is only detected in developing arteries, suggesting a role in arterial differentiation (Jonker and Arthur, 2002; Seki et al., 2003). In the adult, both transcripts are weakly detected in the microvasculature of several organs including the lung (Miller et al., 1999; Panchenko et al., 1996; Seki et al., 2003) but the ENG protein is readily detected in the liver and kidney microvasculature (Minhajat et al., 2006). ENG protein expression is elevated in endothelial cells when angiogenesis is activated during wound repair and chronic inflammation (Torsney et al., 2002). Protein expression of ENG and ALK1 is induced in the endothelium of nearly all solid tumors (Burrows et al., 1995; Hu-Lowe et al., 2011; Miller et al., 1999; Minhajat et al., 2006;

Wang et al., 1993) (Fig. 4). ENG is also detected in cell types other than endothelial cells, such as activated monocytes and at the surface of cancer cells in melanoma and leukemia (Altomonte et al., 1996; Fonsatti et al., 2001; Gougos and Letarte, 1988), while ALK1 is also detected in mesenchymal cells of multiple organs and in trophoblast giant cells during embryogenesis (Roelen et al., 1997).

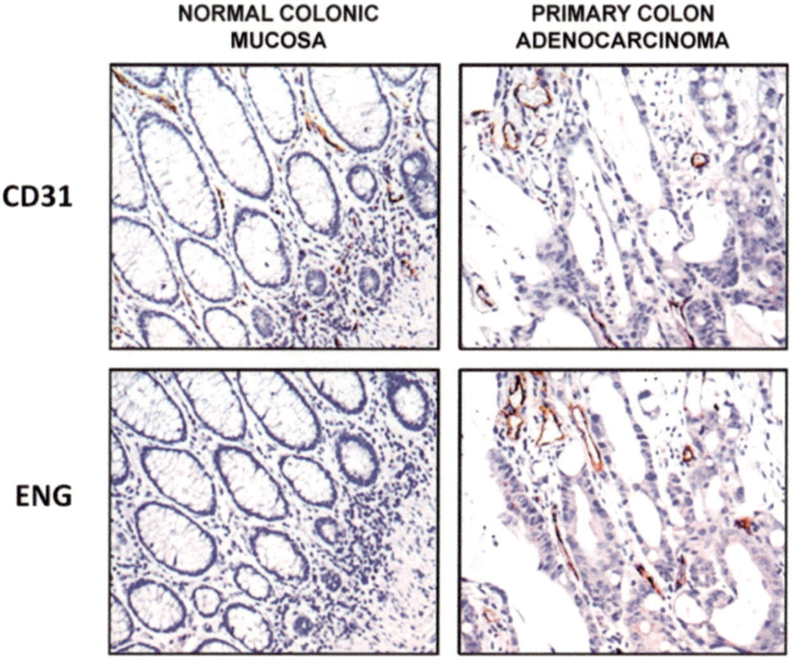

Fig. 4. Differential expression of ENG in tumor endothelial cells.
In contrast to CD31 staining, an endothelial cell marker detected in both the normal colonic mucosa and in the vasculature of colon tumors, ENG is detected at much higher levels in the tumor vasculature and not in the normal colonic vasculature (Dallas et al., 2008). ©Adapted and reprinted by permission from the American Association for Cancer Research: Dallas et al, Endoglin (CD105): A marker of tumor vasculature and potential target for therapy, Clin Cancer Res, 2008, 14(7): 1933.

The relative specificity of ENG and ALK1 expression in endothelial cells and their induction in cancer-associated endothelial cells stem from several mechanisms. First, *ENG* and *ALK1* share a combination of transcription factor binding sites with other endothelial-specific genes such as *PECAM1* and *VEGFR2* representing a possible endothelium transcriptional code (Garrido-Martin et al., 2010). Second, *ENG* is a HIF-1α target gene induced by hypoxia, (Li et al., 2003; Sanchez-Elsner et al., 2002), a near universal hallmark of cancer (Hanahan and Weinberg, 2011), and the *ALK1* promoter contains several HIF-1α binding motifs (Garrido-Martin et al., 2010). Third, ALK1 is induced by BMP4 (Shao et al., 2009), a cytokine required for vascular development (David et al., 2009). Finally, *ENG* transcription is induced by TGFβ (Sanchez-Elsner et al., 2002) and BMP9 signaling (David et al., 2007) through numerous SMAD-binding elements in the *ENG* promoter.

3.2 Hemorrhagic Hereditary Telangectasia: a vascular genetic disorder linked to *ENG* and *ALK1* loss-of-function

Hemorrhagic Hereditary Telangectasia (HHT) is a rare autosomal dominant genetic disorder characterized by vascular abnormalities in the skin, brain, lung, liver and gastro-intestinal tract resulting in the dilatation of post-capillary venules, disappearance of capillary beds, and AVMs (Fig. 5 A-B) (Lebrin and Mummery, 2008). Affected individuals suffer benign skin and mucosal dilatations (telangectasia), nosebleeds and more severe hemorrhage in affected organs (Guttmacher et al., 1995). Most subjects affected with HHT have been linked to heterozygous mutations in *ENG* (McAllister et al., 1994) or *ALK1* (Johnson et al., 1996) and are classified as HHT1 or HHT2 respectively. In most cases of HHT1, mutations generate null alleles of *ENG* leading to reduced expression of the ENG co-receptor, indicating that haploinsufficiency is the underlying genetic mechanism of disease (Fernandez et al., 2005; Pece-Barbara et al., 1999). For HHT2, the affected *ALK1* allele usually contains missense point mutations in the ALK1 kinase domain. The majority of these mutations lead to normal expression of ALK1 but to an absence of signal transduction from the BMP9 cytokine (Ricard et al., 2010) (see Signaling section 3.3). Thus mechanistically, HHT2 is likely caused by *ALK1* haploinsufficiency.

Mouse models carrying heterozygous genetic deletions of *ENG* or *ALK1* genes recapitulate the haploinsufficient pathological features of HHT such as telangectasias and AVMs (Bourdeau et al., 1999; Srinivasan et al., 2003; Torsney et al., 2003). In *ENG* or *ALK1* homozygous mutant embryos, embryonic and yolk sac vascular development proceed normally until day E8.5 (Li et al., 1999; Urness et al., 2000). Hence, neither gene is required for vasculogenesis, the process of endothelial cell differentiation from mesodermal precursors, their assembly into primitive vascular networks and the coalescence of angioblasts to form the endothelial tubes of the dorsal aorta and the cardinal vein (Arthur et al., 2000; Bourdeau et al., 1999; Li et al., 1999; Urness et al., 2000). However, between E9.0 and E9.5, abnormal vascular shunts reminiscent of AVMs appear in both *ALK1* and *ENG* mutant embryos, connecting the dorsal aorta and the cardinal vein and causing blood flow shunts in the embryo (Fig. 5C) (Li et al., 1999; Sorensen et al., 2003; Urness et al., 2000). The maturation of the primitive endothelial network of the yolk sac through angiogenesis also fails to occur in *ENG* or *ALK1* mutant embryos, leading to the disappearance of the vitelline vasculature in both genotypes by E10.5 (Li et al., 1999; Urness et al., 2000). *ENG* and *ALK1* mutant embryos also present severe defects in heart development as both genes are required for heart valve formation (Arthur et al., 2000; Bourdeau et al., 1999). The angiogenesis defects appear to be primary defects and not secondary heart phenotype defects, since the vascular malformations in *ENG* and *ALK1* mutant embryos occur before the onset of heart development phenotypes (Sorensen et al., 2003).

Angiogenesis defects in *ALK1* and *ENG* mutant embryos result from the failure of endothelial cell reorganization leading to abnormal vessel shunting, but also from profound defects in perivascular smooth muscle cells (VSMC) and pericyte recruitment around endothelial cells, leading to vessel fragility and hemorrhaging (Li et al., 1999; Torsney et al., 2003; Urness et al., 2000). Thus, both genes are required for two defining aspects of angiogenesis: endothelial network remodeling and vascular morphogenesis through recruitment of pericytes (Risau, 1997), essential support cells for the formation and maintenance of the vasculature (Bergers and Song, 2005).

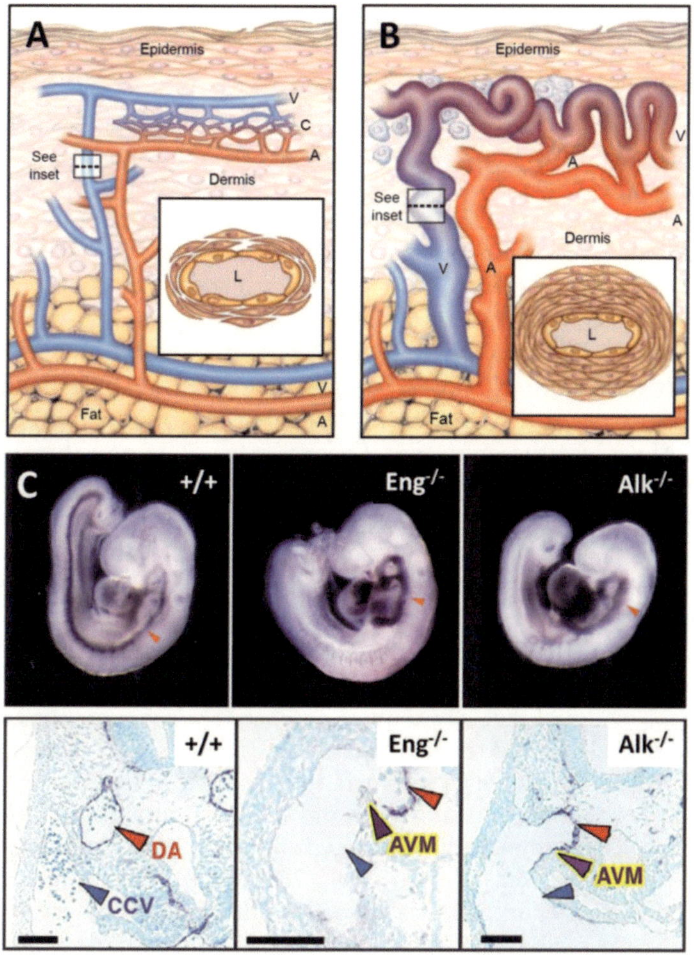

Fig. 5. Phenotypic consequences of loss of *ENG* or *ALK1* function.
A. Normal dermal vasculature: well-differentiated veins and arteries are separated by micro-vascular capillary beds. B. Hereditary Hemorrhagic Telangectasia (HHT) subjects present with enlarged vessels, disappearance of micro-vascular capillary beds and arterio-veinous malformations (AVM) leading to hemorrhage (Guttmacher et al., 1995). C. Mouse embryos carrying *ENG* or *ALK1* mutations present similar defects: shunting of the circulation (upper panels), due to the fusion between the dorsal artery (DA) and the cardinal vein (CCV) (lower panels) (Sorensen et al., 2003). © Adapted and reprinted by permission from the Massachusetts Medical Society: Guttmacher et al, 1995 Hereditary Hemorraghic Telangectasia, NEJM, 1995, (333) 14: 919, and from Elsevier: Sorensen et al, 2003, Loss of distinct arterial and venous boundaries in mice lacking Endoglin, Dev Biol 261: 236-7.

3.3 Signal transduction through ALK1 and ENG

Several alternative models have been proposed regarding the identity of the cytokine capable of triggering physiological ALK1/ENG signaling in endothelial cells, and the type of SMAD response these cytokines trigger. In the following sections, we will review these models and explain why we favor the BMP9/ALK1/ENG/SMAD1-5 signaling model.

3.3.1 "Cross-over" TGFβ/ SMAD1-5 signaling model

Initial studies describing ENG and ALK1 indicated that the two proteins could be part of a TGFβ receptor complex. Over-expressed ENG and ALK1 were found in protein complexes with TGFβ receptor 2 (TBR2) and radio-labeled TGFβ1 (Attisano et al., 1993; Cheifetz et al., 1992) and endogenous complexes containing ENG, TBR2 and radio-labeled TGFβ1 were found in primary endothelial cells (Cheifetz et al., 1992; Yamashita et al., 1994). The finding that TGFβ could induce SMAD1-5 phosphorylation in Mouse Embryonic Endothelial Cells (MEEC) and Bovine Aortic Endothelial Cells (BAEC) through a signaling complex containing ENG, ALK1, ALK5 and TBR2 led to a model of "cross-over" TGFβ signaling, whereby TGFβ/ALK1 signaling antagonized TGFβ/ALK5 signaling in endothelial cells (Fig. 6A) (Goumans et al., 2003; Goumans et al., 2002; Lebrin et al., 2004; Oh et al., 2000). These results were unexpected since TGFβ was thought to be incapable of signaling through BMP Type I receptors such as ALK1. Until then, the "canonical" model of TGFβ signaling axis postulated that ALK5 was the only Type I receptor for TGFβ and that TGFβ exclusively signaled via phosphorylation of SMAD2-3 (Massague, 2000) (Fig. 6B). Several subsequent studies have shown that immortalized or transformed cells could display a non-canonical "cross-over" TGFβ signaling pathway leading to SMAD1-5 phosphorylation via BMP Type I receptors (Daly et al., 2008; Finnson et al., 2008; Liu et al., 2009). This transition to "cross-over" TGFβ/SMAD1-5 signaling from "canonical" TGFβ/SMAD2-3 signaling could explain how cancer cells switch from an anti-proliferative to a pro-invasive TGFβ response in the course of malignant cellular transformation (Liu et al., 2009).

Thus, while there is no doubt that "cross-over" TGFβ/SMAD1-5 signaling has been detected in a number of immortalized and transformed cell lines and in some mesenchymal cell types (Wrighton et al., 2009), the evidence for such a signaling axis existing in endothelial cells rested entirely on results obtained in MEEC and BAEC (Goumans et al., 2002). However, given that MEEC cells are immortalized through infection with a retrovirus encoding the polyoma middle T oncoprotein (Larsson et al., 2001), it is unlikely that they represent a normal and physiological endothelial cell type. In addition, the observation that primary endothelial BAEC cells exhibit TGFβ/SMAD1-5 signaling (Goumans et al., 2002) could not be reproduced (Scharpfenecker et al., 2007; Shao et al., 2009) and TGFβ/SMAD1-5 signaling could not be detected in primary human endothelial cells (David et al., 2007; Shao et al., 2009), suggesting that the "cross-over" TGFβ/SMAD1-5 signaling axis may only be detected in immortalized endothelial cell types.

In vivo evidence also cast doubt on the proposed model of TGFβ as the key cytokine functioning upstream of ALK1/ENG/SMAD1-5 signaling in endothelial cells. Initially, because *ALK1*, *ALK5*, *ENG* and *TBR2* mutant embryos all demonstrated severe vascular phenotypes at day 10.5, including disappearance of the yolk sac vasculature, speculation that they were possibly engaged in the same signaling axis emerged (ten Dijke and Arthur, 2007). However, using genetically engineered mouse strains carrying the *LacZ* reporter gene under the control of the endogenous *ALK1* or *ALK5* promoters, Seki and colleagues demonstrated that *ALK1* was expressed in endothelial cells, whereas *ALK5* was expressed in VSMC (Seki et al., 2006), suggesting distinct *in vivo* functions of the two receptors in vascular development. Moreover, endothelium-specific genetic deletion of *ALK1* during embryogenesis triggered severe vascular defects mimicking pathological features of HHT, whereas endothelium-specific deletion of *TBR2* and *ALK5,* the two main receptors for TGFβ, presented no detectable phenotype in the developing vasculature (Park et al., 2008). These results suggest that the function of ALK1 in the developing endothelium is independent of TGFβ signaling and that TGFβ does not play a role in endothelial signaling functions related to the onset of HHT like phenotypes (Bailly, 2008).

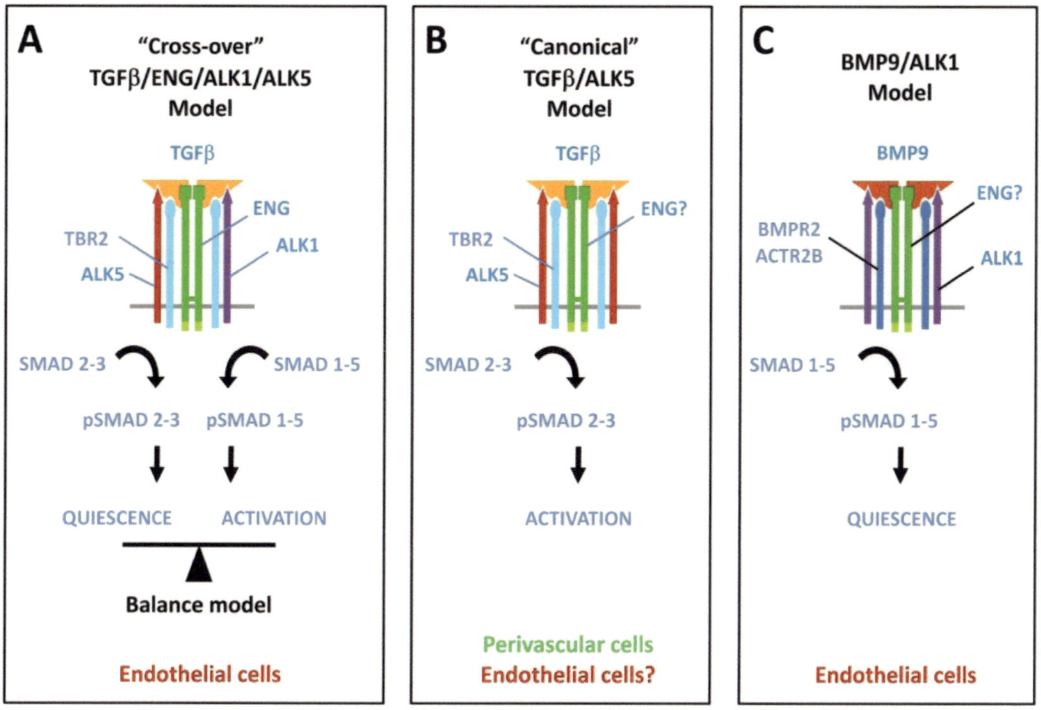

Fig. 6. Models of ALK1 / ENG mediated signaling in endothelial and perivascular cells. A. The "Cross-over" model proposes that TGFβ induces a dual ALK5/SMAD2-3 and ALK1/SMAD1-5 phosphorylation response in endothelial cells, whereby ALK1 signaling induces endothelial cell proliferation and migration, and antagonizes ALK5 signaling. B. The "canonical" TFGβ model proposes that TGFβ-induced SMAD2-3 phosphorylation is central to perivascular cell biology. TGFβ may have endothelial functions unrelated to ALK1 signaling and HHT *in vivo* and ENG may play a role in transducing canonical TGFβ signaling. C. The BMP9 signaling model proposes that BMP9 is a circulating endothelial quiescence factor triggering SMAD1-5 signaling, resulting in endothelial quiescence.

3.3.2 "Canonical" TGFβ / pSMAD2-3 signaling model

In vivo studies have demonstrated a clear role for TGFβ/ALK5 signaling in vascular development (Pardali et al., 2010), but whether TGFβ signaling impacts endothelial cells *in vivo* remain a matter of controversy since endothelium-specific deletion of *ALK5* and *TBR2* do not disrupt the embryonic vasculature (Park et al., 2008). *In vitro* evidence suggests that the "canonical" TGFβ/SMAD2-3 signaling pathway is operative inside primary cultured endothelial cells (Fig. 6B). TGFβ induces SMAD2-3 phosphorylation in cultured endothelial cells (Bostrom et al., 2004; Goumans et al., 2002) and is reported to influence *VEGF-A* and *PDGF-B* transcript levels (Shao et al, 2009; Cunha et al., 2010). Moreover, ENG is detected in association with TBR2 and TGFβ in primary endothelial cells (Cheifetz et al., 1992;

Yamashita et al., 1994); ENG can potentiate "canonical" TGFβ/ALK5/SMAD2-3 signaling (Guerrero-Esteo et al., 2002); and the soluble extra-cellular domain of ENG can inhibit binding of TGFβ to endothelial cells and influence vascular tone (Venkatesha et al., 2006). Taken together, these results indicate that TGFβ may signal in endothelial cells, where it may have ALK1-independent, but ENG-dependent functions in the endothelium unrelated to the onset of HHT and vascular malformations, but related to the regulation of blood pressure (Venkatesha et al., 2006).

3.3.3 BMP9 / SMAD1-5 signaling model

An early study pointed to an unknown ligand present in human serum distinct from TGFβ that could activate ALK1 signaling (Lux et al., 1999). Following a report that BMP9 could be co-crystalized with ALK1 (Brown et al., 2005), other groups demonstrated that BMP9 and 10 were the only cognate ALK1 ligands within the TGFβ super-family (Mitchell et al., 2010) and that BMP9 and 10 triggered ALK1/SMAD1-5 signaling in primary endothelial cells (David et al., 2007; Scharpfenecker et al., 2007). BMP9 is produced by hepatic endothelial and stellate cells and was confirmed to be the ALK1 signaling trigger in human serum (David et al., 2008), while BMP10 is only detected during embryonic heart development (Neuhaus et al., 1999). BMP9 and 10 are the only TGFβ super-family ligands to bind ENG in the absence of other Type I or II receptors (Scharpfenecker et al., 2007), and ENG potentiates BMP9/ALK1/SMAD1-5 signaling in endothelial cells (David et al., 2007). Thus, a new model has emerged to explain the signaling pathway that is likely disrupted in the endothelium of HHT patients, whereby BMP9 triggers SMAD1-5 phosphorylation through a multimeric complex requiring ALK1, BMPR2 or ACTR2B and, possibly, ENG (Fig. 6C).

3.4 Function of BMP9/ALK1/ENG signaling in endothelial cells *in vitro* and *in vivo*

The response of endothelial cells to BMP9 appears to be context-dependent. In primary Human Dermal Microvascular Endothelial Cells (HMVEC-D), obtained from the skin, an organ whose vasculature is clearly affected in HHT patients, activation of ALK1 or stimulation with BMP9 inhibited cell proliferation and migration, while increasing SMAD1-5 target gene expression (David et al., 2007; Lamouille et al., 2002). Over-expression of ALK1 also decreased proliferation of primary HUVEC cells (Ota et al., 2002) and BMP9 blocked the proliferative effect of basic FGF (bFGF) on primary endothelial cells (Scharpfenecker et al., 2007). Based on these *in vitro* results, and on the fact that BMP9 inhibited vessel formation in a bFGF-driven *in vivo* angiogenesis assay (David et al., 2008), BMP9/ALK1 signaling was proposed to function in the resolution phase of angiogenesis, during which endothelial cell proliferation and migration shut down and vessel maturation and differentiation proceeds. According to this model, disruption of ALK1 signaling leads to endothelial cells that cannot stop proliferating and therefore cannot differentiate into mature functional vessels, leading to disruption of angiogenesis (David et al., 2009). Given that BMP9 and ALK1 repress the expression of pro-angiogenic factors *in vitro* (Shao et al., 2009) and *in vivo* (Oh et al., 2000), BMP9/ALK1 signaling may be key to the equilibrium between pro- and anti-angiogenic signals required for the completion of the activation and resolution phases of angiogenesis, which are both required for the formation of a functional vasculature.

Other studies reached opposite conclusions regarding the role of BMP9/ALK1 signaling in endothelial cells, supporting an alternative model in which BMP9 is proangiogenic. Suzuki and colleagues described that BMP9 stimulated the proliferation of MESEC cells (Suzuki et al., 2010), while other groups found that ALK1 and ENG stimulated MEEC proliferation (Goumans et al., 2002; Lebrin et al., 2004). As stated earlier, immortalized endothelial cells such as MESECs or MEECs are probably not the best models to define the physiological function of BMP9 and ALK1. However, the fact that BMP9 stimulated angiogenesis in a matrigel plug assay and a tumor model *in vivo* indicates that assay conditions, such as the concentration of proangiogenic factors, may influence the endothelium's response to BMP9/ALK1 signaling (Suzuki et al., 2010).

3.5 Development of therapeutics targeting ENG and ALK1

Genetic evidence suggests that ENG and ALK1 functionally contribute to tumor angiogenesis. Cancer cells implanted in $ENG^{+/-}$ heterozygous mice produced tumors whose size and vascularization were reduced by 30% compared with tumors implanted in wild-type littermates (Duwel et al., 2007). The growth and vascularization of pancreatic neuro-endocrine tumors were also reduced by ~50% in $ALK1^{+/-}$ mice compared to $ALK1^{+/+}$ mice (Cunha et al., 2010). Together, these studies indicate that blocking ENG or ALK1 function could be an effective anti-tumor therapeutic strategy.

3.5.1 Therapeutic agents targeting ALK1

Agents targeting ALK1 have entered phase 1 clinical trials, including an ALK1-Fc peptibody from Acceleron (RAP-041) (Bendell et al., 2011) and an anti-ALK1 monoclonal antibody from Pfizer (Goff et al., 2010). ALK1-Fc sequesters ALK1 ligands such as BMP9 and BMP10 and inhibits their binding to endothelial ALK1 receptors (Cunha et al., 2010; David et al., 2007; Mitchell et al., 2010). ALK1-Fc prevented tumor growth in a neuro-endocrine pancreatic cancer model, accompanied by a significant decrease in tumor vascularization (Cunha and Pietras, 2011). ALK1-Fc also decreased the tumor burden of breast cancer-implanted mice by 75% (Mitchell et al., 2010), suggesting that RAP-041 may induce an anti-angiogenic response in cancer patients. Phase 1 results indicate preliminary signs of clinical activity but also a potential heart-related toxicity (Bendell et al., 2011).

The Pfizer antibody (PF-03446962) is a fully human monoclonal antibody that blocks serum-induced SMAD1-5 phosphorylation in endothelial cells (Hu-Lowe et al., 2011). A surrogate anti-mouse Alk1 antibody decreased tumor volume by 70% in a breast cancer model and decreased tumor microvascular density, indicating a potent anti-angiogenic effect (Hu-Lowe et al., 2011). This antibody was not tested for its ability to inhibit BMP9 signaling specifically, but since serum-induced SMAD1 phosphorylation is largely due to the presence of circulating BMP9 (David et al., 2008), inhibition of BMP9 signaling is very likely a mechanism of action of this antibody. Importantly, the anti-mouse Alk1 antibody significantly improved the efficacy of VEGF/VEGFR pathway inhibition in a model of VEGF inhibitor-resistant melanoma, indicating the possibility that ALK1 inhibition may overcome mechanisms of resistance to VEGF inhibitors (Hu-Lowe et al., 2011). Preliminary evidence of clinical activity of PF-03446962 has been reported without indications of adverse effects (Goff et al., 2010).

3.5.2 Therapeutic anti-ENG monoclonal antibodies

The clinical evaluation of TRC105, a chimeric human IgG1 anti-ENG antibody derived from the SN6j monoclonal mouse anti-human ENG antibody, has been initiated. SN6j has an anti-proliferative effect on human endothelial cells *in vitro* (She et al., 2004) and decreased tumor growth in several mouse tumor models (Tsujie et al., 2006; Uneda et al., 2009). SN6j also inhibited lung and liver metastases in metastatic cancer models (Uneda et al., 2009). The anti-tumor mechanism of action of SN6j is thought to derive from its anti-angiogenic properties, as SN6j significantly decreased the vascularization of a matrigel plug assay (Tsujie et al., 2006). The SN6j antibody has not been tested for its ability to block BMP9 signaling in endothelial cells, but this possible mechanism of action should be explored. As an IgG1 chimeric antibody (Shiozaki et al., 2006), another possible mechanism of action of TRC105 could be the engagement of an antibody-dependent cell cytotoxic response (ADCC) targeted at the ENG-expressing cancer endothelium (Tsujie et al., 2008).

The results of a phase 1 trial indicate that TRC105 was well tolerated and there was preliminary evidence of clinical responses (Rosen et al., 2010). A phase 1-2 trial conducted in castrate-resistant prostate cancer patients confirmed the evidence of clinical responders, with patients who had progressed on anti-hormone therapies experiencing a significant decrease in PSA levels (Adelberg et al., 2011). Several phase 1 and 2 trials are now planned in Bladder, Breast, Renal and Liver cancer, including a combination trial with bevacizumab, an anti-VEGF-A antibody. This combination could prove efficacious since VEGF-A neutralization induces ENG expression in a pancreatic cancer model (Bockhorn et al., 2003), suggesting that ENG-dependent signaling may be engaged in response to VEGF-A inhibition as a possible adaptation mechanism.

4. Conclusions

In this chapter, we have reviewed signal transduction pathways (NOTCH and BMP9/ALK/ENG) whose key functions affect endothelial cell proliferation and vessel differentiation. As such, both pathways are critical for the resolution phase of angiogenesis, when endothelial cells complete their proliferation and migration in order to form a functional vasculature following recruitment of perivascular cells. NOTCH signaling determines the cell fate of stalk and tip cells, a step to limit vessel sprouting and allow organization into a functional vasculature. Endoglin and ALK1 define a receptor signaling complex which transduces BMP9 signaling in ECs. This signaling axis is critical for endothelial maturation and homeostasis, since even halving the expression or activity of these two proteins leads to hemorrhage and loss of perivascular cells. Both of these processes are distinct from the initiation phase of angiogenesis in which VEGF-A plays a central role. Therefore agents that interfere with NOTCH and ALK1/ENG signaling (1) are predicted to disrupt tumor angiogenesis as monotherapies as suggested by their preclinical activity, (2) may prove useful in combination with anti-VEGF inhibitors by targeting distinct phases of angiogenesis, provided there is no dose limiting toxicity due to the combination, and (3) may be able to overcome intrinsic and acquired resistance mechanisms to anti-VEGF therapeutics. With therapeutics to these pathways now progressing in clinical trials, the ability to target multiple phases of the angiogenic process to provide increased benefit to patients may be tested in the near future.

5. Acknowledgements

The authors thank Drs. Astrid Ruefli-Brasse, Terri Burgess, Dineli Wickramasinghe, Rick Kendall and Glenn Begley for their critical reading of the manuscript. Figures were adapted and reprinted under Creative Common license or with permission from Elsevier, the Massachusetts Medical Society and the American Association for Cancer Research.

6. References

Acar, M., Jafar-Nejad, H., Takeuchi, H., Rajan, A., Ibrani, D., Rana, N.A., Pan, H., Haltiwanger, R.S., and Bellen, H.J. (2008). Rumi is a CAP10 domain glycosyltransferase that modifies Notch and is required for Notch signaling. Cell *132*, 247-258.

Adelberg, D., Apolo, A.B., Madan, R.A., Gulley, J.L., Pierpoint, A., Kohler, D.R., Trepel, J.B., Steinberg, S.M., Figg, W.D., and Dahut, W.L. (2011). A phase I study of TRC105 (anti-CD105 monoclonal antibody) in metastatic castration-resistant prostate cancer (mCRPC). J Clin Oncol *29 s7*, 171.

Altomonte, M., Montagner, R., Fonsatti, E., Colizzi, F., Cattarossi, I., Brasoveanu, L.I., Nicotra, M.R., Cattelan, A., Natali, P.G., and Maio, M. (1996). Expression and structural features of endoglin (CD105), a transforming growth factor beta1 and beta3 binding protein, in human melanoma. Br J Cancer *74*, 1586-1591.

Arthur, H.M., Ure, J., Smith, A.J., Renforth, G., Wilson, D.I., Torsney, E., Charlton, R., Parums, D.V., Jowett, T., Marchuk, D.A., *et al.* (2000). Endoglin, an ancillary TGFbeta receptor, is required for extraembryonic angiogenesis and plays a key role in heart development. Dev Biol *217*, 42-53.

Attisano, L., Carcamo, J., Ventura, F., Weis, F.M., Massague, J., and Wrana, J.L. (1993). Identification of human activin and TGF beta type I receptors that form heteromeric kinase complexes with type II receptors. Cell *75*, 671-680.

Bailly, S. (2008). HHT is not a TGFb disease. Blood *111*, 478.

Beckers, J., Clark, A., Wunsch, K., Hrabe De Angelis, M., and Gossler, A. (1999). Expression of the mouse Delta1 gene during organogenesis and fetal development. Mech Dev *84*, 165-168.

Bendell, J.C., Gordon, M., Hurwitz, H., Yang, Y., Wilson, D.I., Haltom, E., Attie, K.M., Condon, C.H., Sherman, M.L., and Sharma, S. (2011). A Phase 1 dose escalating study with ACE-041, a novel inhibitor of ALK1 mediated angiogenesis, in patients with advanced solid tumors Paper presented at: AACR 102nd Annual Meeting (Orlando, FL, USA).

Benedito, R., Roca, C., Sorensen, I., Adams, S., Gossler, A., Fruttiger, M., and Adams, R.H. (2009). The notch ligands Dll4 and Jagged1 have opposing effects on angiogenesis. Cell *137*, 1124-1135.

Bergers, G., and Hanahan, D. (2008). Modes of resistance to anti-angiogenic therapy. Nat Rev Cancer *8*, 592-603.

Bergers, G., and Song, S. (2005). The role of pericytes in blood-vessel formation and maintenance. Neuro Oncol *7*, 452-464.

Blaumueller, C.M., Qi, H., Zagouras, P., and Artavanis-Tsakonas, S. (1997). Intracellular cleavage of Notch leads to a heterodimeric receptor on the plasma membrane. Cell *90*, 281-291.

Bockhorn, M., Tsuzuki, Y., Xu, L., Frilling, A., Broelsch, C.E., and Fukumura, D. (2003). Differential vascular and transcriptional responses to anti-vascular endothelial growth factor antibody in orthotopic human pancreatic cancer xenografts. Clin Cancer Res *9*, 4221-4226.

Bostrom, K., Zebboudj, A.F., Yao, Y., Lin, T.S., and Torres, A. (2004). Matrix GLA protein stimulates VEGF expression through increased transforming growth factor-beta1 activity in endothelial cells. J Biol Chem *279*, 52904-52913.

Bourdeau, A., Dumont, D.J., and Letarte, M. (1999). A murine model of hereditary hemorrhagic telangiectasia. J Clin Invest *104*, 1343-1351.

Brown, M.A., Zhao, Q., Baker, K.A., Naik, C., Chen, C., Pukac, L., Singh, M., Tsareva, T., Parice, Y., Mahoney, A., *et al.* (2005). Crystal structure of BMP-9 and functional interactions with pro-region and receptors. J Biol Chem *280*, 25111-25118.

Burrows, F.J., Derbyshire, E.J., Tazzari, P.L., Amlot, P., Gazdar, A.F., King, S.W., Letarte, M., Vitetta, E.S., and Thorpe, P.E. (1995). Up-regulation of endoglin on vascular endothelial cells in human solid tumors: implications for diagnosis and therapy. Clin Cancer Res *1*, 1623-1634.

Casanovas, O. (2011). The adaptive stroma joining the antiangiogenic resistance front. J Clin Invest.

Cheifetz, S., Bellon, T., Cales, C., Vera, S., Bernabeu, C., Massague, J., and Letarte, M. (1992). Endoglin is a component of the transforming growth factor-beta receptor system in human endothelial cells. J Biol Chem *267*, 19027-19030.

Chen, F., Yu, G., Arawaka, S., Nishimura, M., Kawarai, T., Yu, H., Tandon, A., Supala, A., Song, Y.Q., Rogaeva, E., *et al.* (2001). Nicastrin binds to membrane-tethered Notch. Nat Cell Biol *3*, 751-754.

Conlon, R.A., Reaume, A.G., and Rossant, J. (1995). Notch1 is required for the coordinate segmentation of somites. Development *121*, 1533-1545.

Crawford, Y., and Ferrara, N. (2009). Tumor and stromal pathways mediating refractoriness/resistance to anti-angiogenic therapies. Trends Pharmacol Sci *30*, 624-630.

Cunha, S.I., Pardali, E., Thorikay, M., Anderberg, C., Hawinkels, L., Goumans, M.J., Seehra, J., Heldin, C.H., ten Dijke, P., and Pietras, K. (2010). Genetic and pharmacological targeting of activin receptor-like kinase 1 impairs tumor growth and angiogenesis. J Exp Med *207*, 85-100.

Cunha, S.I., and Pietras, K. (2011). ALK1 as an emerging target for anti-angiogenic therapy for cancer. Blood *117 (15)*.

Dallas, N.A., Samuel, S., Xia, L., Fan, F., Gray, M.J., Lim, S.J., and Ellis, L.M. (2008). Endoglin (CD105): a marker of tumor vasculature and potential target for therapy. Clin Cancer Res *14*, 1931-1937.

Daly, A.C., Randall, R.A., and Hill, C.S. (2008). Transforming growth factor beta-induced Smad1/5 phosphorylation in epithelial cells is mediated by novel receptor complexes and is essential for anchorage-independent growth. Mol Cell Biol *28*, 6889-6902.

David, L., Feige, J.J., and Bailly, S. (2009). Emerging role of bone morphogenetic proteins in angiogenesis. Cytokine Growth Factor Rev *20*, 203-212.

David, L., Mallet, C., Keramidas, M., Lamande, N., Gasc, J.M., Dupuis-Girod, S., Plauchu, H., Feige, J.J., and Bailly, S. (2008). Bone morphogenetic protein-9 is a circulating vascular quiescence factor. Circulation Research *102*, 914-922.

David, L., Mallet, C., Mazerbourg, S., Feige, J.J., and Bailly, S. (2007). Identification of BMP9 and BMP10 as functional activators of the orphan activin receptor-like kinase 1 (ALK1) in endothelial cells. Blood *109*, 1953-1961.

Djokovic, D., Trindade, A., Gigante, J., Badenes, M., Silva, L., Liu, R., Li, X., Gong, M., Krasnoperov, V., Gill, P.S., *et al.* (2010). Combination of Dll4/Notch and Ephrin-

B2/EphB4 targeted therapy is highly effective in disrupting tumor angiogenesis. BMC Cancer *10*, 641.

Domenga, V., Fardoux, P., Lacombe, P., Monet, M., Maciazek, J., Krebs, L.T., Klonjkowski, B., Berrou, E., Mericskay, M., Li, Z., *et al.* (2004). Notch3 is required for arterial identity and maturation of vascular smooth muscle cells. Genes & Development *18*, 2730-2735.

Duwel, A., Eleno, N., Jerkic, M., Arevalo, M., Bolanos, J.P., Bernabeu, C., and Lopez-Novoa, J.M. (2007). Reduced tumor growth and angiogenesis in endoglin-haploinsufficient mice. Tumour Biol *28*, 1-8.

Eiraku, M., Tohgo, A., Ono, K., Kaneko, M., Fujishima, K., Hirano, T., and Kengaku, M. (2005). DNER acts as a neuron-specific Notch ligand during Bergmann glial development. Nature Neuroscience *8*, 873-880.

Ellis, L.M., and Hicklin, D.J. (2008). VEGF-targeted therapy: mechanisms of anti-tumour activity. Nat Rev Cancer *8*, 579-591.

Fernandez, L.A., Sanz-Rodriguez, F., Zarrabeitia, R., Perez-Molino, A., Hebbel, R.P., Nguyen, J., Bernabeu, C., and Botella, L.M. (2005). Blood outgrowth endothelial cells from Hereditary Haemorrhagic Telangiectasia patients reveal abnormalities compatible with vascular lesions. Cardiovasc Res *68*, 235-248.

Finnson, K.W., Parker, W.L., ten Dijke, P., Thorikay, M., and Philip, A. (2008). ALK1 opposes ALK5/Smad3 signaling and expression of extracellular matrix components in human chondrocytes. J Bone Miner Res *23*, 896-906.

Fonsatti, E., Del Vecchio, L., Altomonte, M., Sigalotti, L., Nicotra, M.R., Coral, S., Natali, P.G., and Maio, M. (2001). Endoglin: An accessory component of the TGF-beta-binding receptor-complex with diagnostic, prognostic, and bioimmunotherapeutic potential in human malignancies. J Cell Physiol *188*, 1-7.

Fryer, C.J., Lamar, E., Turbachova, I., Kintner, C., and Jones, K.A. (2002). Mastermind mediates chromatin-specific transcription and turnover of the Notch enhancer complex. Genes & Development *16*, 1397-1411.

Fryer, C.J., White, J.B., and Jones, K.A. (2004). Mastermind recruits CycC:CDK8 to phosphorylate the Notch ICD and coordinate activation with turnover. Molecular Cell *16*, 509-520.

Funahashi, Y., Hernandez, S.L., Das, I., Ahn, A., Huang, J., Vorontchikhina, M., Sharma, A., Kanamaru, E., Borisenko, V., Desilva, D.M., *et al.* (2008). A notch1 ectodomain construct inhibits endothelial notch signaling, tumor growth, and angiogenesis. Cancer Research *68*, 4727-4735.

Gale, N.W., Dominguez, M.G., Noguera, I., Pan, L., Hughes, V., Valenzuela, D.M., Murphy, A.J., Adams, N.C., Lin, H.C., Holash, J., *et al.* (2004). Haploinsufficiency of delta-like 4 ligand results in embryonic lethality due to major defects in arterial and vascular development. Proceedings of the National Academy of Sciences of the United States of America *101*, 15949-15954.

Garrido-Martin, E.M., Blanco, F.J., Fernandez, L.A., Langa, C., Vary, C.P., Lee, U.E., Friedman, S.L., Botella, L.M., and Bernabeu, C. (2010). Characterization of the human Activin-A receptor type II-like kinase 1 (ACVRL1) promoter and its regulation by Sp1. BMC Mol Biol *11*, 51.

Goff, L.W., De Braud, F.G., Cohen, R.B., Berlin, J., Noberasco, C., Borghaei, H., Wang, E., Hu-Lowe, D., Levin, W.J., and Gallo-Stampino, C. (2010). Phase I study of PF-

03446962, a fully human mab against ALK 1, a TGFß receptor involved in tumor angiogenesis. J Clin Oncol *28*.

Gordon, W.R., Arnett, K.L., and Blacklow, S.C. (2008). The molecular logic of Notch signaling--a structural and biochemical perspective. J Cell Sci *121*, 3109-3119.

Gordon, W.R., Vardar-Ulu, D., Histen, G., Sanchez-Irizarry, C., Aster, J.C., and Blacklow, S.C. (2007). Structural basis for autoinhibition of Notch.[erratum appears in Nat Struct Mol Biol. 2007 May;14(5):455]. Nature Structural & Molecular Biology *14*, 295-300.

Gougos, A., and Letarte, M. (1988). Identification of a human endothelial cell antigen with monoclonal antibody 44G4 produced against a pre-B leukemic cell line. J Immunol *141*, 1925-1933.

Gougos, A., and Letarte, M. (1990). Primary structure of endoglin, an RGD-containing glycoprotein of human endothelial cells. J Biol Chem *265*, 8361-8364.

Goumans, M.J., Valdimarsdottir, G., Itoh, S., Lebrin, F., Larsson, J., Mummery, C., Karlsson, S., and ten Dijke, P. (2003). Activin receptor-like kinase (ALK)1 is an antagonistic mediator of lateral TGFbeta/ALK5 signaling. Mol Cell *12*, 817-828.

Goumans, M.J., Valdimarsdottir, G., Itoh, S., Rosendahl, A., Sideras, P., and ten Dijke, P. (2002). Balancing the activation state of the endothelium via two distinct TGF-beta type I receptors. EMBO J *21*, 1743-1753.

Guerrero-Esteo, M., Sanchez-Elsner, T., Letamendia, A., and Bernabeu, C. (2002). Extracellular and cytoplasmic domains of endoglin interact with the transforming growth factor-beta receptors I and II. J Biol Chem *277*, 29197-29209.

Guttmacher, A.E., Marchuk, D.A., and White, R.I., Jr. (1995). Hereditary hemorrhagic telangiectasia. N Engl J Med *333*, 918-924.

Haines, N., and Irvine, K.D. (2003). Glycosylation regulates Notch signalling. Nat Rev Mol Cell Biol *4*, 786-797.

Hamada, Y., Kadokawa, Y., Okabe, M., Ikawa, M., Coleman, J.R., and Tsujimoto, Y. (1999). Mutation in ankyrin repeats of the mouse Notch2 gene induces early embryonic lethality. Development *126*, 3415-3424.

Hanahan, D., and Weinberg, R.A. (2011). Hallmarks of cancer: the next generation. Cell *144*, 646-674.

Hanlon, L., Avila, J.L., Demarest, R.M., Troutman, S., Allen, M., Ratti, F., Rustgi, A.K., Stanger, B.Z., Radtke, F., Adsay, V., *et al.* (2010). Notch1 functions as a tumor suppressor in a model of K-ras-induced pancreatic ductal adenocarcinoma. Cancer Research *70*, 4280-4286.

Haritunians, T., Boulter, J., Hicks, C., Buhrman, J., DiSibio, G., Shawber, C., Weinmaster, G., Nofziger, D., and Schanen, C. (2002). CADASIL Notch3 mutant proteins localize to the cell surface and bind ligand. Circ Res *90*, 506-508.

Hauschild, A., Agarwala, S.S., Trefzer, U., Hogg, D., Robert, C., Hersey, P., Eggermont, A., Grabbe, S., Gonzalez, R., Gille, J., *et al.* (2009). Results of a phase III, randomized, placebo-controlled study of sorafenib in combination with carboplatin and paclitaxel as second-line treatment in patients with unresectable stage III or stage IV melanoma. J Clin Oncol *27*, 2823-2830.

High, F.A., Lu, M.M., Pear, W.S., Loomes, K.M., Kaestner, K.H., and Epstein, J.A. (2008). Endothelial expression of the Notch ligand Jagged1 is required for vascular smooth muscle development. Proceedings of the National Academy of Sciences of the United States of America *105*, 1955-1959.

Hingorani, S.R., Petricoin, E.F., Maitra, A., Rajapakse, V., King, C., Jacobetz, M.A., Ross, S., Conrads, T.P., Veenstra, T.D., Hitt, B.A., *et al.* (2003). Preinvasive and invasive ductal pancreatic cancer and its early detection in the mouse. Cancer Cell *4*, 437-450.

Hoey, T., Yen, W.C., Axelrod, F., Basi, J., Donigian, L., Dylla, S., Fitch-Bruhns, M., Lazetic, S., Park, I.K., Sato, A., *et al.* (2009). DLL4 blockade inhibits tumor growth and reduces tumor-initiating cell frequency. Cell Stem Cell *5*, 168-177.

Hrabe de Angelis, M., McIntyre, J., 2nd, and Gossler, A. (1997). Maintenance of somite borders in mice requires the Delta homologue DII1. Nature *386*, 717-721.

Hu-Lowe, D.D., Chen, E., Zhang, L., Watson, K.D., Mancuso, P., Lappin, P., Wickman, G., Chen, J.H., Wang, J., Jiang, X., *et al.* (2011). Targeting Activin Receptor-Like Kinase 1 Inhibits Angiogenesis and Tumorigenesis through a Mechanism of Action Complementary to Anti-VEGF Therapies. Cancer Res *71*, 1362-1373.

Hu, Q.D., Ang, B.T., Karsak, M., Hu, W.P., Cui, X.Y., Duka, T., Takeda, Y., Chia, W., Sankar, N., Ng, Y.K., *et al.* (2003). F3/contactin acts as a functional ligand for Notch during oligodendrocyte maturation. Cell *115*, 163-175.

Hurwitz, H., Fehrenbacher, L., Novotny, W., Cartwright, T., Hainsworth, J., Heim, W., Berlin, J., Baron, A., Griffing, S., Holmgren, E., *et al.* (2004). Bevacizumab plus irinotecan, fluorouracil, and leucovorin for metastatic colorectal cancer. N Engl J Med *350*, 2335-2342.

Iso, T., Kedes, L., and Hamamori, Y. (2003). HES and HERP families: multiple effectors of the Notch signaling pathway. J Cell Physiol *194*, 237-255.

Jakobsson, L., Franco, C.A., Bentley, K., Collins, R.T., Ponsioen, B., Aspalter, I.M., Rosewell, I., Busse, M., Thurston, G., Medvinsky, A., *et al.* (2010). Endothelial cells dynamically compete for the tip cell position during angiogenic sprouting. Nat Cell Biol *12*, 943-953.

Jarriault, S., Brou, C., Logeat, F., Schroeter, E.H., Kopan, R., and Israel, A. (1995). Signalling downstream of activated mammalian Notch.[see comment]. Nature *377*, 355-358.

Johnson, D.W., Berg, J.N., Baldwin, M.A., Gallione, C.J., Marondel, I., Yoon, S.J., Stenzel, T.T., Speer, M., Pericak-Vance, M.A., Diamond, A., *et al.* (1996). Mutations in the activin receptor-like kinase 1 gene in hereditary haemorrhagic telangiectasia type 2. Nat Genet *13*, 189-195.

Jonker, L., and Arthur, H.M. (2002). Endoglin expression in early development is associated with vasculogenesis and angiogenesis. Mech Dev *110*, 193-196.

Joutel, A., Andreux, F., Gaulis, S., Domenga, V., Cecillon, M., Battail, N., Piga, N., Chapon, F., Godfrain, C., and Tournier-Lasserve, E. (2000). The ectodomain of the Notch3 receptor accumulates within the cerebrovasculature of CADASIL patients. J Clin Invest *105*, 597-605.

Joutel, A., Corpechot, C., Ducros, A., Vahedi, K., Chabriat, H., Mouton, P., Alamowitch, S., Domenga, V., Cecillion, M., Marechal, E., *et al.* (1996). Notch3 mutations in CADASIL, a hereditary adult-onset condition causing stroke and dementia. Nature *383*, 707-710.

Jubb, A.M., Miller, K.D., Rugo, H.S., Harris, A.L., Chen, D., Reimann, J.D., Cobleigh, M.A., Schmidt, M., Langmuir, V.K., Hillan, K.J., *et al.* (2011). Impact of exploratory biomarkers on the treatment effect of bevacizumab in metastatic breast cancer. Clin Cancer Res *17*, 372-381.

Jubb, A.M., Turley, H., Moeller, H.C., Steers, G., Han, C., Li, J.L., Leek, R., Tan, E.Y., Singh, B., Mortensen, N.J., *et al.* (2009). Expression of delta-like ligand 4 (Dll4) and markers of hypoxia in colon cancer. Br J Cancer *101*, 1749-1757.

Kerbel, R.S. (2008). Tumor angiogenesis. N Engl J Med *358*, 2039-2049.

Kindler, H.L., Niedzwiecki, D., Hollis, D., Oraefo, E., Schrag, D., and Hurwitz, H. (2007). A double-blind, placebo-controlled, randomized phase III trial of gemcitabine plus bevacizumab versus gemcitabine plus placebo in patients with advanced pancreatic cancer. J Clin Oncol *25*, 4508.

Klinakis, A., Lobry, C., Abdel-Wahab, O., Oh, P., Haeno, H., Buonamici, S., van De Walle, I., Cathelin, S., Trimarchi, T., Araldi, E., *et al.* (2011). A novel tumour-suppressor function for the Notch pathway in myeloid leukaemia. Nature *473*, 230-233.

Kopan, R., and Ilagan, M.X. (2009). The canonical Notch signaling pathway: unfolding the activation mechanism. Cell *137*, 216-233.

Kopetz, S., Hoff, P.M., Morris, J.S., Wolff, R.A., Eng, C., Glover, K.Y., Adinin, R., Overman, M.J., Valero, V., Wen, S., *et al.* (2010). Phase II trial of infusional fluorouracil, irinotecan, and bevacizumab for metastatic colorectal cancer: efficacy and circulating angiogenic biomarkers associated with therapeutic resistance. J Clin Oncol *28*, 453-459.

Krebs, L.T., Shutter, J.R., Tanigaki, K., Honjo, T., Stark, K.L., and Gridley, T. (2004). Haploinsufficient lethality and formation of arteriovenous malformations in Notch pathway mutants. Genes & Development *18*, 2469-2473.

Krebs, L.T., Xue, Y., Norton, C.R., Shutter, J.R., Maguire, M., Sundberg, J.P., Gallahan, D., Closson, V., Kitajewski, J., Callahan, R., *et al.* (2000). Notch signaling is essential for vascular morphogenesis in mice. Genes & Development *14*, 1343-1352.

Krebs, L.T., Xue, Y., Norton, C.R., Sundberg, J.P., Beatus, P., Lendahl, U., Joutel, A., and Gridley, T. (2003). Characterization of Notch3-deficient mice: normal embryonic development and absence of genetic interactions with a Notch1 mutation. Genesis *37*, 139-143.

Lamouille, S., Mallet, C., Feige, J.J., and Bailly, S. (2002). Activin receptor-like kinase 1 is implicated in the maturation phase of angiogenesis. Blood *100*, 4495-4501.

Larsson, J., Goumans, M.J., Sjostrand, L.J., van Rooijen, M.A., Ward, D., Leveen, P., Xu, X., ten Dijke, P., Mummery, C.L., and Karlsson, S. (2001). Abnormal angiogenesis but intact hematopoietic potential in TGF-beta type I receptor-deficient mice. EMBO J *20*, 1663-1673.

Lebrin, F., Goumans, M.J., Jonker, L., Carvalho, R.L., Valdimarsdottir, G., Thorikay, M., Mummery, C., Arthur, H.M., and ten Dijke, P. (2004). Endoglin promotes endothelial cell proliferation and TGF-beta/ALK1 signal transduction. EMBO J *23*, 4018-4028.

Lebrin, F., and Mummery, C.L. (2008). Endoglin-mediated vascular remodeling: mechanisms underlying hereditary hemorrhagic telangiectasia. Trends Cardiovasc Med *18*, 25-32.

Li, C., Issa, R., Kumar, P., Hampson, I.N., Lopez-Novoa, J.M., Bernabeu, C., and Kumar, S. (2003). CD105 prevents apoptosis in hypoxic endothelial cells. J Cell Sci *116*, 2677-2685.

Li, D.Y., Sorensen, L.K., Brooke, B.S., Urness, L.D., Davis, E.C., Taylor, D.G., Boak, B.B., and Wendel, D.P. (1999). Defective angiogenesis in mice lacking endoglin. Science *284*, 1534-1537.

Lieber, T., Kidd, S., Alcamo, E., Corbin, V., and Young, M.W. (1993). Antineurogenic phenotypes induced by truncated Notch proteins indicate a role in signal transduction and may point to a novel function for Notch in nuclei. Genes & Development *7*, 1949-1965.

Limbourg, A., Ploom, M., Elligsen, D., Sorensen, I., Ziegelhoeffer, T., Gossler, A., Drexler, H., and Limbourg, F.P. (2007). Notch ligand Delta-like 1 is essential for postnatal arteriogenesis. Circ Res *100*, 363-371.

Limbourg, F.P., Takeshita, K., Radtke, F., Bronson, R.T., Chin, M.T., and Liao, J.K. (2005). Essential role of endothelial Notch1 in angiogenesis. Circulation *111*, 1826-1832.

Liu, I.M., Schilling, S.H., Knouse, K.A., Choy, L., Derynck, R., and Wang, X.F. (2009). TGFbeta-stimulated Smad1/5 phosphorylation requires the ALK5 L45 loop and mediates the pro-migratory TGFbeta switch. EMBO J *28*, 88-98.

Liu, Z., Turkoz, A., Jackson, E.N., Corbo, J.C., Engelbach, J.A., Garbow, J.R., Piwnica-Worms, D.R., and Kopan, R. (2011). Notch1 loss of heterozygosity causes vascular tumors and lethal hemorrhage in mice. J Clin Invest *121*, 800-808.

Llovet, J.M., Ricci, S., Mazzaferro, V., Hilgard, P., Gane, E., Blanc, J.F., de Oliveira, A.C., Santoro, A., Raoul, J.L., Forner, A., *et al.* (2008). Sorafenib in advanced hepatocellular carcinoma. N Engl J Med *359*, 378-390.

Lobov, I.B., Renard, R.A., Papadopoulos, N., Gale, N.W., Thurston, G., Yancopoulos, G.D., and Wiegand, S.J. (2007). Delta-like ligand 4 (Dll4) is induced by VEGF as a negative regulator of angiogenic sprouting. Proceedings of the National Academy of Sciences of the United States of America *104*, 3219-3224.

Logeat, F., Bessia, C., Brou, C., LeBail, O., Jarriault, S., Seidah, N.G., and Israel, A. (1998). The Notch1 receptor is cleaved constitutively by a furin-like convertase. Proceedings of the National Academy of Sciences of the United States of America *95*, 8108-8112.

Loges, S., Schmidt, T., and Carmeliet, P. (2010). Mechanisms of resistance to anti-angiogenic therapy and development of third generation anti-angiogenic drug candidates. Genes Cancer *1*, 12-25.

Loomes, K.M., Taichman, D.B., Glover, C.L., Williams, P.T., Markowitz, J.E., Piccoli, D.A., Baldwin, H.S., and Oakey, R.J. (2002). Characterization of Notch receptor expression in the developing mammalian heart and liver. Am J Med Genet *112*, 181-189.

Lux, A., Attisano, L., and Marchuk, D.A. (1999). Assignment of transforming growth factor beta1 and beta3 and a third new ligand to the type I receptor ALK-1. J Biol Chem *274*, 9984-9992.

Massague, J. (2000). How cells read TGF-beta signals. Nat Rev Mol Cell Biol *1*, 169-178.

McAllister, K.A., Grogg, K.M., Johnson, D.W., Gallione, C.J., Baldwin, M.A., Jackson, C.E., Helmbold, E.A., Markel, D.S., McKinnon, W.C., Murrell, J., *et al.* (1994). Endoglin, a TGF-beta binding protein of endothelial cells, is the gene for hereditary haemorrhagic telangiectasia type 1. Nat Genet *8*, 345-351.

McCright, B., Gao, X., Shen, L., Lozier, J., Lan, Y., Maguire, M., Herzlinger, D., Weinmaster, G., Jiang, R., and Gridley, T. (2001). Defects in development of the kidney, heart and eye vasculature in mice homozygous for a hypomorphic Notch2 mutation. Development *128*, 491-502.

McCright, B., Lozier, J., and Gridley, T. (2002). A mouse model of Alagille syndrome: Notch2 as a genetic modifier of Jag1 haploinsufficiency. Development *129*, 1075-1082.

Miller, D.W., Graulich, W., Karges, B., Stahl, S., Ernst, M., Ramaswamy, A., Sedlacek, H.H., Muller, R., and Adamkiewicz, J. (1999). Elevated expression of endoglin, a component of the TGF-beta-receptor complex, correlates with proliferation of tumor endothelial cells. Int J Cancer *81*, 568-572.

Miller, K., Wang, M., Gralow, J., Dickler, M., Cobleigh, M., Perez, E.A., Shenkier, T., Cella, D., and Davidson, N.E. (2007). Paclitaxel plus bevacizumab versus paclitaxel alone for metastatic breast cancer. N Engl J Med *357*, 2666-2676.

Minhajat, R., Mori, D., Yamasaki, F., Sugita, Y., Satoh, T., and Tokunaga, O. (2006). Organ-specific endoglin (CD105) expression in the angiogenesis of human cancers. Pathol Int *56*, 717-723.

Mitchell, D., Pobre, E.G., Mulivor, A.W., Grinberg, A.V., Castonguay, R., Monnell, T.E., Solban, N., Ucran, J.A., Pearsall, R.S., Underwood, K.W., *et al.* (2010). ALK1-Fc inhibits multiple mediators of angiogenesis and suppresses tumor growth. Mol Cancer Ther *9*, 379-388.

Mohr, O.L. (1919). Character Changes Caused by Mutation of an Entire Region of a Chromosome in Drosophila. Genetics *4*, 275-282.

Moloney, D.J., Panin, V.M., Johnston, S.H., Chen, J., Shao, L., Wilson, R., Wang, Y., Stanley, P., Irvine, K.D., Haltiwanger, R.S., *et al.* (2000). Fringe is a glycosyltransferase that modifies Notch.[see comment]. Nature *406*, 369-375.

Morgan, T.H., and Bridges, C.B. (1916). Sex-linked inheritance in Drosophila (Carnegie Institution of Washington).

Motzer, R.J., Hutson, T.E., Tomczak, P., Michaelson, M.D., Bukowski, R.M., Oudard, S., Negrier, S., Szczylik, C., Pili, R., Bjarnason, G.A., *et al.* (2009). Overall survival and updated results for sunitinib compared with interferon alfa in patients with metastatic renal cell carcinoma. J Clin Oncol *27*, 3584-3590.

Neuhaus, H., Rosen, V., and Thies, R.S. (1999). Heart specific expression of mouse BMP-10 a novel member of the TGF-beta superfamily. Mech Dev *80*, 181-184.

Nicolas, M., Wolfer, A., Raj, K., Kummer, J.A., Mill, P., van Noort, M., Hui, C.C., Clevers, H., Dotto, G.P., and Radtke, F. (2003). Notch1 functions as a tumor suppressor in mouse skin. Nat Genet *33*, 416-421.

Noguera-Troise, I., Daly, C., Papadopoulos, N.J., Coetzee, S., Boland, P., Gale, N.W., Lin, H.C., Yancopoulos, G.D., and Thurston, G. (2006). Blockade of Dll4 inhibits tumour growth by promoting non-productive angiogenesis.[see comment]. Nature *444*, 1032-1037.

Oberg, C., Li, J., Pauley, A., Wolf, E., Gurney, M., and Lendahl, U. (2001). The Notch intracellular domain is ubiquitinated and negatively regulated by the mammalian Sel-10 homolog. J Biol Chem *276*, 35847-35853.

Oh, S.P., Seki, T., Goss, K.A., Imamura, T., Yi, Y., Donahoe, P.K., Li, L., Miyazono, K., ten Dijke, P., Kim, S., *et al.* (2000). Activin receptor-like kinase 1 modulates transforming growth factor-beta 1 signaling in the regulation of angiogenesis. Proc Natl Acad Sci U S A *97*, 2626-2631.

Ohtsuka, T., Ishibashi, M., Gradwohl, G., Nakanishi, S., Guillemot, F., and Kageyama, R. (1999). Hes1 and Hes5 as notch effectors in mammalian neuronal differentiation. EMBO Journal *18*, 2196-2207.

Ong, C.-T., Cheng, H.-T., Chang, L.-W., Ohtsuka, T., Kageyama, R., Stormo, G.D., and Kopan, R. (2006). Target selectivity of vertebrate notch proteins. Collaboration between discrete domains and CSL-binding site architecture determines activation probability. J Biol Chem *281*, 5106-5119.

Ota, T., Fujii, M., Sugizaki, T., Ishii, M., Miyazawa, K., Aburatani, H., and Miyazono, K. (2002). Targets of transcriptional regulation by two distinct type I receptors for transforming growth factor-beta in human umbilical vein endothelial cells. J Cell Physiol *193*, 299-318.

Panchenko, M.P., Williams, M.C., Brody, J.S., and Yu, Q. (1996). Type I receptor serine-threonine kinase preferentially expressed in pulmonary blood vessels. Am J Physiol *270*, L547-558.

Pardali, E., Goumans, M.J., and ten Dijke, P. (2010). Signaling by members of the TGF-beta family in vascular morphogenesis and disease. Trends Cell Biol *20*, 556-567.

Park, S.O., Lee, Y.J., Seki, T., Hong, K.H., Fliess, N., Jiang, Z., Park, A., Wu, X., Kaartinen, V., Roman, B.L., *et al.* (2008). ALK5- and TGFBR2-independent role of ALK1 in the pathogenesis of hereditary hemorrhagic telangiectasia type 2. Blood *111*, 633-642.

Patel, N.S., Dobbie, M.S., Rochester, M., Steers, G., Poulsom, R., Le Monnier, K., Cranston, D.W., Li, J.L., and Harris, A.L. (2006). Up-regulation of endothelial delta-like 4 expression correlates with vessel maturation in bladder cancer. Clinical Cancer Research *12*, 4836-4844.

Patel, N.S., Li, J.L., Generali, D., Poulsom, R., Cranston, D.W., and Harris, A.L. (2005). Up-regulation of delta-like 4 ligand in human tumor vasculature and the role of basal expression in endothelial cell function. Cancer Research *65*, 8690-8697.

Pece-Barbara, N., Cymerman, U., Vera, S., Marchuk, D.A., and Letarte, M. (1999). Expression analysis of four endoglin missense mutations suggests that haploinsufficiency is the predominant mechanism for hereditary hemorrhagic telangiectasia type 1. Hum Mol Genet *8*, 2171-2181.

Ricard, N., Bidart, M., Mallet, C., Lesca, G., Giraud, S., Prudent, R., Feige, J.J., and Bailly, S. (2010). Functional analysis of the BMP9 response of ALK1 mutants from HHT2 patients: a diagnostic tool for novel ACVRL1 mutations. Blood *116*, 1604-1612.

Ridgway, J., Zhang, G., Wu, Y., Stawicki, S., Liang, W.C., Chanthery, Y., Kowalski, J., Watts, R.J., Callahan, C., Kasman, I., *et al.* (2006). Inhibition of Dll4 signalling inhibits tumour growth by deregulating angiogenesis.[see comment]. Nature *444*, 1083-1087.

Rini, B.I., and Atkins, M.B. (2009). Resistance to targeted therapy in renal-cell carcinoma. Lancet Oncol *10*, 992-1000.

Risau, W. (1997). Mechanisms of angiogenesis. Nature *386*, 671-674.

Roelen, B.A., van Rooijen, M.A., and Mummery, C.L. (1997). Expression of ALK-1, a type 1 serine/threonine kinase receptor, coincides with sites of vasculogenesis and angiogenesis in early mouse development. Dev Dyn *209*, 418-430.

Rosen, L.S., Gordon, M.S., Hurwitz, H.I., Wong, M., Adams, B.J., Alvarez, D., Seon, B.K., Leigh, B.R., and Theuer, C.P. (2010). A first in human phase 1 study of Anti-CD105 (Anti-endoglin) antibody therapy with TRC105 in patients with advanced solid tumors. Paper presented at: 22nd EORTC-NCI-AACR Symposium on Molecular Targets and Cancer Therapeutics (Berlin, Germany).

Sanchez-Elsner, T., Botella, L.M., Velasco, B., Langa, C., and Bernabeu, C. (2002). Endoglin expression is regulated by transcriptional cooperation between the hypoxia and transforming growth factor-beta pathways. J Biol Chem *277*, 43799-43808.

Sanchez-Irizarry, C., Carpenter, A.C., Weng, A.P., Pear, W.S., Aster, J.C., and Blacklow, S.C. (2004). Notch subunit heterodimerization and prevention of ligand-independent proteolytic activation depend, respectively, on a novel domain and the LNR repeats. Molecular & Cellular Biology *24*, 9265-9273.

Sandler, A., Gray, R., Perry, M.C., Brahmer, J., Schiller, J.H., Dowlati, A., Lilenbaum, R., and Johnson, D.H. (2006). Paclitaxel-carboplatin alone or with bevacizumab for non-small-cell lung cancer. N Engl J Med *355*, 2542-2550.

Scharpfenecker, M., van Dinther, M., Liu, Z., van Bezooijen, R.L., Zhao, Q., Pukac, L., Lowik, C.W., and ten Dijke, P. (2007). BMP-9 signals via ALK1 and inhibits bFGF-induced endothelial cell proliferation and VEGF-stimulated angiogenesis. J Cell Sci *120*, 964-972.

Schroeter, E.H., Kisslinger, J.A., and Kopan, R. (1998). Notch-1 signalling requires ligand-induced proteolytic release of intracellular domain.[see comment]. Nature *393*, 382-386.

Seki, T., Hong, K.H., and Oh, S.P. (2006). Nonoverlapping expression patterns of ALK1 and ALK5 reveal distinct roles of each receptor in vascular development. Lab Invest *86*, 116-129.

Seki, T., Yun, J., and Oh, S.P. (2003). Arterial endothelium-specific activin receptor-like kinase 1 expression suggests its role in arterialization and vascular remodeling. Circ Res *93*, 682-689.

Shao, E.S., Lin, L., Yao, Y., and Bostrom, K.I. (2009). Expression of vascular endothelial growth factor is coordinately regulated by the activin-like kinase receptors 1 and 5 in endothelial cells. Blood *114*, 2197-2206.

She, X., Matsuno, F., Harada, N., Tsai, H., and Seon, B.K. (2004). Synergy between anti-endoglin (CD105) monoclonal antibodies and TGF-beta in suppression of growth of human endothelial cells. Int J Cancer *108*, 251-257.

Shiozaki, K., Harada, N., Greco, W.R., Haba, A., Uneda, S., Tsai, H., and Seon, B.K. (2006). Antiangiogenic chimeric anti-endoglin (CD105) antibody: pharmacokinetics and immunogenicity in nonhuman primates and effects of doxorubicin. Cancer Immunol Immunother *55*, 140-150.

Shutter, J.R., Scully, S., Fan, W., Richards, W.G., Kitajewski, J., Deblandre, G.A., Kintner, C.R., and Stark, K.L. (2000). Dll4, a novel Notch ligand expressed in arterial endothelium. Genes & Development *14*, 1313-1318.

Sorensen, I., Adams, R.H., and Gossler, A. (2009). DLL1-mediated Notch activation regulates endothelial identity in mouse fetal arteries. Blood *113*, 5680-5688.

Sorensen, L.K., Brooke, B.S., Li, D.Y., and Urness, L.D. (2003). Loss of distinct arterial and venous boundaries in mice lacking endoglin, a vascular-specific TGFbeta coreceptor. Dev Biol *261*, 235-250.

Srinivasan, S., Hanes, M.A., Dickens, T., Porteous, M.E., Oh, S.P., Hale, L.P., and Marchuk, D.A. (2003). A mouse model for hereditary hemorrhagic telangiectasia (HHT) type 2. Hum Mol Genet *12*, 473-482.

Struhl, G., and Greenwald, I. (1999). Presenilin is required for activity and nuclear access of Notch in Drosophila.[see comment]. Nature *398*, 522-525.

Suzuki, Y., Ohga, N., Morishita, Y., Hida, K., Miyazono, K., and Watabe, T. (2010). BMP-9 induces proliferation of multiple types of endothelial cells in vitro and in vivo. J Cell Sci *123*, 1684-1692.

Swiatek, P.J., Lindsell, C.E., del Amo, F.F., Weinmaster, G., and Gridley, T. (1994). Notch1 is essential for postimplantation development in mice. Genes & Development *8*, 707-719.

ten Dijke, P., and Arthur, H.M. (2007). Extracellular control of TGFbeta signalling in vascular development and disease. Nat Rev Mol Cell Biol *8*, 857-869.

Torsney, E., Charlton, R., Diamond, A.G., Burn, J., Soames, J.V., and Arthur, H.M. (2003). Mouse model for hereditary hemorrhagic telangiectasia has a generalized vascular abnormality. Circulation *107*, 1653-1657.

Torsney, E., Charlton, R., Parums, D., Collis, M., and Arthur, H.M. (2002). Inducible expression of human endoglin during inflammation and wound healing in vivo. Inflamm Res *51*, 464-470.

Tsujie, M., Tsujie, T., Toi, H., Uneda, S., Shiozaki, K., Tsai, H., and Seon, B.K. (2008). Anti-tumor activity of an anti-endoglin monoclonal antibody is enhanced in immunocompetent mice. Int J Cancer *122*, 2266-2273.

Tsujie, M., Uneda, S., Tsai, H., and Seon, B.K. (2006). Effective anti-angiogenic therapy of established tumors in mice by naked anti-human endoglin (CD105) antibody: differences in growth rate and therapeutic response between tumors growing at different sites. Int J Oncol *29*, 1087-1094.

Uneda, S., Toi, H., Tsujie, T., Tsujie, M., Harada, N., Tsai, H., and Seon, B.K. (2009). Anti-endoglin monoclonal antibodies are effective for suppressing metastasis and the primary tumors by targeting tumor vasculature. Int J Cancer *125*, 1446-1453.

Urness, L.D., Sorensen, L.K., and Li, D.Y. (2000). Arteriovenous malformations in mice lacking activin receptor-like kinase-1. Nat Genet *26*, 328-331.

Venkatesha, S., Toporsian, M., Lam, C., Hanai, J., Mammoto, T., Kim, Y.M., Bdolah, Y., Lim, K.H., Yuan, H.T., Libermann, T.A., *et al.* (2006). Soluble endoglin contributes to the pathogenesis of preeclampsia. Nat Med *12*, 642-649.

Vooijs, M., Ong, C.T., Hadland, B., Huppert, S., Liu, Z., Korving, J., van den Born, M., Stappenbeck, T., Wu, Y., Clevers, H., *et al.* (2007). Mapping the consequence of Notch1 proteolysis in vivo with NIP-CRE. Development *134*, 535-544.

Wallberg, A.E., Pedersen, K., Lendahl, U., and Roeder, R.G. (2002). p300 and PCAF act cooperatively to mediate transcriptional activation from chromatin templates by notch intracellular domains in vitro. Molecular & Cellular Biology *22*, 7812-7819.

Wang, J.M., Kumar, S., Pye, D., van Agthoven, A.J., Krupinski, J., and Hunter, R.D. (1993). A monoclonal antibody detects heterogeneity in vascular endothelium of tumours and normal tissues. Int J Cancer *54*, 363-370.

Wrighton, K.H., Lin, X., Yu, P.B., and Feng, X.H. (2009). Transforming Growth Factor {beta} Can Stimulate Smad1 Phosphorylation Independently of Bone Morphogenic Protein Receptors. J Biol Chem *284*, 9755-9763.

Wu, Y., Cain-Hom, C., Choy, L., Hagenbeek, T.J., de Leon, G.P., Chen, Y., Finkle, D., Venook, R., Wu, X., Ridgway, J., *et al.* (2010). Therapeutic antibody targeting of individual Notch receptors. Nature *464*, 1052-1057.

Xu, J., Krebs, L.T., and Gridley, T. (2010). Generation of mice with a conditional null allele of the Jagged2 gene. Genesis *48*, 390-393.

Xue, Y., Gao, X., Lindsell, C.E., Norton, C.R., Chang, B., Hicks, C., Gendron-Maguire, M., Rand, E.B., Weinmaster, G., and Gridley, T. (1999). Embryonic lethality and vascular defects in mice lacking the Notch ligand Jagged1. Human Molecular Genetics *8*, 723-730.

Yamashita, H., Ichijo, H., Grimsby, S., Moren, A., ten Dijke, P., and Miyazono, K. (1994). Endoglin forms a heteromeric complex with the signaling receptors for transforming growth factor-beta. J Biol Chem *269*, 1995-2001.

Yan, M., Callahan, C.A., Beyer, J.C., Allamneni, K.P., Zhang, G., Ridgway, J.B., Niessen, K., and Plowman, G.D. (2010). Chronic DLL4 blockade induces vascular neoplasms. Nature *463*, E6-7.

Yang, L.T., Nichols, J.T., Yao, C., Manilay, J.O., Robey, E.A., and Weinmaster, G. (2005). Fringe glycosyltransferases differentially modulate Notch1 proteolysis induced by Delta1 and Jagged1. Mol Biol Cell *16*, 927-942.

Zeng, Q., Li, S., Chepeha, D.B., Giordano, T.J., Li, J., Zhang, H., Polverini, P.J., Nor, J., Kitajewski, J., and Wang, C.Y. (2005). Crosstalk between tumor and endothelial cells promotes tumor angiogenesis by MAPK activation of Notch signaling. Cancer Cell *8*, 13-23.

Zhou, S., Fujimuro, M., Hsieh, J.J., Chen, L., Miyamoto, A., Weinmaster, G., and Hayward, S.D. (2000). SKIP, a CBF1-associated protein, interacts with the ankyrin repeat domain of NotchIC To facilitate NotchIC function. Molecular & Cellular Biology *20*, 2400-2410.

5

Platelet Regulation of Angiogenesis, Tumor Growth and Metastasis

Jessica Cedervall and Anna-Karin Olsson
Uppsala University,
Sweden

1. Introduction

Angiogenesis - formation of new capillary blood vessels - is essential during development and physiological conditions, such as wound healing and the reproductive cycle. Prolonged and excessive angiogenesis has been implicated in a number of pathological processes, for instance rheumatoid arthritis, retinopathy and tumor growth. The normal vasculature is tightly regulated by a balance between pro- and anti-angiogenic factors. The most well studied pro-angiogenic factor - vascular endothelial growth factor-A(VEGF-A) – is required for development of a vascular system during embryogenesis and is also a central regulator of adult neovascularization (Olsson et al., 2006).

Angiogenesis is a multistep process involving oxygen sensing, growth factor signaling, matrix degradation, endothelial cell proliferation, migration and differentiation into a functional blood vessel. This process - formation of new blood vessels from pre-existing ones - must take place without compromising blood flow.

Platelets are central players in maintaining hemostasis of the blood. At sites of blood vessel injury, platelets are activated to induce blood coagulation and form aggregates at the site of the damaged endothelium to prevent hemorrhage and thereby protects us from fatal bleedings. Besides their role in hemostasis, platelets have been shown to contribute to non-hemostatic processes such as wound healing, immunity, angiogenesis, cardiovascular disease and tumor metastasis (Felding-Habermann et al., 1996; Jurk and Kehrel, 2005).

A connection between platelets and malignant disease has been recognized since the end of the 19th century, when Armand Trousseau observed increased thrombotic events in patients that were later diagnosed with cancer (Trousseau, 1865). This enhanced tendency to form blood clots, or hypercoagulability, is named Trousseau's syndrome (Varki, 2007) and is especially pronounced in certain forms of cancer such as pancreatic and lung cancer.

Growth of solid tumors, like all expanding tissues, is dependent on angiogenesis for oxygen and nutrient supply, as well as for removal of waste products. The hypotheses that platelets contribute to tumor-induced angiogenesis was put forward by Pinedo and collegues in 1998 (Pinedo et al., 1998). During the last decade, this hypotheses has been experimentally supported by several independent research groups, demonstrating that platelets can regulate endothelial cell behavior and angiogenesis. Platelets are now recognized as the major source of VEGF-A in the body (Holmes et al., 2008; Peterson et al., 2010; Verheul et al., 1997). In addition to stimulation of tumor growth and angiogenesis, platelets have also been found to regulate metastasis. Possible explanations involve protection of the tumor cells from immune recognition and shear stress in the circulation. Platelets may also enable easier tumor cell adherence and subsequent extravasation through the vessel wall.

The current chapter will review the role of platelets in regulation of angiogenesis, tumor growth and metastasis. We do not claim a full coverage of the existing literature, but wish to highlight certain aspects of these processes.

2. Platelet regulation of hemostasis and thrombosis

Platelets are anuclear cellular fragments, derived from megakaryocytes in the bone marrow (Lecine et al., 1998). These cell fragments play a crucial role in regulating blood hemostasis and thrombosis. At sites of blood vessel injury, platelets are activated and aggregate at the site of the damaged endothelium to prevent hemorrhage. Although platelets lack nuclei, they are highly organized and contain different organelles such as granula, mitochondria and the cytoskeletal components microtubules and actin filaments. Platelets contain three different types of granules; dense granules, lysosomes, α-granules (Rendu and Brohard-Bohn, 2001). Dense granules are involved in recruitment of other platelets by release of small, non-protein molecules, lysosomes play a role in eliminating circulating platelet aggregates by secretion of hydrolases and α-granules contain proteins involved in the healing reaction (Rendu and Brohard-Bohn, 2001).

Upon blood vessel injury, exposure of sub-endothelial molecules such as von Willebrand factor (vWF) and collagen trigger adhesion, activation, aggregation and degranulation of platelets (Jackson, 2007; Varga-Szabo et al., 2008). Released adenosine diphosphate (ADP) reinforce the activation by binding to P2Y receptors on the platelet, which in turn induce activation of the fibrinogen receptor GPIIb/IIIa. Fibrinogen can bridge between platelets, forming a temporary plug. This is converted to a more stable fibrin clot by cleavage of fibrinogen by the serine protease thrombin, which is activated in the coagulation cascade (Jackson, 2007; Varga-Szabo et al., 2008). The fibrin clot will be enzymatically degraded by plasminogen when the damaged vessel is repaired (Cesarman-Maus and Hajjar, 2005).

In addition to prevent bleeding, platelets can also promote wound healing. Gastric ulcer healing, a process known to be dependent on VEGF-A and angiogenesis, can be regulated by platelets (Ma et al., 2001; Ma et al., 2005). Similarly, healing of diabetic wounds can be enhanced by platelet rich plasma (Pietramaggiori et al., 2008).

3. The role of platelets in tumor angiogenesis and growth

It is well recognized that cancer patients commonly suffer from problems with thrombotic occlusion of vessels as well as other abnormalities of their coagulation system such as high platelet turnover, elevated platelet counts and bleeding disorders (Dvorak, 1994; Sun et al., 1979). The prothrombotic environment of tumors can induce platelets to form microthrombi and to release endothelial stimulating factors from their granules, such as VEGF-A (Mohle et al., 1997; Pinedo et al., 1998). As will be described below, several lines of evidence suggest that platelets promote tumor growth by stimulating its vasculature by different mechanisms.

As mentioned in section 2. above, platelets play a role during wound healing. Indeed, tumors have been described as "wounds that do not heal", due to the chronic inflammation of the cancer tissue (Dvorak, 1986). In a normal wound, platelets provide important growth factors for recruitment of myofibroblasts and stimulation of tissue regeneration. In this physiological situation platelet activation is terminated when the wound is healed. In cancer however, platelets are continuously activated via for instance tumor cell expression of tissue factor (TF), which activates thrombin, a potent platelet activator. This can be parallelled to the capacity of tumor cells to attract various cell types to their stroma, such as fibroblasts and macrophages, and to stimulate these to secrete factors that maintain survival and proliferation of the tumor cells. Similarly, malignant cells may take advantage of the physiological function of platelets during wound healing to support the continued expansion of the tumor mass.

Platelets contain a variety of both pro- and anti-angiogenic molecules, which can be released upon activation. Examples of positive regulators of angiogenesis found in platelets are vascular endothelial growth factor (Mohle et al., 1997), platelet-derived growth factor (Heldin et al., 1981) and basic fibroblast growth factor (Brunner et al., 1993), while negative regulators include thrombospondin, platelet factor-4 (PF-4), endostatin and plasminogen activator inhibitor type-1 (PAI-1) (Browder et al., 2000; Staton and Lewis, 2005). Despite their content of both positive and negative regulators of blood vessel formation, platelets have in several different experimental settings been shown to stimulate angiogenesis. Early studies identified platelets as a source of endothelial stimulating factors (Busch et al., 1977). Rafii and collegues showed that megakaryocytes contain high levels of VEGF-A and that bone marrow microvascular endothelial cells can be maintained in serum-free medium if cocultured with megakaryocytes (Mohle et al., 1997). This effect was attributed to the release of VEGF-A from the megakaryocytes. In another *in vitro* study, purified human platelets were shown to promote tube formation of human umbilical vein endothelial cells (HUVECs) in Matrigel (Pipili-Synetos et al., 1998). The platelet stimulating effect on endothelial cell differentiation was not dependent on activation and granule release from the platelets, since unstimulated platelets were equally potent in this respect. Instead, direct adhesion of platelets to the endothelial cells was suggested as the event promoting tube formation in this assay (Pipili-Synetos et al., 1998). Along the same lines, Verheul et al showed that activation of cultured endothelial cells with VEGF-A promoted adhesion of unstimulated platelets (Verheul et al., 2000). This adhesion was dependent on VEGF-A-induced expression of TF by the endothelial cells, which in turn generated thrombin and subsequent activation and adhesion of the previously non-activated platelets. These three *in vitro* studies together nicely illustrate the reciprocal relationship between activated platelets and endothelial cells.

The concept of platelet-regulated angiogenesis is further supported by a number of *in vivo* studies. In a mouse model of hypoxia-induced retinal angiogenesis, inhibition of platelet aggregation as well as thrombocytopenia was demonstrated to reduce vascularization (Rhee et al., 2004). Using two other *in vivo* models of angiogenesis; the cornea micropocket assay and the Matrigel plug assay, Kisucka et al showed that platelets contribute significantly to angiogenesis (Kisucka et al., 2006). In addition, platelet-derived CD40L has been suggested to play a central role in stimulating tumor angiogenes via CD40-expressing endothelial cells in a transgenic mouse model for breast cancer (Chiodoni et al., 2006).

What is the reason for this primarily stimulating effect on vascularization by platelets, considering that they contain both anti-angiogenic as well as pro-angiogenic factors in their granules? This apparent contradiction may be explained by recent data showing that pro- and anti-angiogenic factors are stored in separate α-granules in the same platelet and that these granules can release their content in a regulated manner by selective stimulation of the thrombin protease activated receptors PAR-1 and PAR-4 (Italiano et al., 2008; Ma et al., 2005). These data demonstrate a more fine-tuned regulation of platelet degranulation than was previously known. Similarly, ADP stimulation of platelets resulted in release of VEGF-A, but not of endostatin (Bambace et al., 2010; Battinelli et al., 2011), while thromboxane A2 released endostatin but not VEGF-A (Battinelli et al., 2011). Furthermore, Batinelli et al could show that the breast cancer cell line MCF-7 stimulated platelets to release pro-angiogenic factors (Battinelli et al., 2011). However, it remains to be addressed under which *in vivo* conditions a selective stimulation of different platelet receptors such as PAR-1 and PAR-4 could occur. The concept of functionally co-clustering of proteins in distinct granules was also recently challenged. Using different quantitative immunofluorescence microscopy techniques, Kamykowski et al reported that they did not obtain data in support of this model (Kamykowski et al., 2011).

Another less complex explanation for the stimulating effect on endothelial cells could be that the platelet-derived pro-angiogenic factors simply predominate among the released factors, resulting in a net effect of platelet activation on angiogenesis. In support of this hypotheses are data from Brill et al showing that platelet relesate is able to support angiogenesis *in vitro* and *in vivo*, despite the presence of anti-angiogenic factors such as platelet factor-4. If however the action of PF-4 was blocked by an antibody, the angiogenic response to the platelet relesate was potentiated (Brill et al., 2004). Thrombospondins (TSPs), well-studied inhibitors of angiogenesis, are the most abundant proteins in the platelet α-granules (Baenziger et al., 1972). Although TSPs are expressed in several cell types, Rafii and co-workers have elegantly shown that TSP-1 and TSP-2 derived from megakaryocytes and platelets function as a major anti-angiogenic switch (Kopp et al., 2006). The proposed mechanism involves binding and sequestration of stromal cell-derived factor 1 (SDF-1), a potent pro-angiogenic factor. Platelets from TSP-1 and TSP-2 double knock-out mice were also more efficient stimulators of angiogenes in Matrigel plugs compared to platelets from wild-type mice (Kopp et al., 2006), supporting the concept that pro- and anti-angiogenic factors released from platelets balance each other.

Factors that regulate angiogenesis can also be generated during platelet activation. One example is the angiogenesis inhibitor angiostatin, which is generated from proteolytic cleavage of plasminogen. Platelets release functional angiostatin, but the inhibitor is also generated during platelet activation and aggregation. Platelets contain plasminogen and enzymes like matrix metalloproteinases (MMPs) and urokinase plasminogen activator (uPA), that are capable of generating angiostatin by cleavage of plasminogen (Jurasz et al., 2003). In addition to release and generation, a third mechanism to locally increase the concentration of an angiogenesis inhibitor during platelet activation has been described. This mechanism involves creation of a microenvironment that favors retention of the anti-angiogenic molecule at sites of platelet degranulation (Thulin et al., 2009). This finding may reflect a host response to counteract angiogenesis during pathological conditions where platelets are activated.

In addition to various growth factors, platelets can release proteases such as MMPs (Jain et al., 2010) as well as phospholipids (English et al., 2001) that have the capacity to promote neovascularization by different mechanisms. Moreover, recent data point to a novel role for platelets in hypoxia-induced angiogenesis. Using three different tumor models and the hindlimb ischemia assay, platelet secretion from α-granules were shown to recruit bone marrow-derived cells into the growing neovasculature (Feng et al., 2011). These findings suggest a role for platelets as a way for communication between hypoxic tissue and the bone marrow during angiogenesis.

Platelets can stimulate endothelial cells by other mechanisms than release of pro-angiogenic factors from their granules. Fibrin, a product of coagulation and platelet activation, is commonly found deposited in tumors (Dvorak, 1994). This provisional matrix can support endothelial cell adhesion, survival and migration and hence promote angiogenesis (Dvorak et al., 1995; Qi et al., 1997). Also, platelets are also able to stimulate angiogenesis via shedding of microparticles (reviewed below in a separate section).

At which stage of angiogenesis do platelets have an influence? Studies by Kisucka et al using the cornea micropocket assay in thrombocytopenic mice indicate that it is primarily the early stages in neovascularization that are affected by platelets (Kisucka et al., 2006). Moreover, mice lacking the endogenous angiogenesis inhibitor histidine-rich glycoprotein (HRG) have a coagulation defect and enhanced activation of platelets (Tsuchida-Straeten et al., 2005; Ringvall et al., 2011). HRG-deficient Rip1-Tag2 mice, a transgenic model of insulinoma, have a significantly increased number of angiogenic islets of Langerhans in their pancreas (Thulin et al., 2009). This elevated angiogenic switch can be suppressed by induction of thrombocytopenia, i.e. reduced platelet count, two weeks before onset of the switch. However, thrombocytopenia had no effect on angiogenesis at a later stage when the angiogenic islets had developed into invasive carcinomas (Ringvall et al., 2011). In addition, negative regulation of angiogenesis by platelet-derived TSP was demonstrated to play a role during early stages of tumor vascularization (Zaslavsky et al., 2010). Together these data support a role for platelets early in the angiogenic process. Later, when the tumor cell mass has expanded and a new microenvironment been created, with for example recruited inflammatory cells, the contribution of platelets may be of less significance.

Platelet-derived factors have not only been shown to regulate angiogenesis, but also to play a critical role in preventing hemorrhage from angiogenic (Kisucka et al., 2006) and inflamed microvessels (Goerge et al., 2008). Interestingly, this ability to support the integrity of blood vessels is not dependent on the capacity of platelets to form thrombi. Instead it seems to rely on the secretion of their granule content (Ho-Tin-Noe et al., 2008).

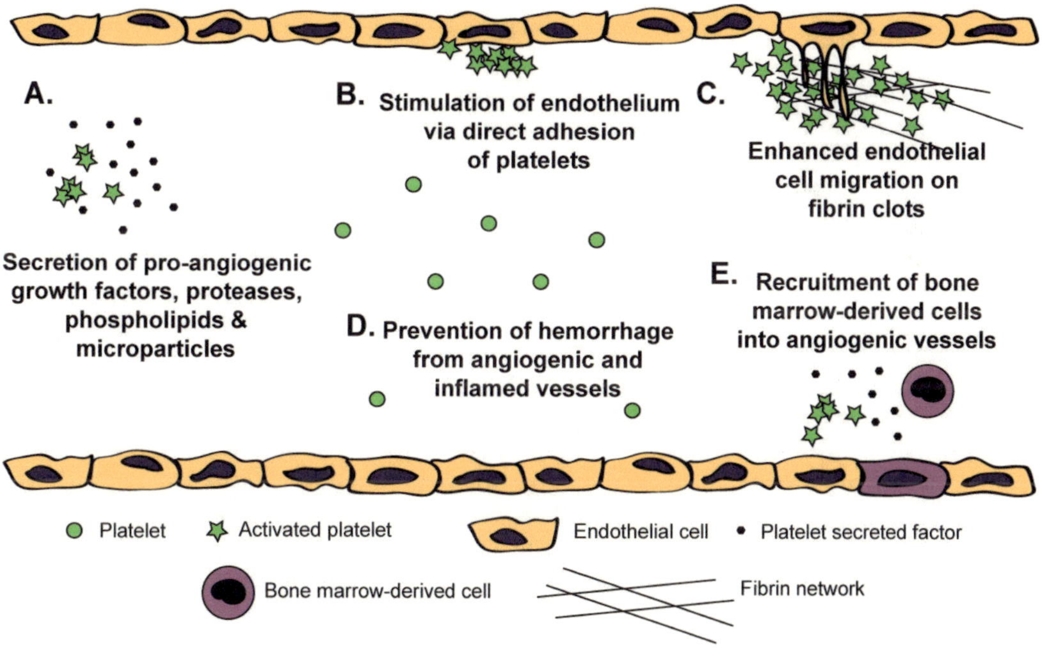

Fig. 1. Schematic illustration showing how platelets can stimulate angiogenesis.

Another interesting feature of platelets is their reported ability to selectively take up and sequester angiogenic regulators (Klement et al., 2009). Even a very small amount of VEGF-A secreted by microscopic subcutaneous tumors was reported to result in elevated levels of platelet VEGF-A. The "angiogenic profile" of platelets was therefore suggested as a possible early marker of malignant disease. It was recently shown that the TSP-1 protein present in platelets is derived from megakaryocytes (Zaslavsky et al., 2010), highlighting that not only platelet uptake but also endocytosis or increased production in the bone marrow precursor cells may account for the protein content of platelets.
Besides being a potent activator of platelets, thrombin can also have direct effects on tumor cells. Thrombin-treated tumor cells show an enhanced adhesion to endothelial cells and secrete endothelial growth factors such as VEGF-A and growth regulated oncogene alpha (GRO-α). In addition, thrombin can stimulate chemokinesis and possibly proliferation via the receptor PAR-1 on tumor cells (Nierodzik and Karpatkin, 2006). TF expression by tumor cells - which may be a thousand-fold higher than the amount expressed by their normal counterpart - generates thrombin, as described in a previous section. However, TF may also support tumor progression by formation of a cancer stem cell niche. In tumors a small subset of CD133-positive cells can be found, which are known as cancer stem cells or tumor-initiating cells. These cells have the ability to generate new tumors, either by relapse or metastasis. Interestingly, CD133-positive tumor cells have been found to express sinificantly higher levels of TF than the corresponding CD133-negative cells (Milsom and Rak, 2008).
In addition to the platelet-endothelial cell interactions that have been the focus of this section, platelet-tumor cell interactions significantly affect the capacity of tumor cells to form distant metastases, as discussed below.

4. The role of platelets in tumor metastasis

In addition to regulating tumor angiogenesis and growth, there is also experimental evidence that platelets are involved in the metastatic process. This has been shown by several independent research groups using various approaches. Experimental studies revealed that tumor cells with the ability to activate platelets *in vitro*, form more metastases upon xenografting in mice, than tumor cells lacking that capacity (Gasic et al., 1973; Pearlstein et al., 1980). Furthermore, it has been shown that thrombocytopenia is closely associated with reduced metastasis in various mouse models (Gasic et al., 1968). In yet another study, addition of platelets to thrombocytopenic mice restored the capacity for metastases formation to levels corresponding to non-thrombocytopenic control mice (Karpatkin et al., 1988). However, by interfering with platelet adhesion via inhibition of vWF or GpIIb/IIIa, the rescuing effect was lost. Intervening with the production of platelets by disturbing the maturation of megakaryocytes resulted in an almost complete inhibition of metastasis in an experimental mouse model (Camerer et al., 2004). Another study has revealed that intravenous injection of tumor cells in mice may lead to thrombocytopenia, giving further proof for the important tumor-platelet interplay (Karpatkin et al., 1981). Today, it is known that platelets can affect the metastatic process in several ways; by physical coverage of the tumor cells in the blood stream, by aiding in tethering and adhesion to the vessel wall, and by activation-induced secretion of various factors involved in invasion and migration.
Survival of tumor cells in the blood stream is essential for metastasis. Experimental mouse models of metastasis show that the metastatic process is highly inefficient, and that the

majority of tumor cells do not survive in the hostile microenvironment after intravasation. Natural Killer (NK) cells, cytotoxic lymphocytes capable of inducing tumor cell lysis, exert the major threat to tumor cells in the blood stream (Gorelik et al., 1982; Hanna, 1985). Elimination of NK-cells has repeatedly been shown to increase metastases formation in experimental mouse models. Platelets are suggested to serve as a physical guard for the tumor cells in the blood circulation, allowing protection against immune elimination. A study published by Nieswandt et al. showed that xenografts derived from several NK-sensitive tumor cell lines exhibited decreased metastatic potential after platelet depletion (Nieswandt et al., 1999) . The same study did also show that aggregation of platelets on the tumor surface protected the tumor cells from NK-cell induced cytotoxicity *in vitro*. This observation was confirmed a few years later by another research group, showing that mice with platelets unable to undergo activation, have decreased numbers of experimental as well as spontaneous metastases (Palumbo et al., 2005). Further investigation revealed that the effect was due to lower NK-cell cytotoxicity. However, there are studies indicating that platelets may inhibit NK-cell cytotoxic activity independent of direct contact, e.g. via soluble factors. For example, a study performed by Skov Madsen et al. suggested that supernatant from activated platelets are able to reduce NK-cell dependent lysis of human leukemia cells *in vitro* (Skov Madsen et al., 1986). More recently, a possible mechanism for this effect was presented, suggesting that platelet-derived TGFβ may down-regulate the cytokine NKG2D (Natural Killer Group 2, member D) on the NK-cell surface, resulting in decreased NK-cell cytotoxicity (Kopp et al., 2009).

Intervening directly with the platelet-tumor cell interaction affects metastasis in a similar way. Several lines of evidence confirm that intervening with receptors or ligands of importance for this interplay have significant impact on the tumors capacity to disseminate. Activated platelets bind to tumors via fibrinogen, using the fibrinogen receptor GpIIb/IIIa. Studies performed in mouse models reveal that inhibition of the fibrinogen receptor on platelets result in reduced numbers of metastases in the lungs (Amirkhosravi et al., 2003). Results from fibrinogen-deficient mice reveal diminished experimental metastasis, spontaneous hematogenous metastasis and lymphatic metastasis (Camerer et al., 2004; Palumbo et al., 2000; Palumbo et al., 2002). Interacting with the function of thrombin also affects the binding of platelets to the tumor cells. It has been shown *in vitro* that treating platelets with thrombin can enhance their binding to tumor cells by several times (Nierodzik et al., 1991). In line with this, thrombin-activated tumor cells have been shown to generate up to 150 times higher incidence of experimental metastasis, as detected using cell lines derived from murine melanoma and colon carcinoma (Nierodzik et al., 1996). P-selectin is expressed on the surface of activated platelets and is involved in platelet aggregation as well as platelet-tumor cell complex-formation. It has been shown that P-selectin deficient mice have decreased metastasis, a result obtained using both human and mouse carcinoma cells in immunodeficient and immunocompetent mice, respectively (Borsig et al., 2002; Kim et al., 1998). P-selectin dependent binding between platelets and tumor cells can be inhibited by heparin and results from syngenic mouse models reveal that heparin-dependent inhibition of P-selectin results in impaired experimental metastasis (Borsig et al., 2001).

Tissue factor expressed by platelets or tumor cells can induce formation of platelet-tumor cell aggregates. Furthermore, it is capable of enhancing fibrin-binding of tumor cells, facilitating tumor cell adhesion to the endothelium. This indicates that TF, due to its pro-coagulant function, might be of importance for tumor progression. Several studies do indeed show that TF is involved in the metastatic process. For example, inhibition of TF resulted in decreased metastasis in a mouse model for pulmonary metastasis (Amirkhosravi et al., 2002; Mueller et al., 1992; Mueller and Ruf, 1998). Results from clinical studies are also in line with the results obtained using animal models. Increased levels of TF correlates to an increased risk for metastasis and decreased overall survival in patients with colorectal cancer (Seto et al., 2000). However, it has been suggested that TF affects the metastatic potential of tumor cells, independent of its role as an initiator of the coagulation cascade. One study showed that its cytoplasmic domain, a part that is not involved in the coagulation process, could exert the pro-metastatic function of TF. Modulation of the pro-coagulant part of TF in melanoma cells did not show any effect on the metastatic potential, further suggesting that TF might affect metastasis also via coagulation-independent mechanisms (Bromberg et al., 1995; Paborsky et al., 1991).

Another group of molecules that have the capacity to affect hematogenous metastasis are the PARs. In mice, *in vivo* grafting of B16 mouse melanoma cells overexpressing PAR-1 was shown to result in significantly increased numbers of experimental metastases compared to cells with normal levels of PAR-1 (Nierodzik et al., 1998). Similarly, PAR-2 expression has been shown to affect spontaneous metastasis in a mouse model for mammary adenocarcinoma (Versteeg et al., 2008). In the clinic, a direct correlation between PAR-1 expression and breast cancer invasiveness has been detected (Even-Ram et al., 1998). PAR-4 knock-out mice, lacking the capacity for platelet aggregation in response to thrombin, have reduced metastasis compared to wild type PAR-4 positive mice (Camerer et al., 2004). GPVI, an adhesion-receptor on platelets responsible for the binding of collagen, has been shown to be of importance for metastatic spread in a study using GPVI knock out-mice (Jain et al., 2009). Intravenous injection of metastatic tumor cells of both melanoma and lung cancer origin in GPVI-deficient mice resulted in a 50% reduction of observable tumor formation, as compared to injection of the same cell lines in wild-type mice with normal GPVI function.

Platelets can also affect the metastatic capacity of tumor cells by secretion of pro-metastatic as well as metastasis-preventing factors. These factors are released upon activation, for example during tumor cell induced platelet aggregation, facilitating or inhibiting further tumor progression. For example, matrix-degrading proteases, such as matrix metalloproteinase -1, -2 and -9, are stored in α-granules and released upon platelet activation, facilitating invasion and migration (Fernandez-Patron et al., 1999; Sawicki et al., 1997). Another factor stored in platelet α-granules is the protein vWF, which participates in platelet aggregation after binding to the GP1b-V-IX complex, suggesting it to have metastasis-preventing effects. This has also been confirmed in a study where melanoma and lung tumor cells were grafted in mice lacking vWF (Terraube et al., 2006). Indeed, these mice had significantly higher numbers of pulmonary metastases than vWF-expressing mice. This phenotype could be corrected by restoring the vWF levels in the knock-out mice. The difference in metastatic burden was suggested to depend on increased survival of the metastatic tumor cells in the lungs during the first 24 hours. Fibronectin, another extracellular matrix-protein involved in platelet aggregation and stored in platelet α-granules, seem to have pro-metastatic effects, reverting the metastasis-preventing effects of clot formation (Malik et al., 2010). Fibronectin binds to αvβ3 integrin and forms complex with fibrin during clot formation. Mice lacking fibronectin have reduced numbers of experimental melanoma metastases spreading to the lungs.

Platelets are able to facilitate the metastatic process by affecting the vascular permeability. For example, secretion of growth factors such as PDGF, TGFβ, EGF or VEGF-A, influences the integrity of the endothelium. Release of serotonin and histamin, stored in the dense-granules in platelets, might also affect the metastatic process by enhancing the vascular permeability and thereby facilitate transport over the vascular endothelium. It has been shown that introduction of tumor cells into the circulation of mice results in significant increase of serotonin in the blood, and inhibition of serotonin receptors or calcium channels results in diminished metastasis to the liver (Skolnik et al., 1989; Skolnik et al., 1984). The vascular permeability may also be regulated by the signalling molecules sphingosine-1 phosphate (S1P) and lysophosphatidic acid (LPA), which are stored in platelet α-granules. Both S1P and LPA are capable of regulating the vascular integrity, S1P as an inhibitor of vascular leakage and LPA as a stabilizer for certain endothelial cell types (Sarker et al.; 2010 Schaphorst et al., 2003; Yin and Watsky, 2005).

Finally, platelets are suggested to support rolling and tethering of tumor cells on the vessel wall. This is a prerequisite for subsequent firm adhesion to the vessel wall, which is necessary for extravasation from the circulatory system into tissues for establishment of metastatic foci. Activated platelets secrete several factors that can activate endothelial cells in the vasculature and enable binding of platelets and tumor cells. Several studies indicate that platelets can support a transient tumor cell interaction with the vascular endothelium and that this is partly mediated via selectins (Laubli and Borsig, 2010). Selectins are expressed by endothelial cells and leukocytes and enables migration of leukocytes during inflammation by promoting their adhesion to the vessels wall. In a similar manner, selectins on the platelet-surface seem to be able to support transient tumor cell adhesion to the vessel wall (Laubli and Borsig, 2010). The adhesion formed between platelets and tumor cells has been suggested to depend on CD44 expressed on the tumor cell surface, interacting with fibrin (Alves et al., 2008). Selectin-dependent interactions between tumor cells, platelets and leukocytes might also have indirect metastasis-promoting effects, by inducing CCL5-release from endothelial cells (Laubli et al., 2009). This results in recruitment of monocytes leading to further increase in metastatic capacity. The low affinity binding supplied by selectins has to be replaced by high affinity adhesion, to enable extravasation. The platelet integrin that mainly contributes to firm arrest of tumor cells within the vasculature is integrin αIIbβ3 (Shattil et al., 2010). In addition, interaction between endothelial vWF and the Gp1bα receptor on platelets is important for platelet tethering to the endothelium during thrombus formation. Several studies confirm the involvement of both vWF and Gp1bα in the metastatic process, suggesting that this mechanism might be of importance also during cancer progression (Jain et al., 2007; Kitagawa et al., 1989). Prevailing adhesion, invasion and migration needed for extravasation, are further supported by tumor cell expression of integrin αvβ3, in interaction with platelets (Desgrosellier and Cheresh, 2010; Felding-Habermann et al., 1996).

5. Platelet-derived microparticles

Platelets also affect tumor progression indirectly by shedding of microparticles, containing fragments of the platelet plasma membrane and α-granules. Microparticles are small vesicles, sized between 0,1-1 μm and derived from a variety of healthy as well as malignant cells upon activation or apoptosis. They are present in the blood of healthy individuals, and are suggested to be involved in thrombosis, inflammation and angiogenesis (Burnier et al., 2009; Morel et al., 2006; Nieuwland and Sturk, 2010). Microparticles facilitates communication between neighbouring cells via several different mechanisms; by affecting direct cell-cell contacts, by their function as transport vesicles carrying and transferring

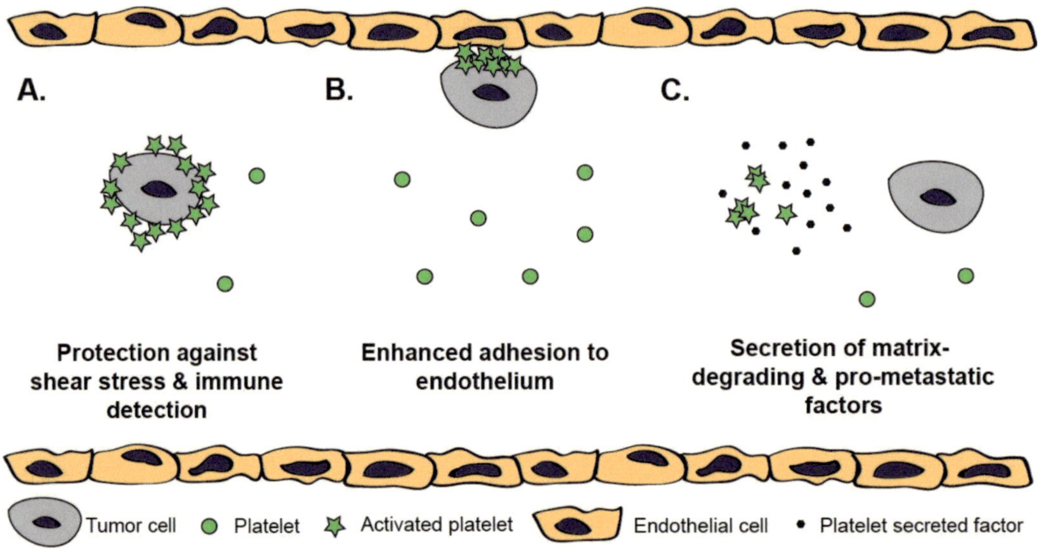

Fig. 2. Schematic illustration showing how platelets can affect tumor metastasis.

proteins and mRNA between cells and by direct regulation of cell signalling (Baj-Krzyworzeka et al., 2006; Essayagh et al., 2007; Mack et al., 2000; Simak and Gelderman, 2006). The levels of microparticles in the blood are increased in several diseased states, including cardiovascular disease, inflammation but also cancer (Piccin et al., 2007). Increased numbers of microparticles in the circulation of cancer patients also correlates with the risk for thrombosis (Khorana et al., 2008; Zwicker, 2010).

The majority of the microparticles in the blood stream are derived from megakaryocytes or platelets (Diamant et al., 2004). Platelet-derived microparticles have a negatively charged surface allowing binding of factors involved in clotting, and contain a specific set of proteins reflecting their platelet origin (Zwicker, 2008). The size and the major components of the platelet-derived microvesicles differ; large microparticles derived from the platelet plasma membrane contain platelet surface protein such as integrin αIIbβIII, Gp1b, TF, PECAM and P-selectin, while others are of subcellular-origin containing α-granules or platelet organelles (Denzer et al., 2000; Gracia Ballarin, 2005; Jin et al., 2005; Perez-Pujol et al., 2007). Pro-coagulant microparticles containing TF may not only be derived from platelets, but also from tumor cells. TF-bearing microparticles have a central role in regulating the coagulation cascade and they tend to accumulate during clot formation induced by cellular injury, resulting in increased risk for thrombosis (Diamant et al., 2004).

As described, platelet-derived microparticles affect blood coagulation, but they are also involved in processes of importance for tumor progression, such as angiogenesis (Kim et al., 2004). Platelet-derived microparticles carry adhesion-molecules as well as growth factors and proteases, which are needed for angiogenesis. *In vitro* studies indicate that microparticles from platelets stimulate mRNA-expression of pro-angiogenic factors, such as MMP-9, VEGF-A and HGF, in tumor cells (Janowska-Wieczorek et al., 2005). It has also been shown, both *in vitro* and *in vivo*, that platelet-derived microparticles are capable of inducing angiogenic sprouting to a similar extent as whole platelets (Brill et al., 2005). Furthermore, another study shows that platelet-derived microparticles can stimulate angiogenic tube formation from endothelial progenitor cells (Prokopi et al., 2009).

Several studies have shown associations between platelet-derived microparticles and tumor progression. Higher levels of platelet-derived microparticles in blood from prostate cancer patients have been correlated to aggressive disease and poor clinical outcome (Helley et al., 2009). Similarly, platelet-derived microparticle levels were suggested to be good predictors for tumor metastasis in patients with gastric cancer (Kim et al., 2003). The mechanisms behind these effects are not fully understood and still under investigation. However, it has been suggested that platelet-derived microparticles might induce tumor secretion of various matrix-metalloproteinases, facilitating the metastatic process (Dashevsky et al., 2009) (Janowska-Wieczorek et al., 2005). A study on the role of platelet-derived microparticles for metastatic capacity in lung cancer revealed that there might as well be direct effects on both tumor cell proliferation and adhesion to fibrinogen and endothelial cells (Janowska-Wieczorek et al., 2005).

As mentioned above, microparticles derived from other types of cells than platelets also have pro-coagulant functions. This means that microparticles can affect tumor progression via platelets in an indirect manner. It has been shown that TF-bearing microparticles originating from the tumor cells *per se* are present in the circulation of cancer patients (Tesselaar and Osanto, 2007; Zwicker, 2008). In general the levels of TF-bearing microparticles, independent of origin, have been associated with a more progressed cancer. For example, breast- and pancreatic cancer patients with metastatic disease have significantly higher levels of TF-bearing microparticles, as compared to healthy individuals and patients with non-metastatic cancer (Tesselaar and Osanto, 2007). In the same study, a negative correlation was found between microparticle-associated TF-activity and overall survival, further indicating the importance of TF-bearing microparticles in cancer. Results obtained from clinical studies are supported by studies performed in experimental mouse models. It has been shown that the amount of tumor-derived TF-bearing microparticles in the circulation correlates with tumor burden (Davila et al., 2008). Resection of tumors of several different sorts, including glioblastoma, pancreatic carcinoma and prostate cancer, has also resulted in decreased levels of TF-positive microparticles in several independent studies (Haubold et al., 2009; Sartori et al.; Zwicker et al., 2009). As expected, higher levels of TF-bearing microparticles have been associated with higher risk for cancer-associated venous thromboembolism (Tesselaar et al., 2009).

6. Therapeutic implications

Targeting the platelet-tumor interplay to inhibit tumor progression and metastasis is not used as a cancer therapy in the clinic today, but is an interesting strategy. Growing evidence indicate that the platelet-tumor cell interplay has an important role for tumor progression in several different ways. Hence, therapeutic approaches striking against this interaction might be an option for future development of cancer drugs. Such treatment would need further studies and potential targets identified in animal trials, such as P-selectin, GpVI or modulation of NK-cell reactivity, have to be validated in the clinical situation. Moreover, targeting platelet-endothelial interactions may be of equal importance in preventing malignant growth, since a significant part of the tumor-promoting effect of platelets seem to be via stimulation of tumor angiogenesis. The challenge in developing drugs that inhibit platelet function is to avoid the risk of bleedings. However, the recent findings that platelet-mediated protection of tumor vessel integrity requires platelet degranulation, but not plug formation, may allow for specific targeting of the two processes (Ho-Tin-Noe et al., 2009).

Species-specific differences concerning platelet biology and function makes it difficult to predict how well results obtained in mice would reflect the situation in humans (Schmitt et al., 2001). However, results from studies on clinical material confirm a strong connection between platelets and tumor growth and progression, suggesting platelets to be promising targets also in human cancer.

7. Conclusion

The literature describing tumor-promoting effects of platelets is significant and rapidly growing. Despite the extent of our current knowledge of these processes, many questions remain to be answered. How is differential release of separate platelet α-granules regulated in a mechanistic manner and which are the underlying signal transduction pathways? Do platelets contribute at a specific stage of tumor development, or are they equally important throughout cancer progression? Could targeting of platelet interactions with the vessel wall inhibit angiogenesis? Is it possible to target a distinct platelet process, such as degranulation, without affecting others, like clot formation? Considering the rapid development of this field of research and the continued efforts of several laboratories around the world, answers - as well as new questions - will surely come in a near future.

8. References

Alves, C.S., Burdick, M.M., Thomas, S.N., Pawar, P., & Konstantopoulos, K. (2008). The dual role of CD44 as a functional P-selectin ligand and fibrin receptor in colon carcinoma cell adhesion. *Am J Physiol Cell Physiol* 294, C907-916. ISSN 0363-6143.

Amirkhosravi, A., Meyer, T., Chang, J.Y., Amaya, M., Siddiqui, F., Desai, H., & Francis, J.L. (2002). Tissue factor pathway inhibitor reduces experimental lung metastasis of B16 melanoma. *Thromb Haemost* 87, 930-936. ISSN 0340-6245.

Amirkhosravi, A., Mousa, S.A., Amaya, M., Blaydes, S., Desai, H., Meyer, T., & Francis, J.L. (2003). Inhibition of tumor cell-induced platelet aggregation and lung metastasis by the oral GpIIb/IIIa antagonist XV454. *Thromb Haemost* 90, 549-554. ISSN 0340-6245.

Baenziger, N.L., Brodie, G.N., & Majerus, P.W. (1972). Isolation and properties of a thrombin-sensitive protein of human platelets. *J Biol Chem* 247, 2723-2731. ISSN 0021-9258.

Baj-Krzyworzeka, M., Szatanek, R., Weglarczyk, K., Baran, J., Urbanowicz, B., Branski, P., Ratajczak, M.Z., & Zembala, M. (2006). Tumour-derived microvesicles carry several surface determinants and mRNA of tumour cells and transfer some of these determinants to monocytes. *Cancer Immunol Immunother* 55, 808-818. ISSN 0340-7004.

Bambace, N.M., Levis, J.E., & Holmes, C.E. (2010). The effect of P2Y-mediated platelet activation on the release of VEGF and endostatin from platelets. *Platelets* 21, 85-93. ISSN 1369-1635.

Battinelli, E.M., Markens, B.A., & Italiano, J.E., Jr. (2011). Release of angiogenesis regulatory proteins from platelet alpha granules: modulation of physiological and pathological angiogenesis. *Blood*. Epub ahead of print. ISSN 1528-0020.

Borsig, L., Wong, R., Feramisco, J., Nadeau, D.R., Varki, N.M., & Varki, A. (2001). Heparin and cancer revisited: mechanistic connections involving platelets, P-selectin, carcinoma mucins, and tumor metastasis. *Proc Natl Acad Sci U S A* 98, 3352-3357. ISSN 0027-8424.

Borsig, L., Wong, R., Hynes, R.O., Varki, N.M., & Varki, A. (2002). Synergistic effects of L- and P-selectin in facilitating tumor metastasis can involve non-mucin ligands and implicate leukocytes as enhancers of metastasis. *Proc Natl Acad Sci U S A* 99, 2193-2198. ISSN 0027-8424.

Brill, A., Dashevsky, O., Rivo, J., Gozal, Y., & Varon, D. (2005). Platelet-derived microparticles induce angiogenesis and stimulate post-ischemic revascularization. *Cardiovasc Res* 67, 30-38. ISSN 0008-6363.

Brill, A., Elinav, H., & Varon, D. (2004). Differential role of platelet granular mediators in angiogenesis. *Cardiovasc Res* 63, 226-235. ISSN 0008-6363.

Bromberg, M.E., Konigsberg, W.H., Madison, J.F., Pawashe, A., & Garen, A. (1995). Tissue factor promotes melanoma metastasis by a pathway independent of blood coagulation. *Proc Natl Acad Sci U S A* 92, 8205-8209. ISSN 0027-8424.

Browder, T., Folkman, J., & Pirie-Shepherd, S. (2000). The hemostatic system as a regulator of angiogenesis. *J Biol Chem* 275, 1521-1524. ISSN 0021-9258.

Brunner, G., Nguyen, H., Gabrilove, J., Rifkin, D.B., & Wilson, E.L. (1993). Basic fibroblast growth factor expression in human bone marrow and peripheral blood cells. *Blood* 81, 631-638. ISSN 0006-4971.

Burnier, L., Fontana, P., Kwak, B.R., & Angelillo-Scherrer, A. (2009). Cell-derived microparticles in haemostasis and vascular medicine. *Thromb Haemost* 101, 439-451. ISSN 0340-6245.

Busch, C., Heldin, C.H., Wasteson, A., & Westermark, B. (1977). Stimulation of endothelial cell proliferation by a factor released from human platelets. *Bibl Anat*, 219-222. ISSN 0067-7833.

Camerer, E., Qazi, A.A., Duong, D.N., Cornelissen, I., Advincula, R., & Coughlin, S.R. (2004). Platelets, protease-activated receptors, and fibrinogen in hematogenous metastasis. *Blood* 104, 397-401. ISSN 0006-4971.

Cesarman-Maus, G., & Hajjar, K.A. (2005). Molecular mechanisms of fibrinolysis. *Br J Haematol* 129, *307-321*. ISSN 0007-1048.

Chiodoni, C., Iezzi, M., Guiducci, C., Sangaletti, S., Alessandrini, I., Ratti, C., Tiboni, F., Musiani, P., Granger, D.N., & Colombo, M.P. (2006). Triggering CD40 on endothelial cells contributes to tumor growth. *J Exp Med* 203, 2441-2450. ISSN 0022-1007.

Dashevsky, O., Varon, D., & Brill, A. (2009). Platelet-derived microparticles promote invasiveness of prostate cancer cells via upregulation of MMP-2 production. *Int J Cancer* 124, 1773-1777. ISSN 1097-0215.

Davila, M., Amirkhosravi, A., Coll, E., Desai, H., Robles, L., Colon, J., Baker, C.H., & Francis, J.L. (2008). Tissue factor-bearing microparticles derived from tumor cells: impact on coagulation activation. *J Thromb Haemost* 6, 1517-1524. ISSN 1538-7836.

Denzer, K., Kleijmeer, M.J., Heijnen, H.F., Stoorvogel, W., & Geuze, H.J. (2000). Exosome: from internal vesicle of the multivesicular body to intercellular signaling device. *J Cell Sci* 113 Pt 19, 3365-3374. ISSN 0021-9533.

Desgrosellier, J.S., & Cheresh, D.A. (2010). Integrins in cancer: biological implications and therapeutic opportunities. *Nat Rev Cancer* 10, 9-22. ISSN 1474-1768.

Diamant, M., Tushuizen, M.E., Sturk, A., & Nieuwland, R. (2004). Cellular microparticles: new players in the field of vascular disease? *Eur J Clin Invest* 34, 392-401. ISSN 0014-2972.

Dvorak, H. (1994). Abnormalities of hemostasis in malignancy. In: *Hemostasis and thrombosis: basic principles and clinical practice, 3rd edn,* Colman, R.W., Hirsch, J., Marder, V.J., Saltzman, E.W., pp 1238-1254, *Philadelphia: JB Lipincott Company.*

Dvorak, H.F. (1986). Tumors: wounds that do not heal. Similarities between tumor stroma generation and wound healing. *N Engl J Med* 315, 1650-1659. ISSN 0028-4793.

Dvorak, H.F., Brown, L.F., Detmar, M., & Dvorak, A.M. (1995). Vascular permeability factor/vascular endothelial growth factor, microvascular hyperpermeability, and angiogenesis. *Am J Pathol* 146, 1029-1039. ISSN 0002-9440.

English, D., Garcia, J.G., & Brindley, D.N. (2001). Platelet-released phospholipids link haemostasis and angiogenesis. *Cardiovasc Res* 49, 588-599.

Essayagh, S., Xuereb, J.M., Terrisse, A.D., Tellier-Cirioni, L., Pipy, B., & Sie, P. (2007). Microparticles from apoptotic monocytes induce transient platelet recruitment and tissue factor expression by cultured human vascular endothelial cells via a redox-sensitive mechanism. *Thromb Haemost* 98, 831-837. ISSN 0340-6245.

Even-Ram, S., Uziely, B., Cohen, P., Grisaru-Granovsky, S., Maoz, M., Ginzburg, Y., Reich, R., Vlodavsky, I., & Bar-Shavit, R. (1998). Thrombin receptor overexpression in malignant and physiological invasion processes. *Nat Med* 4, 909-914. ISSN 1078-8956.

Felding-Habermann, B., Habermann, R., Saldivar, E., & Ruggeri, Z.M. (1996). Role of beta3 integrins in melanoma cell adhesion to activated platelets under flow. *J Biol Chem* 271, 5892-5900. ISSN 0021-9258.

Feng, W., Madajka, M., Kerr, B.A., Mahabeleshwar, G.H., Whiteheart, S.W., & Byzova, T.V. (2011). A novel role for platelet secretion in angiogenesis: mediating bone marrow-derived cell mobilization and homing. *Blood* 117, 3893-3902. ISSN 1528-0020.

Fernandez-Patron, C., Martinez-Cuesta, M.A., Salas, E., Sawicki, G., Wozniak, M., Radomski, M.W., & Davidge, S.T. (1999). Differential regulation of platelet aggregation by matrix metalloproteinases-9 and -2. *Thromb Haemost* 82, 1730-1735. ISSN 0340-6245.

Gasic, G.J., Gasic, T.B., Galanti, N., Johnson, T., & Murphy, S. (1973). Platelet-tumor-cell interactions in mice. The role of platelets in the spread of malignant disease. *Int J Cancer* 11, 704-718. ISSN 0020-7136.

Gasic, G.J., Gasic, T.B., & Stewart, C.C. (1968). Antimetastatic effects associated with platelet reduction. *Proc Natl Acad Sci U S A* 61, 46-52. ISSN 0027-8424.

Goerge, T., Ho-Tin-Noe, B., Carbo, C., Benarafa, C., Remold-O'Donnell, E., Zhao, B.Q., Cifuni, S.M., & Wagner, D.D. (2008). Inflammation induces hemorrhage in thrombocytopenia. *Blood* 111, 4958-4964. ISSN 1528-0020.

Gorelik, E., Wiltrout, R.H., Okumura, K., Habu, S., & Herberman, R.B. (1982). Role of NK cells in the control of metastatic spread and growth of tumor cells in mice. *Int J Cancer* 30, 107-112. ISSN 0020-7136.

Gracia Ballarin, R. (2005). Communication with patient, family and community in the rural world. *Rural Remote Health* 5, 424. ISSN 1445-6354.

Hanna, N. (1985). The role of natural killer cells in the control of tumor growth and metastasis. *Biochim Biophys Acta* 780, 213-226. ISSN 0006-3002.

Haubold, K., Rink, M., Spath, B., Friedrich, M., Chun, F.K., Marx, G., Amirkhosravi, A., Francis, J.L., Bokemeyer, C., Eifrig, B., & Langer, F. (2009). Tissue factor procoagulant activity of plasma microparticles is increased in patients with early-stage prostate cancer. *Thromb Haemost* 101, 1147-1155. ISSN 0340-6245.

Heldin, C.H., Westermark, B., & Wasteson, A. (1981). Platelet-derived growth factor. Isolation by a large-scale procedure and analysis of subunit composition. *Biochem J* 193, 907-913. ISSN 0264-6021.

Helley, D., Banu, E., Bouziane, A., Banu, A., Scotte, F., Fischer, A.M., & Oudard, S. (2009). Platelet microparticles: a potential predictive factor of survival in hormone-refractory prostate cancer patients treated with docetaxel-based chemotherapy. *Eur Urol* 56, 479-484. ISSN 1873-7560.

Ho-Tin-Noe, B., Goerge, T., Cifuni, S.M., Duerschmied, D., & Wagner, D.D. (2008). Platelet granule secretion continuously prevents intratumor hemorrhage. *Cancer Res* 68, 6851-6858. ISSN 1538-7445.

Ho-Tin-Noe, B., Goerge, T., & Wagner, D.D. (2009). Platelets: guardians of tumor vasculature. *Cancer Res* 69, 5623-5626. ISSN 1538-7445.

Holmes, C.E., Huang, J.C., Pace, T.R., Howard, A.B., & Muss, H.B. (2008). Tamoxifen and aromatase inhibitors differentially affect vascular endothelial growth factor and endostatin levels in women with breast cancer. *Clin Cancer Res* 14, 3070-3076. ISSN 1078-0432.

Italiano, J.E., Jr., Richardson, J.L., Patel-Hett, S., Battinelli, E., Zaslavsky, A., Short, S., Ryeom, S., Folkman, J., & Klement, G.L. (2008). Angiogenesis is regulated by a novel mechanism: pro- and antiangiogenic proteins are organized into separate platelet alpha granules and differentially released. *Blood* 111, 1227-1233. ISSN 0006-4971.

Jackson, S.P. (2007). The growing complexity of platelet aggregation. Blood *109*, 5087-5095. ISSN 0006-4971.

Jain, S., Harris, J., & Ware, J. (2010). Platelets: linking hemostasis and cancer. *Arterioscler Thromb Vasc Biol* 30, 2362-2367. ISSN 1524-4636.

Jain, S., Russell, S., & Ware, J. (2009). Platelet glycoprotein VI facilitates experimental lung metastasis in syngenic mouse models. *J Thromb Haemost* 7, 1713-1717. ISSN 1538-7836.

Jain, S., Zuka, M., Liu, J., Russell, S., Dent, J., Guerrero, J.A., Forsyth, J., Maruszak, B., Gartner, T.K., Felding-Habermann, B., & Ware, J. (2007). Platelet glycoprotein Ib alpha supports experimental lung metastasis. *Proc Natl Acad Sci U S A* 104, 9024-9028. ISSN 0027-8424.

Janowska-Wieczorek, A., Wysoczynski, M., Kijowski, J., Marquez-Curtis, L., Machalinski, B., Ratajczak, J., & Ratajczak, M.Z. (2005). Microvesicles derived from activated platelets induce metastasis and angiogenesis in lung cancer. *Int J Cancer* 113, 752-760. ISSN 0020-7136.

Jin, M., Drwal, G., Bourgeois, T., Saltz, J., & Wu, H.M. (2005). Distinct proteome features of plasma microparticles. *Proteomics* 5, 1940-1952. ISSN 1615-9853.

Jurasz, P., Alonso, D., Castro-Blanco, S., Murad, F., & Radomski, M.W. (2003). Generation and role of angiostatin in human platelets. *Blood* 102, 3217-3223. ISSN 0006-4971.

Jurk, K., & Kehrel, B.E. (2005). Platelets: physiology and biochemistry. *Semin Thromb Hemost* 31, 381-392. ISSN 0094-6176.

Kamykowski, J., Carlton, P., Sehgal, S., & Storrie, B. (2011). Quantitative immunofluorescence mapping reveals little functional co-clustering of proteins within platelet {alpha}-granules. *Blood*. Epub ahead of print. ISSN 1528-0020.

Karpatkin, S., Pearlstein, E., Ambrogio, C., & Coller, B.S. (1988). Role of adhesive proteins in platelet tumor interaction in vitro and metastasis formation in vivo. *J Clin Invest* 81, 1012-1019. ISSN 0021-9738.

Karpatkin, S., Pearlstein, E., Salk, P.L., & Yogeeswaran, G. (1981). Role of platelets in tumor cell metastases. *Ann N Y Acad Sci* 370, 101-118. ISSN 0077-8923.

Khorana, A.A., Francis, C.W., Menzies, K.E., Wang, J.G., Hyrien, O., Hathcock, J., Mackman, N., & Taubman, M.B. (2008). Plasma tissue factor may be predictive of venous thromboembolism in pancreatic cancer. *J Thromb Haemost* 6, 1983-1985. ISSN 1538-7836.

Kim, H.K., Song, K.S., Chung, J.H., Lee, K.R., & Lee, S.N. (2004). Platelet microparticles induce angiogenesis in vitro. *Br J Haematol* 124, 376-384. ISSN 0007-1048.

Kim, H.K., Song, K.S., Park, Y.S., Kang, Y.H., Lee, Y.J., Lee, K.R., Ryu, K.W., Bae, J.M., & Kim, S. (2003). Elevated levels of circulating platelet microparticles, VEGF, IL-6 and RANTES in patients with gastric cancer: possible role of a metastasis predictor. *Eur J Cancer* 39, 184-191. ISSN 0959-8049.

Kim, Y.J., Borsig, L., Varki, N.M., & Varki, A. (1998). P-selectin deficiency attenuates tumor growth and metastasis. *Proc Natl Acad Sci U S A* 95, 9325-9330. ISSN 0027-8424.

Kisucka, J., Butterfield, C.E., Duda, D.G., Eichenberger, S.C., Saffaripour, S., Ware, J., Ruggeri, Z.M., Jain, R.K., Folkman, J., & Wagner, D.D. (2006). Platelets and platelet adhesion support angiogenesis while preventing excessive hemorrhage. *Proc Natl Acad Sci U S A* 103, 855-860. ISSN 0027-8424.

Kitagawa, H., Yamamoto, N., Yamamoto, K., Tanoue, K., Kosaki, G., & Yamazaki, H. (1989). Involvement of platelet membrane glycoprotein Ib and glycoprotein IIb/IIIa complex in thrombin-dependent and -independent platelet aggregations induced by tumor cells. *Cancer Res* 49, 537-541. ISSN 0008-5472.

Klement, G.L., Yip, T.T., Cassiola, F., Kikuchi, L., Cervi, D., Podust, V., Italiano, J.E., Wheatley, E., Abou-Slaybi, A., Bender, E., Almog, N., Kieran, M.W., & Folkman, J. (2009). Platelets actively sequester angiogenesis regulators. *Blood* 113, 2835-2842. ISSN 1528-0020.

Kopp, H.G., Hooper, A.T., Broekman, M.J., Avecilla, S.T., Petit, I., Luo, M., Milde, T., Ramos, C.A., Zhang, F., Kopp, T., Bornstein, P., Jon, D.K., Marcus, A.J., & Rafii, S. (2006). Thrombospondins deployed by thrombopoietic cells determine angiogenic switch and extent of revascularization. *J Clin Invest* 116, 3277-3291. ISSN 0021-9738.

Kopp, H.G., Placke, T., & Salih, H.R. (2009). Platelet-derived transforming growth factor-beta down-regulates NKG2D thereby inhibiting natural killer cell antitumor reactivity. *Cancer Res* 69, 7775-7783. ISSN 1538-7445.

Laubli, H., & Borsig, L. (2010). Selectins promote tumor metastasis. *Semin Cancer Biol* 20, 169-177. ISSN 1096-3650.

Laubli, H., Spanaus, K.S., & Borsig, L. (2009). Selectin-mediated activation of endothelial cells induces expression of CCL5 and promotes metastasis through recruitment of monocytes. *Blood* 114, 4583-4591. ISSN 1528-0020.

Lecine, P., Villeval, J.L., Vyas, P., Swencki, B., Xu, Y., & Shivdasani, R.A. (1998). Mice lacking transcription factor NF-E2 provide in vivo validation of the proplatelet model of thrombocytopoiesis and show a platelet production defect that is intrinsic to megakaryocytes. *Blood* 92, 1608-1616. ISSN 0006-4971.

Ma, L., Elliott, S.N., Cirino, G., Buret, A., Ignarro, L.J., & Wallace, J.L. (2001). Platelets modulate gastric ulcer healing: role of endostatin and vascular endothelial growth factor release. *Proc Natl Acad Sci U S A* 98, 6470-6475. ISSN 0027-8424.

Ma, L., Perini, R., McKnight, W., Dicay, M., Klein, A., Hollenberg, M.D., & Wallace, J.L. (2005). Proteinase-activated receptors 1 and 4 counter-regulate endostatin and VEGF release from human platelets. *Proc Natl Acad Sci U S A* 102, 216-220. ISSN 0027-8424.

Mack, M., Kleinschmidt, A., Bruhl, H., Klier, C., Nelson, P.J., Cihak, J., Plachy, J., Stangassinger, M., Erfle, V., & Schlondorff, D. (2000). Transfer of the chemokine receptor CCR5 between cells by membrane-derived microparticles: a mechanism for cellular human immunodeficiency virus 1 infection. *Nat Med* 6, 769-775. ISSN 1078-8956.

Malik, G., Knowles, L.M., Dhir, R., Xu, S., Yang, S., Ruoslahti, E., & Pilch, J. (2010). Plasma fibronectin promotes lung metastasis by contributions to fibrin clots and tumor cell invasion. *Cancer Res* 70, 4327-4334. ISSN 1538-7445.

Milsom, C., & Rak, J. (2008). Tissue factor and cancer. *Pathophysiol Haemost Thromb* 36, 160-176. ISSN 1424-8840.

Mohle, R., Green, D., Moore, M.A., Nachman, R.L., & Rafii, S. (1997). Constitutive production and thrombin-induced release of vascular endothelial growth factor by human megakaryocytes and platelets. *Proc Natl Acad Sci U S A* 94, 663-668. ISSN 0027-8424.

Morel, O., Toti, F., Hugel, B., Bakouboula, B., Camoin-Jau, L., Dignat-George, F., & Freyssinet, J.M. (2006). Procoagulant microparticles: disrupting the vascular homeostasis equation? *Arterioscler Thromb Vasc Biol* 26, 2594-2604. ISSN 1524-4636.

Mueller, B.M., Reisfeld, R.A., Edgington, T.S., & Ruf, W. (1992). Expression of tissue factor by melanoma cells promotes efficient hematogenous metastasis. *Proc Natl Acad Sci U S A* 89, 11832-11836. ISSN 0027-8424.

Mueller, B.M., & Ruf, W. (1998). Requirement for binding of catalytically active factor VIIa in tissue factor-dependent experimental metastasis. *J Clin Invest* 101, 1372-1378. ISSN 0021-9738.

Nierodzik, M.L., Bain, R.M., Liu, L.X., Shivji, M., Takeshita, K., & Karpatkin, S. (1996). Presence of the seven transmembrane thrombin receptor on human tumour cells: effect of activation on tumour adhesion to platelets and tumor tyrosine phosphorylation. *Br J Haematol* 92, 452-457. ISSN 0007-1048.

Nierodzik, M.L., Chen, K., Takeshita, K., Li, J.J., Huang, Y.Q., Feng, X.S., D'Andrea, M.R., Andrade-Gordon, P., & Karpatkin, S. (1998). Protease-activated receptor 1 (PAR-1) is required and rate-limiting for thrombin-enhanced experimental pulmonary metastasis. *Blood* 92, 3694-3700. ISSN 0006-4971.

Nierodzik, M.L., & Karpatkin, S. (2006). Thrombin induces tumor growth, metastasis, and angiogenesis: Evidence for a thrombin-regulated dormant tumor phenotype. *Cancer Cell* 10, 355-362. ISSN 1535-6108.

Nierodzik, M.L., Plotkin, A., Kajumo, F., & Karpatkin, S. (1991). Thrombin stimulates tumor-platelet adhesion in vitro and metastasis in vivo. *J Clin Invest* 87, 229-236. ISSN 0021-9738.

Nieswandt, B., Hafner, M., Echtenacher, B., & Mannel, D.N. (1999). Lysis of tumor cells by natural killer cells in mice is impeded by platelets. *Cancer Res* 59, 1295-1300. ISSN 0008-5472.

Nieuwland, R., & Sturk, A. (2010). Why do cells release vesicles? *Thromb Res* 125 Suppl 1, S49-51. ISSN 1879-2472.

Olsson, A.K., Dimberg, A., Kreuger, J., & Claesson-Welsh, L. (2006). VEGF receptor signalling - in control of vascular function. *Nat Rev Mol Cell Biol* 7, 359-371. ISSN 1471-0072.

Paborsky, L.R., Caras, I.W., Fisher, K.L., & Gorman, C.M. (1991). Lipid association, but not the transmembrane domain, is required for tissue factor activity. Substitution of the transmembrane domain with a phosphatidylinositol anchor. *J Biol Chem* 266, 21911-21916. ISSN 0021-9258.

Palumbo, J.S., Kombrinck, K.W., Drew, A.F., Grimes, T.S., Kiser, J.H., Degen, J.L., & Bugge, T.H. (2000). Fibrinogen is an important determinant of the metastatic potential of circulating tumor cells. *Blood* 96, 3302-3309. ISSN 0006-4971.

Palumbo, J.S., Potter, J.M., Kaplan, L.S., Talmage, K., Jackson, D.G., & Degen, J.L. (2002). Spontaneous hematogenous and lymphatic metastasis, but not primary tumor growth or angiogenesis, is diminished in fibrinogen-deficient mice. *Cancer Res* 62, 6966-6972. ISSN 0008-5472.

Palumbo, J.S., Talmage, K.E., Massari, J.V., La Jeunesse, C.M., Flick, M.J., Kombrinck, K.W., Jirouskova, M., & Degen, J.L. (2005). Platelets and fibrin(ogen) increase metastatic potential by impeding natural killer cell-mediated elimination of tumor cells. *Blood* 105, 178-185. ISSN 0006-4971.

Pearlstein, E., Salk, P.L., Yogeeswaran, G., & Karpatkin, S. (1980). Correlation between spontaneous metastatic potential, platelet-aggregating activity of cell surface extracts, and cell surface sialylation in 10 metastatic-variant derivatives of a rat renal sarcoma cell line. *Proc Natl Acad Sci U S A* 77, 4336-4339. ISSN 0027-8424.

Perez-Pujol, S., Marker, P.H., & Key, N.S. (2007). Platelet microparticles are heterogeneous and highly dependent on the activation mechanism: studies using a new digital flow cytometer. *Cytometry* A 71, 38-45. ISSN 1552-4922.

Peterson, J.E., Zurakowski, D., Italiano, J.E., Jr., Michel, L.V., Fox, L., Klement, G.L., & Folkman, J. (2010). Normal ranges of angiogenesis regulatory proteins in human platelets. *Am J Hematol* 85, 487-493. ISSN 1096-8652.

Piccin, A., Murphy, W.G., & Smith, O.P. (2007). Circulating microparticles: pathophysiology and clinical implications. *Blood Rev* 21, 157-171. ISSN 0268-960X.

Pietramaggiori, G., Scherer, S.S., Cervi, D., Klement, G., & Orgill, D.P. (2008). Tumors stimulate platelet delivery of angiogenic factors in vivo: an unexpected benefit. *Am J Pathol* 173, 1609-1616. ISSN 1525-2191.

Pinedo, H.M., Verheul, H.M., D'Amato, R.J., & Folkman, J. (1998). Involvement of platelets in tumour angiogenesis? *Lancet* 352, 1775-1777. ISSN 0140-6736.

Pipili-Synetos, E., Papadimitriou, E., & Maragoudakis, M.E. (1998). Evidence that platelets promote tube formation by endothelial cells on matrigel. *Br J Pharmacol* 125, 1252-1257. ISSN 0007-1188.

Prokopi, M., Pula, G., Mayr, U., Devue, C., Gallagher, J., Xiao, Q., Boulanger, C.M., Westwood, N., Urbich, C., Willeit, J., Steiner, M., Breuss, J., Xu, Q., Kiechi, S., & Mayr, M. (2009). Proteomic analysis reveals presence of platelet microparticles in endothelial progenitor cell cultures. *Blood* 114, 723-732. ISSN 1528-0020.

Qi, J., Goralnick, S., & Kreutzer, D.L. (1997). Fibrin regulation of interleukin-8 gene expression in human vascular endothelial cells. *Blood* 90, 3595-3602. ISSN 0006-4971.

Rendu, F., & Brohard-Bohn, B. (2001). The platelet release reaction: granules' constituents, secretion and functions. *Platelets* 12, 261-273. ISSN 0953-7104.

Rhee, J.S., Black, M., Schubert, U., Fischer, S., Morgenstern, E., Hammes, H.P., & Preissner, K.T. (2004). The functional role of blood platelet components in angiogenesis. *Thromb Haemost* 92, 394-402. ISSN 0340-6245.

Ringvall, M., Thulin, A., Zhang, L., Cedervall, J., Tsuchida-Straeten, N., Jahnen-Dechent, W., Siegbahn, A., & Olsson, A.K. (2011). Enhanced platelet activation mediates the accelerated angiogenic switch in mice lacking histidine-rich glycoprotein. *PLoS One* 6, e14526. ISSN 1932-6203.

Sarker, M.H., Hu, D.E., & Fraser, P.A. (2010). Regulation of cerebromicrovascular permeability by lysophosphatidic acid. *Microcirculation* 17, 39-46. ISSN 1549-8719.

Sartori, M.T., Della Puppa, A., Ballin, A., Saggiorato, G., Bernardi, D., Padoan, A., Scienza, R., d'Avella, D., & Cella, G. (2010). Prothrombotic state in glioblastoma multiforme: an evaluation of the procoagulant activity of circulating microparticles. *J Neurooncol*. Epub ahead of print. ISSN 1573-7373.

Sawicki, G., Salas, E., Murat, J., Miszta-Lane, H., & Radomski, M.W. (1997). Release of gelatinase A during platelet activation mediates aggregation. *Nature* 386, 616-619. ISSN 0028-0836.

Schaphorst, K.L., Chiang, E., Jacobs, K.N., Zaiman, A., Natarajan, V., Wigley, F., & Garcia, J.G. (2003). Role of sphingosine-1 phosphate in the enhancement of endothelial barrier integrity by platelet-released products. *Am J Physiol Lung Cell Mol Physiol* 285, L258-267. ISSN 1040-0605.

Schmitt, A., Guichard, J., Masse, J.M., Debili, N., & Cramer, E.M. (2001). Of mice and men: comparison of the ultrastructure of megakaryocytes and platelets. *Exp Hematol* 29, 1295-1302. ISSN 0301-472X.

Seto, S., Onodera, H., Kaido, T., Yoshikawa, A., Ishigami, S., Arii, S., & Imamura, M. (2000). Tissue factor expression in human colorectal carcinoma: correlation with hepatic metastasis and impact on prognosis. *Cancer* 88, 295-301. ISSN 0008-543X.

Shattil, S.J., Kim, C., & Ginsberg, M.H. (2010). The final steps of integrin activation: the end game. *Nat Rev Mol Cell Biol* 11, 288-300. ISSN 1471-0080.

Simak, J., & Gelderman, M.P. (2006). Cell membrane microparticles in blood and blood products: potentially pathogenic agents and diagnostic markers. *Transfus Med Rev* 20, 1-26. ISSN 0887-7963.

Skolnik, G., Bagge, U., Blomqvist, G., Djarv, L., & Ahlman, H. (1989). The role of calcium channels and serotonin (5-HT2) receptors for tumour cell lodgement in the liver. *Clin Exp Metastasis* 7, 169-174. ISSN 0262-0898.

Skolnik, G., Bagge, U., Dahlstrom, A., & Ahlman, H. (1984). The importance of 5-HT for tumor cell lodgement in the liver. *Int J Cancer* 33, 519-523. ISSN 0020-7136.

Skov Madsen, P., Hokland, P., & Hokland, M. (1986). Secretory products from thrombin-stimulated human platelets exert an inhibitory effect on NK-cytotoxic activity. *Acta Pathol Microbiol Immunol Scand* C 94, 193-200. ISSN 0108-0202.

Staton, C.A., & Lewis, C.E. (2005). Angiogenesis inhibitors found within the haemostasis pathway. *J Cell Mol Med* 9, 286-302. ISSN 1582-1838.

Sun, N.C., McAfee, W.M., Hum, G.J., & Weiner, J.M. (1979). Hemostatic abnormalities in malignancy, a prospective study of one hundred eight patients. Part I. Coagulation studies. *Am J Clin Pathol* 71, 10-16. ISSN 0002-9173.

Terraube, V., Pendu, R., Baruch, D., Gebbink, M.F., Meyer, D., Lenting, P.J., & Denis, C.V. (2006). Increased metastatic potential of tumor cells in von Willebrand factor-deficient mice. *J Thromb Haemost* 4, 519-526. ISSN 1538-7933.

Tesselaar, M.E., & Osanto, S. (2007). Risk of venous thromboembolism in lung cancer. *Curr Opin Pulm Med* 13, 362-367. ISSN 1070-5287.

Tesselaar, M.E., Romijn, F.P., van der Linden, I.K., Bertina, R.M., & Osanto, S. (2009). Microparticle-associated tissue factor activity in cancer patients with and without thrombosis. *J Thromb Haemost* 7, 1421-1423. ISSN 1538-7836.

Thulin, A., Ringvall, M., Dimberg, A., Karehed, K., Vaisanen, T., Vaisanen, M.R., Hamad, O., Wang, J., Bjerkvig, R., Nilsson, B., Pihlajaniemi, T., Akerud, H., Pietras, K., Jahnen-Dechent, W., Siegbahn, A., & Olsson A.K. (2009). Activated platelets provide a functional microenvironment for the antiangiogenic fragment of histidine-rich glycoprotein. *Mol Cancer Res* 7, 1792-1802. ISSN 1557-3125.

Trousseau, A. (1865). Phlegmasia alba dolens. *Clinique Medicale de l'Hotel-Dieu de Paris, The Syndenham Society 94-96.*

Tsuchida-Straeten, N., Ensslen, S., Schafer, C., Woltje, M., Denecke, B., Moser, M., Graber, S., Wakabayashi, S., Koide, T., & Jahnen-Dechent, W. (2005). Enhanced blood coagulation and fibrinolysis in mice lacking histidine-rich glycoprotein (HRG). *J Thromb Haemost* 3, 865-872. ISSN 1538-7933.

Varga-Szabo, D., Pleines, I., & Nieswandt, B. (2008). Cell adhesion mechanisms in platelets. *Arterioscler Thromb Vasc Biol* 28, 403-412. ISSN 1524-4636.

Varki, A. (2007). Trousseau's syndrome: multiple definitions and multiple mechanisms. *Blood* 110, 1723-1729. ISSN 0006-4971.

Verheul, H.M., Hoekman, K., Luykx-de Bakker, S., Eekman, C.A., Folman, C.C., Broxterman, H.J., & Pinedo, H.M. (1997). Platelet: transporter of vascular endothelial growth factor. *Clin Cancer Res* 3, 2187-2190. ISSN 1078-0432.

Verheul, H.M., Jorna, A.S., Hoekman, K., Broxterman, H.J., Gebbink, M.F., & Pinedo, H.M. (2000). Vascular endothelial growth factor-stimulated endothelial cells promote adhesion and activation of platelets. *Blood* 96, 4216-4221. ISSN 0006-4971.

Versteeg, H.H., Schaffner, F., Kerver, M., Ellies, L.G., Andrade-Gordon, P., Mueller, B.M., & Ruf, W. (2008). Protease-activated receptor (PAR) 2, but not PAR1, signaling promotes the development of mammary adenocarcinoma in polyoma middle T mice. *Cancer Res* 68, 7219-7227. ISSN 1538-7445.

Yin, F., & Watsky, M.A. (2005). LPA and S1P increase corneal epithelial and endothelial cell transcellular resistance. *Invest Ophthalmol Vis Sci* 46, 1927-1933. ISSN 0146-0404.

Zaslavsky, A., Baek, K.H., Lynch, R.C., Short, S., Grillo, J., Folkman, J., Italiano, J.E., Jr., & Ryeom, S. (2010). Platelet-derived thrombospondin-1 is a critical negative regulator and potential biomarker of angiogenesis. *Blood* 115, 4605-4613. ISSN 1528-0020.

Zwicker, J.I. (2008). Tissue factor-bearing microparticles and cancer. *Semin Thromb Hemost* 34, 195-198. ISSN 0094-6176.

Zwicker, J.I. (2010). Predictive value of tissue factor bearing microparticles in cancer associated thrombosis. *Thromb Res* 125 Suppl 2, S89-91. ISSN 1879-2472.

Zwicker, J.I., Liebman, H.A., Neuberg, D., Lacroix, R., Bauer, K.A., Furie, B.C., & Furie, B. (2009). Tumor-derived tissue factor-bearing microparticles are associated with venous thromboembolic events in malignancy. *Clin Cancer Res* 15, 6830-6840. ISSN 1078-0432.

6

Malignant Transformation in Skin is Associated with the Loss of T-Cadherin Expression in Human Keratinocytes and Heterogeneity in T-Cadherin Expression in Tumor Vasculature

Kseniya Rubina[1], Veronika Sysoeva[1], Ekaterina Semina[1], Natalia Kalinina[1], Ekaterina Yurlova[1], Albina Khlebnikova[2] and Vladimir Molochkov[2]
[1]*Department of Biological and Medical Chemistry, Faculty of Basic Medicine, Lomonosov Moscow State University*
[2]*Dermatology Department, First Moscow State Medical University, Russian Federation*

1. Introduction

A tumor is an abnormal mass of cells, the growth of which exceeds that of the normal tissue. Although most of the skin tumors retain a resemblance to the normal tissues from which they arise, they can show variations in their structure which cause difficulties in establishing pathological diagnosis. In contrast to benign skin tumors, which in most cases remain at the site of their origin and form compact mass of tumor cells, malignant tumors are composed of cells with the ability to invade the basement membrane and metastasize to other organs through blood and lymphatic vessels. Moreover, malignant tumors are often characterized by a more rapid growth and less differentiation, which histologically is characterized by a higher mitotic index and cellular and nuclear pleomorphism (Quinn & Perkins, 2010). Differentiation between benign and malignant skin tumors is one of important questions in terms of diagnostics, prognosis and treatment of the skin lesions.

Recently, a variety of molecular markers were shown to be promising in correlation with aggressive and invasive behavior of skin cancers. These involve aberrant expression of p53 (Verdolini et al., 2001), increased expression of transcription factors (Keehn et al., 2004), metalloproteinases (MMPs) (Verdolini et al., 2001), and proliferation markers mib1, Ki-67 (Oh & Penneys, 2004), stem cell markers c-kit, p63 (Laskin & Miettinen, 2003), increased phosphorylation of regulatory proteins and up-regulation of receptors of growth factors (Weigelt et al., 2005).

Tumor growth and invasiveness is accompanied by altered cell-cell communications. Thus, aggressive cancers are associated with decreased expression of E-cadherin which correlates with increased expression of desmosomal junction protein desmoglein (Kurzen et al., 2003) and N-cadherin (Gloushankova, 2008; Berx & van Roy, 2009).

T-cadherin, a non-classical member of cadherin family, was also suggested to play a role in cancer progression (Andreeva & Kutuzov, 2010; Philippova et al., 2009).

2. T-cadherin structure and intracellular signaling

T-cadherin is an atypical member of the cadherin superfamily. While possessing the general extracellular structure of classical cadherins, T-cadherin lacks transmembrane and cytoplasmic domains and is anchored to the plasma membrane by a glycosylphosphatidylinositol (GPI) moiety (Ranscht & Dours-Zimmermann, 1991). Since transmembrane and cytoplasmic domains of classical cadherins are generally recognized to be crucial in maintaining stable cell-cell contacts (Gumbiner, 2005), it is considered that the main function of T-cadherin is not cell-cell adhesion (Rubina et al., 2005a; Rubina & Tkachuk, 2004). Like other GPI-anchored proteins, T-cadherin is located in lipid rafts/caveolae (Philippova et al., 1998). Lipid rafts are cholesterol and sphingolipid rich domains of plasma membrane, which contain GPI-anchored proteins and signal transduction molecules such as Src-family kinases (Brown & London, 2000; Maxfield, 2002).

Indeed, T-cadherin was shown to be involved in regulation of cell adhesion, migration, proliferation and survival via activation of intracellular signaling. By using dominant negative and constitutively active forms of Rho, Rac and Cdc42 it was shown that Rho GTPases act downstream of T-cadherin and the activation of Rac1 and Cdc42 GTPases results in increased phosphorylation of LIMK1 kinase, actin and microtubule cytoskeleton rearrangements, activation of endothelial cell migration and increased permeability of endothelial cell monolayer (Philippova et al., 2005; Semina et al., 2009). Overexpression of T-cadherin in endothelial cells led to higher phosphorylation levels for phosphatidylinositol-3-kinase (PI3K) target Akt and mTOR target $p70^{S6K}$ involved in survival pathway in endothelial cells, but lower levels for p38MAPK (death pathway) (Joshi et al., 2005). In line with that, it was shown that T-cadherin mediated activation of PI3K/Akt/GSK3β signaling which protects endothelial cells from oxidative stress-induced apoptosis (Joshi et al., 2005). The effects of T-cadherin on Akt activation and survival require T-cadherin interacting partner Grp78, which is also known to be up-regulated in cancers (Andreeva et al., 2010; Philippova et al., 2008). High molecular weight adiponectin activates NF-kB and inhibits endothelial cell apoptosis suggesting that T-cadherin binding to adiponectin could prevent apoptosis of endothelial cells in tumor vessels (Adachi et al., 2006). Overexpression of T-cadherin in human aortic smooth muscle cells and in HUVECs increases cell proliferation (Ivanov et al., 2004). However, T-cadherin overexpression in HUVECs also results in an increased number of multinuclear cells, whereas its downregulaion results in increased amount of cells with multiple centrosomes (Andreeva et al., 2009). Stimulation of vascular endothelial cells and T-cadherin overexpressing HEK293 cells with plasma low density lipoproteins demonstrated the T-cadherin-induced signaling involving phospholipase C and IP3 formation, intracellular Ca^{2+} mobilization, activation of tyrosine kinases Erk 1/2, and nuclear translocation of NF-kB (Kipmen-Korgun et al., 2005; Rubina et al., 2005b).

However, in contrast to endothelial cells, overexpression of T-cadherin in C6 glioma (Huang et al., 2003) hepatocellular carcinoma cells (Chan et al., 2008), in immortalized keratinocytes (Mukoyama et al., 2005) and in p53(-/-) mouse embryonic fibroblasts (Chan et al., 2008) suppresses proliferation by delaying the G_2/M phase progression. In hepatocellular carcinoma cells T-cadherin expression also increases sensitivity to TNFα-induced apoptosis (Chan et al., 2008). Hence, in different studies T-cadherin was shown to be involved in regulation of proliferation, apoptosis and angiogenesis in normal tissues and tumor growth.

3. T-cadherin mediates homophilic interaction and vessel repulsion in angiogenesis

It is worth noting that in most experimental studies, the main attention is usually paid to the expression of T-cadherin in endothelial cells of the vessels while the role of T-cadherin expression by stromal cells in neoangiogenesis is rarely considered. In contrast, we used the Matrigel model, where Matrigel plugs containing L929 fibroblasts (control or overexpressing T-cadherin) where injected subcutaneously into nu/nu mice. In this settings, migrating endothelial cells, naturally expressing T-cadherin, contacted with T-cadherin positive fibroblasts and this interaction resulted in suppressed blood vessel growth. This effect of T-cadherin was dependent upon the concentration of T-cadherin expressing cells injected into the Matrigel. Moreover, small vessels and capillaries which invaded the Matrigel plug with high level of T-cadherin, did not express T-cadherin. Conceivably, high expression of T-cadherin inhibited the growth of the blood vessels. Furthermore, T-cadherin overexpression in the stroma regulated qualitative composition of blood vessels infiltrating the tissue either by negative guiding of T-cadherin expressing vascular endothelial cells or by downregulation of T-cadherin expression in the growing vessels, or both (Rubina et al., 2007).

It was shown that the general mechanism of T-cadherin mediated repulsion could involve homophilic T-cadherin interaction and contact inhibition as it was revealed for the growth of axons in the embryonic nervous system (Fredette et al., 1996). The same mechanism was shown to be responsible for regulation of the trajectory of the growing vessels. The first set of evidence came from in vitro experiments utilizing immobilized N-terminal EC1 domain of T-cadherin (Ivanov et al., 2004), which was responsible for homophilic T-cadherin interaction of contacting cells (Rubina et al., 2007). In vitro in Boyden chamber, ring aorta and capillary tube assays, we have shown that migration of endothelial cells, which endogenously express T-cadherin (Philippova et al., 2003), was inhibited by immobilized EC1 domain.

Thus, the most likely mechanism of T-cadherin-mediated suppression of blood vessel ingrowth is the interaction between T-cadherin molecules on endothelial and surrounding cells. This interaction leads to initiation of intracellular signaling cascades, which presumably are similar to ephrin's signaling, followed by cell-cell repulsion.

4. T-cadherin and tumor growth and vascularization

It has been proposed that T-cadherin functions as a tumor suppressor factor and its downregulation due to allelic loss or hypermethylation in the promoter region of the gene or some other reasons is related to tumor growth and metastasis in certain cancers (Takeuchi et al., 2002b; Andreeva & Kutuzov, 2010). Downregulation of T-cadherin was shown to be associated with malignant phenotype and tumorigenecity in breast (Riener et al., 2008), lung (Sato et al., 1998), and gallbladder cancers (Adachi et al., 2009). However, in other cancers such as ovarian, endometrial (Widschwendter et al., 2004; Suehiro et al., 2008) and osteosarcoma (Zucchini et al., 2004) T-cadherin decreased expression correlated positively with patient survival. T-cadherin overexpression was found to be a common feature of human invasive hepatocellular carcinomas (Riou et al., 2006) and high grade astrocytomas, where it was associated with malignant transformation of astrocytes. Hetezygosity for NF1 (neurofibromatosis 1) tumor suppressor resulting in reduced attachment and spreading and increased motility also coincided with upregulated T-cadherin expression (Gutmann et al., 2001).

Data on non-melanoma skin cancers and related premalignant lesions are also contradicting. In normal skin T-cadherin is expressed in keratinocyte basal cell layer (Zhou et al., 2002). In actinic keratosis T-cadherin expression is pronounced on the atypical keratinocytes, while in Bowen disease expression of T-cadherin varies and is in general weaker than in normal skin (Pfaff et al., 2010). Expression of T-cadherin is reduced in psoriasis (Zhou et al., 2003), is absent in invasive cutaneous squamous cell carcinoma due to aberrant methylation and gene deletion (Takeuchi et al., 2002a) and is down-regulated in basal cell carcinoma of the skin (Takeuchi et al., 2002b).

While in some studies the authors investigated the correlation between the hypermetylation of T-cadherin promoter or allelic loss, the others addressed the effect of T-cadherin re-expression on the malignant properties of cancer cells upon injection of cells in vivo in mouse models. Melanoma cells (Kuphal et al., 2009), hepatocellular carcinoma cells (Chan et al., 2008) and human breast carcinoma cells (Lee et al., 1998) showed a reduced tumor growth upon re-expression of T-cadherin. The transfection of mammary gland cells with cDNA of T-cadherin resulted in suppression of the cell proliferation in culture, which was also accompanied by transformation of the cancer cells from the invasive to the normal phenotype (Lee, 1996). The overexpression of T-cadherin in the neuroblastoma cells led to the suppression of invasion of the cells and the loss of their ability to respond to the addition of epidermal growth factor (EGF) with increased proliferation (Takeuchi et al., 2000). The overexpression of T-cadherin in the cells of glioma C6 was accompanied by the decrease of cell migration and suppression of the growth and proliferation in those cells due to blockade of the cell cycle on the stage G_2 (Huang et al., 2003). In immortalized keratinocyte cell lines derived from squamous cell carcinoma forced over-expression of T-cadherin resulted in decreased cell proliferation (Mukoyama et al., 2005).

These in vivo and in vitro data suggest that T-cadherin could be an endogenous negative regulator of keratinocyte proliferation. However, proliferating basal keratinocytes of the epidermis also express T-cadherin, leading to the conclusion that the role of T-cadherin in regulation of tumor cell growth and invasion is more complex.

Angiogenesis is necessary for tumor growth, invasion and metastases, therefore it has prognostic value and can be a therapeutic target. Angiogenesis is the process in which endothelial cells divide and migrate to form new capillaries, which support the continued growth of tumor through blood flow (Hasan et al., 2002; Sasano et al., 1998). Cancer-induced angiogenesis in general results from increased expression of angiogenic factors by tumor and/or stromal cells such as VEGF-A or decreased expression of anti-angiogenic factors, or a combination of both events (Hasan et al., 2002). Numerous authors reported that angiogenesis plays an important role in tumor progression and metastasis of the great majority of human solid tumors (Hasan et al., 2002; Offersen et al., 2002; Rubin et al., 1999; Vieira et al., 2004). During tumor angiogenesis, a certain sequence of events occurs resulting in directional migration of endothelial cells through the basement membrane and perivascular stromal cells toward angiogenic stimuli produced by tumor cells. In normal angiogenesis after endothelial cell migration and proliferation mural cells (smooth muscle cells and pericytes) enable stabilization of the nascent vessels. However, the newly formed tumor vessels are usually thin-walled capillaries or sinusoids with little more than an endothelial lining stabilized by a basement membrane and are susceptible to spontaneous hemorrhage and thrombosis (Carmeliet, 2000; Jain & Carmeliet, 2001; Yancopoulos et al., 2000).

Increasing evidence supports the essential role of VE and N-cadherin in the assembly of the vascular network. The adhesive properties of these cadherins are important for their angiogenic function, as far as they control both endothelial cell–cell interactions and the interaction of endothelial cells with stroma. The application of antibody against N-terminal repeat of VE-cadherin established this cadherin as a possible target for inhibiting angiogenesis in tumors (Cavallaro et al., 2006).

It is quite possible that T-cadherin affects carcinogenesis not only due to its aberrant expression in cancer cells, but also because it affects tumor neovascularization. Thus, in normal blood vessels T-cadherin is expressed in endothelial and mural cells (smooth muscle cells and pericytes) (Ivanov et al., 2001). However, as shown in numerous studies, T-cadherin expression is altered in tumor vessels: in Lewis carcinoma lung metastasis and F9 teratocarcinoma, PC-3 prostate cancer, in A673 rhabdomyosarcoma the expression of T-cadherin is upregulated on endothelial cells of the blood vessels penetrating the tumor (Riou et al., 2006; Wyder et al., 2000), while no T-cadherin could be detected in the blood vessels of B16F10 melanoma lung metastasis (Wyder et al., 2000). Using mouse mammary tumor virus (MMTV)-polyoma virus middle T (PyV-mT) transgenic model with inactivated T-cadherin gene it was shown that T-cadherin deficiency limits mammary tumor vascularization and reduces tumor growth (Hebbard et al., 2008).

In tumor neovascularization of hepatocellular carcinoma (HCC) T-cadherin is also upregulated in intratumoral capillary endothelial cells, whereas in surrounding tumor tissue as well as in normal liver no T-cadherin could be detected (Adachi et al., 2006). The increase in T-cadherin expression in endothelial cells of HCC was shown to correlate with tumor progression (Adachi et al., 2006). The involvement of T-cadherin in melanoma angiogenesis was demonstrated using an in vitro tumor spheroid model in co-culture with endothelial cells where T-cadherin upregulation in endothelial cells potentiated intratumoral angiogenesis (Ghosh et al., 2007). These data indicate that the contradictory results on tumor progression could be due to the complex cancer, stromal and endothelial cell intracellular interactions inside the growing tumor. The possible mechanism underlying the function of T-cadherin in angiogenesis could be the regulation of the trajectory of the growing blood vessels, thus T-cadherin acts as a navigating receptor (Rubina et al., 2007).

A diversity of navigating receptors has been already identified and shown to be involved in regulation of angiogenesis during embryogenesis and regeneration. These include semaphorins and their receptors (plexins and neuropilins), neutrins and their receptors (DCC/neogenine and Unc5), slit-ligands and their receptors Robo, and ephrins and their receptors (Adams et al., 1999; Weinstein, 2005). It is also known that ephrins and their receptors are navigation molecules regulating the trajectory of migration and differentiation of the cells in cardiovascular system (Adams et al., 1999); they have also been linked to the regulation of tumor angiogenesis (Ogawa et al., 2000).

To address the influence of T-cadherin overexpression in tumor cells on the ingrowth of the blood vessels into the tumor we used in vivo model of chorioallantoic membrane. For that the melanoma B16F10 cells overexpressing T-cadherin were injected under the chorioallantoic membrane in chick embryo, thus creating the microenvironment with high content of T-cadherin. This resulted in the reduction of the amount of blood vessels growing into the tumor with high expression of T-cadherin in comparison to the control (Yurlova et al., 2010). Presumably, the homophilic interaction and "repulsion" between molecules of T-cadherin on the surface of endothelial cells and tumor cells occurred at the contact of migrating endothelial cells which endogenously express T-cadherin with the tumor cells of melanoma, thereby resulting in the suppression of angiogenesis.

5. Stroma plays an active role in tumor growth and progression

In normal tissues stromal fibroblasts are responsible for the synthesis, deposition and remodeling of the extracellular matrix, as well as for the production of the soluble paracrine factors that regulate (promote or inhibit) cell proliferation, morphology and migration, survival and apoptosis (Klopp et al., 2011; Tlsty & Coussens, 2006). Tumor fibroblasts are derived, in part, from mesenchymal stem cells that may be recruited regionally or from circulating populations from the bone marrow (Mishra et al., 2008; Spaeth et al., 2008). Tumor fibroblasts isolated from malignant tissues exhibit altered phenotypes, mostly because of the aberrant production of the extracellular matrix proteins and growth factors (Bauer et al., 1979; Knudson et al., 1984; Tlsty & Coussens, 2006), disorganized patterns of growth, and enhanced proliferation (Rasmussen & Cullen, 1998; van den Hooff, 1988). Such phenotypes promote tumor progression (Klopp et al., 2011).

Tissue combination experiments using normal human prostatic epithelial cells with stromal cells obtained from prostatic adenocarcinoma demonstrated an interaction that limited growth potential of the epithelial cells while re-establishing their ability to form ductal structures resembling prostatic intraepithelial neoplasia. Engrafting of the stromal cells isolated from tumors together with immortalized human prostatic epithelial cells led to tumor formation exceeding by 500 fold the weight of control grafts (Olumi et al., 1999). Remarkably, isolation of pure human epithelial cell populations from these tumors and subsequent grafting into animals demonstrated that the epithelial cells were then able to form tumors while tumor fibroblasts presence and activity was no longer necessary (Olumi et al., 1999). Histological analysis of these tumors showed their characteristic features of malignant neoplasms with enhanced cell proliferation, reduced apoptosis, active angiogenesis, and genomic instability. Tumor fibroblasts isolated from human tumors also facilitate the growth of human breast and ovarian cancers when co-injected into immunosuppressed mice (Orimo et al., 2005).

These studies demonstrate that tumor stromal cells can produce oncogenic signals that can transform normal epithelial cells and induce them towards malignant state, thus establishing an active role of stromal cells in tumorigenic processes. Reciprocally, when placed in co-culture, tumor cells can directly induce stromal cells to convert into α–smooth muscle actin positive cells and express vimentin and stromal derived factor 1 (SDF-1), common to cancer associated fibroblasts. Transforming growth factor β (TGF–β) often produced by tumor cells was shown to induce conversion of adjacent stromal cells into α–smooth muscle actin expressing cells (Mishra et al., 2008; Spaeth et al., 2009; Tlsty & Coussens, 2006).

Thus, stromal cells together with cancer cells regulate tumor neoangiogenesis, in part, by local changes in the balance between soluble and insoluble molecules that elicit either pro- or antiangiogenic effects (Cavallaro et al., 2006; Takeuchi & Ohtsuki, 2001; Wyder et al., 2000). Mesenchymal stromal cells are known to secrete different proangiogenic factors, such as vascular endothelial growth factor (VEGF-A), fibroblast-derived growth factor (FGF), platelet-derived growth factor (PDGF), and SDF-1 (Efimenko et al., 2010; Rubina et al., 2009). These cytokines promote endothelial and smooth muscle migration and proliferation at the tumor site, facilitating angiogenesis (Kinnaird et al, 2004; Potapova et al., 2007). Other growth factors responsible for mesenchymal stromal cell effects on tumor vasculature include hepatocyte growth factor (HGF), cyclooxygenase, insulin-like growth factor 1 (IGF-1), PDGF-a, and TGF–α (Beckermann et al., 2008).

6. T-cadherin expression in precancerous lesions and malignant neoplasm of the skin

To define the role of T-cadherin in the pathogenesis of skin lesions we performed a comparative study of T-cadherin expression in normal skin samples, in non-melanoma skin cancer and related premalignant lesions. Cryosections of human skin biopsies from healthy donors, patients with keratoacanthoma in growth and stabilization stages, patients with keratosis, patients with superficial, nodular and infiltrative types of basal cell carcinoma, patients with basosquamous cell carcinoma and patients with squamous cell carcinoma were immunostained with antibodies against T-cadherin and vascular cell markers and analysed using fluorescent microscope.

6.1 Immunofluorescent staining

Human skin biopsies from 6 healthy donors, 10 patients with keratoacanthoma, 3 patients with keratosis, 30 patients with basal cell carcinoma, 5 patients with basosquamous cell carcinoma and 5 patients with squamous cell carcinoma were obtained from Dermatology Department of First Moscow State Medical University. Consequent cryosections of skin biopsies (7μm thick) were fixed in 4% paraformaldehyde (PRS Panreac, Spain) for 10 min. After several washes with phosphate buffer saline (PBS, Sigma-Aldrich, USA) sections were incubated in PBS/0.1% bovine serum albumine (BSA, Sigma-Aldrich, USA) containing 10% normal donkey serum (Sigma-Aldrich, USA) to block non-specific binding of antibodies. This was followed by incubation in a mixture of primary antibodies against T-cadherin (rabbit anti-human, ProSci, USA) and endothelial cell markers - vWF (Von Willebrand factor, mouse anti-human, BD Biosciences, USA) or CD31 (mouse anti-human, BD Biosciences, USA), or marker of smooth muscle cells and pericytes - α–actin (rabbit anti-human, Epitomics, USA) for 1 hour and subsequent extensive washing in PBS. Then sections were incubated in a mixture of secondary antibodies Alexa488-conjugated donkey anti-mouse and Alexa594-conjugated donkey anti-rabbit or Alexa488-conjugated donkey anti-rabbit and Alexa594-conjugated donkey anti-mouse (Molecular Probes, USA) (1μg/ml in PBS). Cell nuclei were counterstained with DAPI (Molecular Probes, USA). Sections were mounted in Vectashield mounting media (Vector Laboratories Inc., USA). For negative controls mouse or rabbit non-specific IgGs were used in appropriate concentration. Images were obtained using Zeiss Axiovert 200M microscope equipped with CCD camera AxioCam HRc and Axiovision software (Zeiss, Germany) and further processed using Adobe PhotoShop software (Adobe Systems, USA).

6.1.1 Normal skin

In normal skin the strongest T-cadherin expression was found in basal keratinocytes, stromal cells and in all blood vessels located in the underlying derma as observed by staining with antibody against endothelial marker vWF and marker of smooth muscle cells and/or pericytes - α–actin (Fig.1).

This data are in line with the previous observations (Takeuchi et al., 2002b). And yet, for the first time we have identified T-cadherin expression in hair follicles and sebaceous glands (Fig.1). In contrast to other studies (Zhou et al., 2002; Pfaff et al., 2010), we have found T-cadherin expression in the suprabasal layers of epidermal keratinocytes, although weaker than in the basal layer.

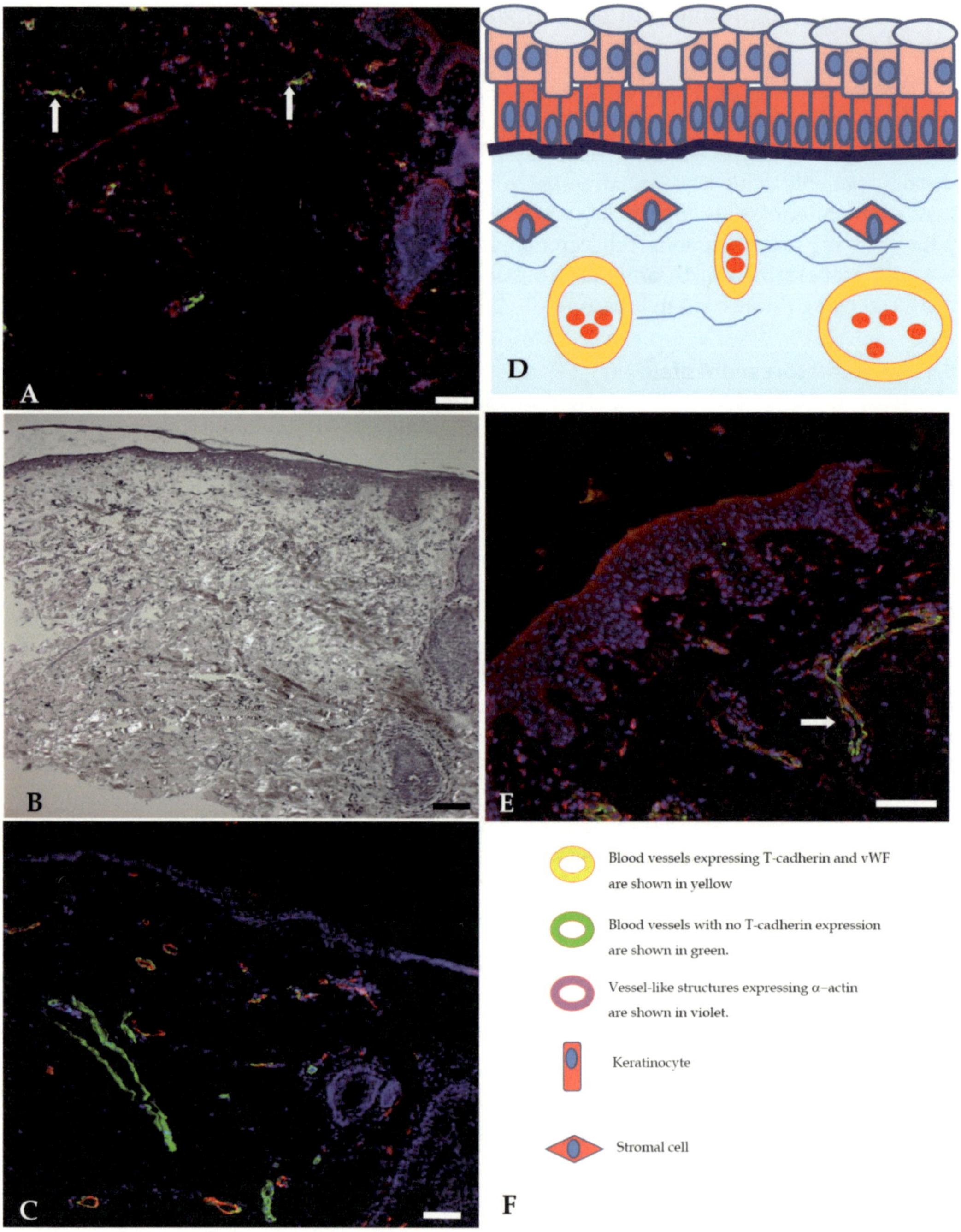

Fig. 1. Double immunofluorescent staining of normal skin samples with antibodies against T-cadherin (red) and vWF (green) (A, E) or vWF (red) and α–actin (green) (C). Figures A, B, C represent parallel frozen sections of the same sample. T-cadherin expression was detected in basal keratinocytes, suprabasal layers, stromal cells and in hair follicles and sebaceous glands. Nuclei were counterstained with DAPI (blue). Figure B depicts phase contrast image. Uniform

expression of T-cadherin in small and large blood vessels was noted (yellow), colocalization of T-cadherin and vWF is showed by the arrow. Stabilized vessels were located in derma and were double positive for vWF and α–actin; stromal cells were also α–actin-positive (C). Bars, 100 μm. Figure D represents the diagram explaining strong T-cadherin expression in basal cell layer (red) and stromal cells, moderate T-cadherin expression (pink) in suprabasal layers and T-cadherin expression in all vWF-positive blood vessels (yellow). F figure legend.

Premalignant epithelial lesions are conditions that have certain clinical and histopathological features and are associated with an increased risk of cancer development (Quinn and Perkins, 2010). Premalignant lesions frequently have many histopathological changes in common with invasive cancers; however, this doesn't imply that the premalignat lesions will change into neoplastic process. Therefore, it is important to identify the diagnostic markers which will allow better accuracy in diagnostics of premalignant lesions and cancer and their treatment.

6.1.2 Psoriasis

Psoriasis is a chronic condition that causes keratinocytes proliferate much faster that in normal skin and move to the skin surface forming sharply demarcated erythematous plaques or thick patches (Godic, 2004). Such pathology reflects the abnormal epidermal keratinocyte proliferation and differentiation and delayed apoptosis. Histological characteristics of psoriasis are hyperkeratosis, parakeratosis, acanthosis of the epidermis, tortuous and dilated capillary vessels and an inflammatory infiltrate composed mainly of lymphocytes, which is located in the upper dermis. The underlying mechanism of increased keratinocyte growth remains controversial. It is considered to be genetically determined and have a strong autoimmune component implicating activated T-lymphocytes and excessive production of inflammatory cytokines (Godic, 2004). However, psoriasis is unique because it exhibits excessive but controlled keratinocyte proliferation. Recent study demonstrated that there is downregulation of T-cadherin expression in epidermal keratinocytes in psoriatic samples compared to normal skin. The immunostaining against T-cadherin in psoriasis vulgaris as shown in this paper is restricted to the keratinocyte basal cell layer (Zhou et al., 2003). In contrast, our results indicate that T-cadherin expression in psoriatic skin is comparable to normal skin (Fig.1 and Fig.2). Our data have been acquired at a fixed exposure period and the intensity of the immunifluorescent staining in both types of samples was the same. In psoriatic skin T-cadherin expression was found in all keratinocyte cell layers with a stronger expression in basal keratinocytes than in hyperproliferating suprabasal layers, also in stromal cells and in all blood vessels located in the underlying derma. Strikingly, in contrast to normal skin samples, in psoriatic skin the abnormal location of blood vessels within the epidermal layer was also found (Fig.1 and Fig.2). Noteworthy, these vessels, as verified by endothelial marker vWF, also uniformly expressed T-cadherin (Fig.2).

6.1.3 Actinic Keratosis (AK)

AK is a common sun-induced skin lesion. Actinic keratosis is usually characterized as scaly or keratotic papules with a diffuse erythematous base, usually less than 1-2 cm in diameter. Historically, AK has been described as a pre-cancerous lesion (Quinn and Perkins, 2010). Many authors consider these lesions as pre-malignant epithelial tumors that have the potential to develop into squamous cell carcinoma (SCC) (Epstein, 2004; Jorizzo et al., 2004; Yu et al., 2003). However, a number of studies indicate that progression of AK to invasive SCC may be rather exception than a rule and that AKs can undergo spontaneous regression

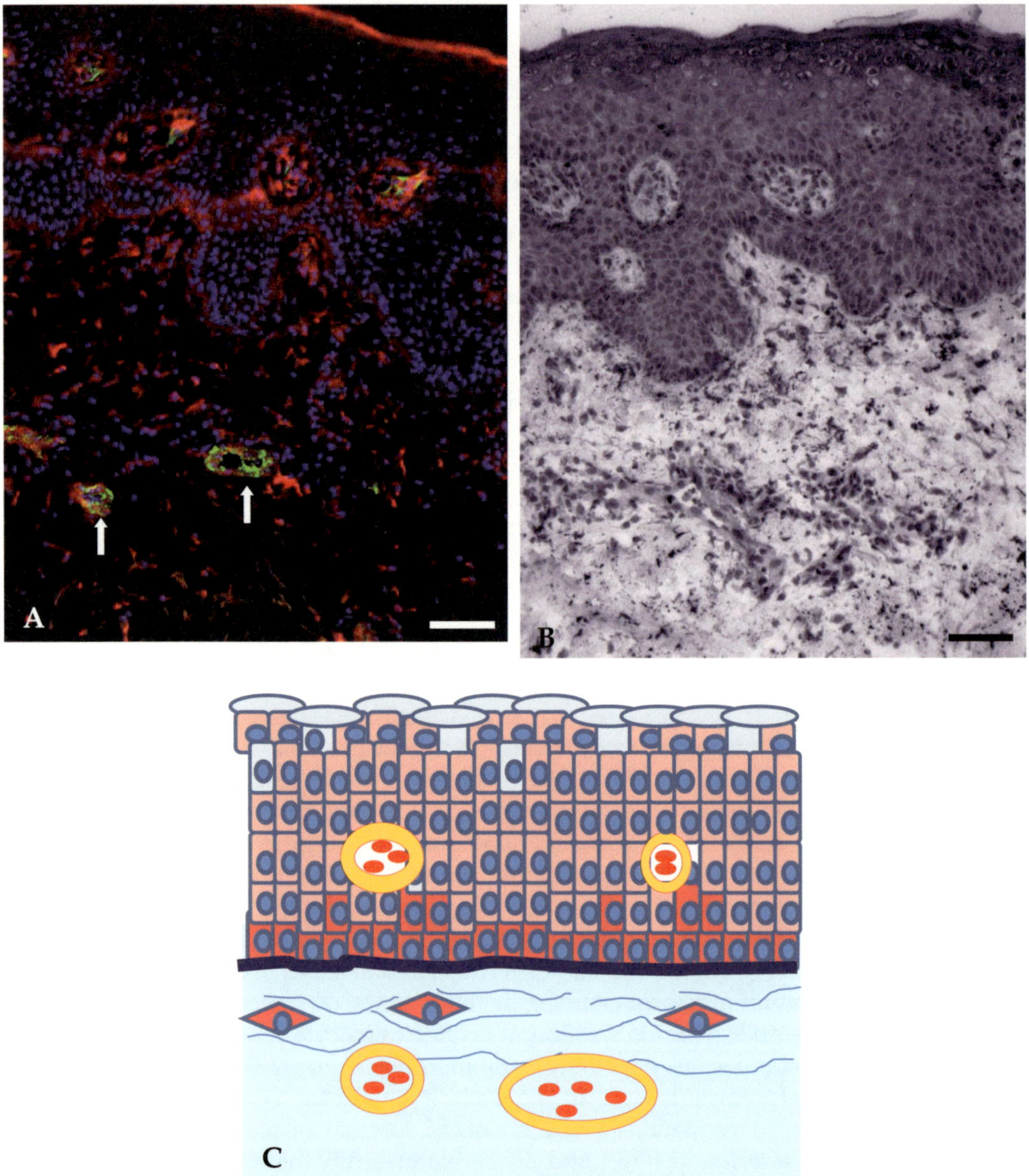

Fig. 2. Double immunofluorescent staining of psoriatic skin sample with antibodies against T-cadherin (red) and vWF (green) (A). Nuclei were counterstained with DAPI (blue). Figure B represents hematoxylin staining of the parallel section. Strong T-cadherin expression was found in basal keratinocytes, in hyperproliferating suprabasal layers, stromal cells and blood vessels located in the underlying derma and within the epidermal layer. Uniform expression of T-cadherin in small and large blood vessels was observed (yellow), colocalization of T-cadherin and vWF is showed by the arrows. Bars, 100 μm. The diagram (C) explaining strong T-cadherin expression in basal cell layer (red), moderate T-cadherin expression in suprabasal layers and stromal cells (pink) and T-cadherin expression in all and all vWF-positive blood vessels (yellow).

(as cited in Quinn & Perkins, 2010). Other authors have stated that there is no patho-biological difference between AK and SCC and that AK itself represents SCC variant (Ackerman & Mones, 2006; Freeman et al., 1984; Lebwohl et al., 2004). Without treatment, AK can develop into invasive SCC and has the potential to metastasise and cause death.

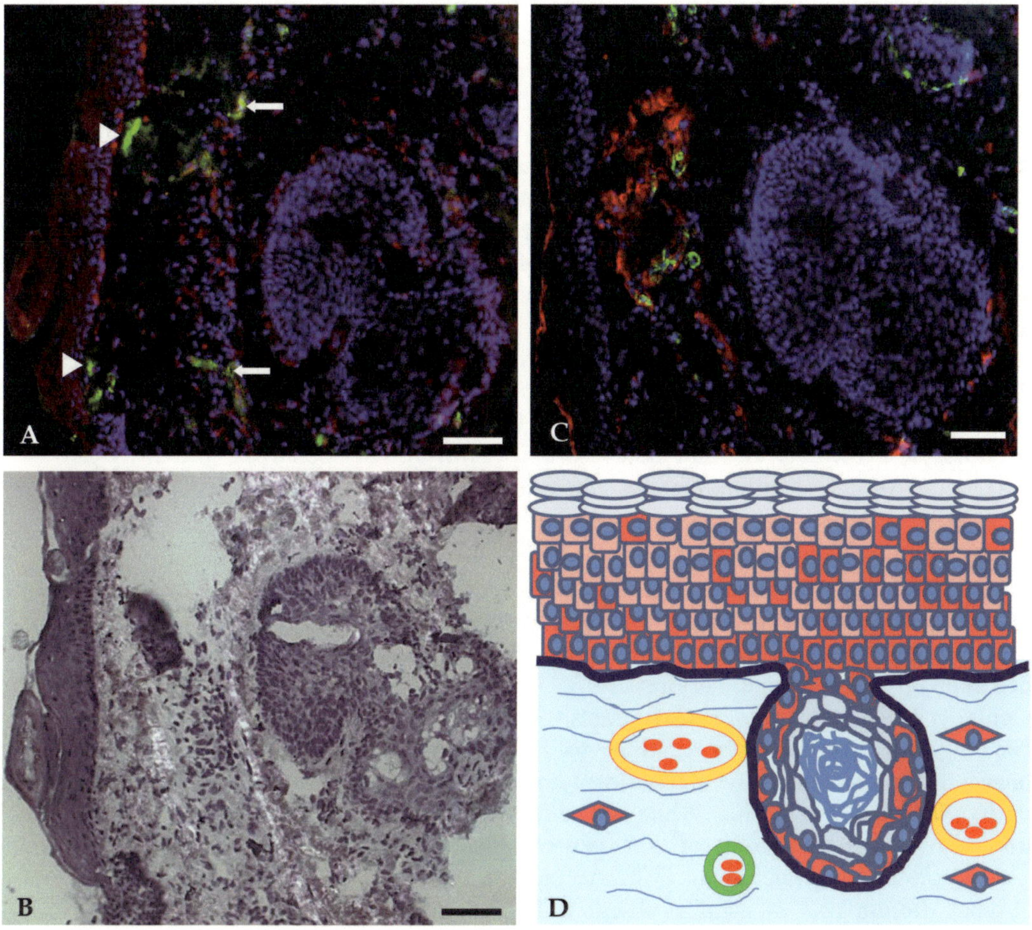

Fig. 3. Double immunofluorescent staining of actinic keratosis sample with antibodies against T-cadherin (red) and vWF (green) (A) or vWF (green) and α–actin (red) (C). Nuclei were counterstained with DAPI (blue). Figure B represents hematoxylin staining of the parallel section. T-cadherin expression was observed in basal keratinocytes, including suprabasal layers, with a more pronounced staining in the basal cell layer. Not all blood vessels as detected by vWF staining were positive for T-cadherin. Colocalization of T-cadherin and vWF is shown by the arrows, blood vessels which do not express T-cadherin - by arrowheads. Stabilized vessels were located in derma and were double positive for vWF and α–actin; (C). Bars, 100 μm. The diagram (D) explaining strong T-cadherin expression in basal cell layer (red), moderate T-cadherin expression in suprabasal layers and stromal cells (pink). Blood vessels expressing T-cadherin and vWF are shown in yellow, blood vessels with no T-cadherin expression are shown in green.

In AK the boundary between unaffected and affected epidermis is sharp. The affected zone grows under the normal epidermis and around the ductal epithelium. Histologically, AK is characterized by the presence of atypical keratinocytes at the epidermal basal cell layer, which in advanced lesions may extend into the entire epidermis (Röwert-Huber et al., 2007). There is epidermal hypertrophy with hyperkeratosis and parakeratosis. The basement membrane is intact but basaloid cells may form multiple buds. Within the epidermis there may be a simple dysplasia or a range of abnormalities. The underlying papillary vessels are irregularly increased. There is degeneration of dermal collagen and deposition of material staining like elastin in the upper half of the dermis (Quinn & Perkins, 2010). In addition to the epidermal changes, a common feature of AK is the presence of a chronic inflammation in the papillary dermis of the abnormal epidermis (Pinkus et al., 1963).
Figure 3 presents the hematoxylin and immunofluorescent stainings of AK sections with antibody against T-cadherin, vWF and α–actin. The lesion is characterized by the presence of atypical keratinocytes at the epidermal basal cell layer and loss of orderly maturation of keratinocytes. The affected zone has grown under the epidermis and is separated from it by the cleft. T-cadherin is uniformly expressed in all layers of keratinocytes, including suprabasal layers, with a slightly increased staining in the basal cell layer (Fig.3), which correlates with literature data (Pfaff et al., 2010). T-cadherin expression was also verified in the dermal blood vessels (in endothelial and mural cells) and in the stromal cells, in the vicinity of atypical keratinocytes. However, not all blood vessels which were vWF positive expressed T-cadherin, which puts AK in line with malignant skin lesions such as squamous cells carcinoma (Fig.6).

6.1.4 Keratoacanthoma (KA)

Keratoacanthoma (KA) is a low-grade malignancy skin lesion with rapid growth, followed by a slow spontaneous resolution. KA is composed of keratinizing squamous cells originating in pilosebaceous follicles and histopathologically resembles squamous cells carcinoma (SCC) (Quinn & Perkins, 2010). However, it is well known that the morphological similarity between KA and SCC contrasts with their different biological behavior.
Histologically, the squamous keratinocytes in KAs are enlarged, pale, eosinophilic, and often have a hyalinized or "glassy"-appearing cytoplasm. Inflammatory infiltrates are present in the underlying papillary dermis. While superficially infiltrative and mitotically active, especially in early lesions, the cells of KA generally show no pronounced atypia or cellular pleomorphism of conventional SCC. Atypical mitoses are not found in KA. Additionally, stromal desmoplasia is usually absent unlike invasive SCC, and the nests are typically rounded and sharply demarcated from the surrounding stroma (Cassarino et al., 2006b).
SCC is a malignant tumor with the potential to grow, metastasize and cause death, while KA usually undergoes regression, thus representing a self-limiting or "biologically benign" variant of SCC (Zalaudek et al., 2009). KA progression could be divided into 3 phases: growth, stabilization and involution. The first phase is characterized by a rapid increase in size within a few weeks or months followed by stabilization and spontaneous resolution over 4-6 months. However, occasionally KA may enlarge up to 5 cm and become locally aggressive (Quinn & Perkins, 2010). Lesions typically begin as firm skin papules that progress to nodules with a central crateriform ulceration or keratin plug that may project like a horn. The histological features vary with the stage of evolution. The early lesion is composed of a mass of rapidly proliferating squamous cells. The marginal cells aggressively invade the surrounding derma, while those in the center keratinize to form a core of keratin that communicates with the surface. Resolution occurs through maturation of the hyperplastic cell masses and lesion

opening to the surface. When the horn is finally shed, the irregular epithelium under the lesion is formed. KA leaves a residual scar, if not excised (Quinn & Perkins, 2010).

Figure 4 and Figure 5 represents KA in the stage of growth and stabilization, correspondingly. As a whole, our histological data indicate that the cells in KA are mature and the epithelium exhibit differentiation from the basal layer to the surface keratinocytes.

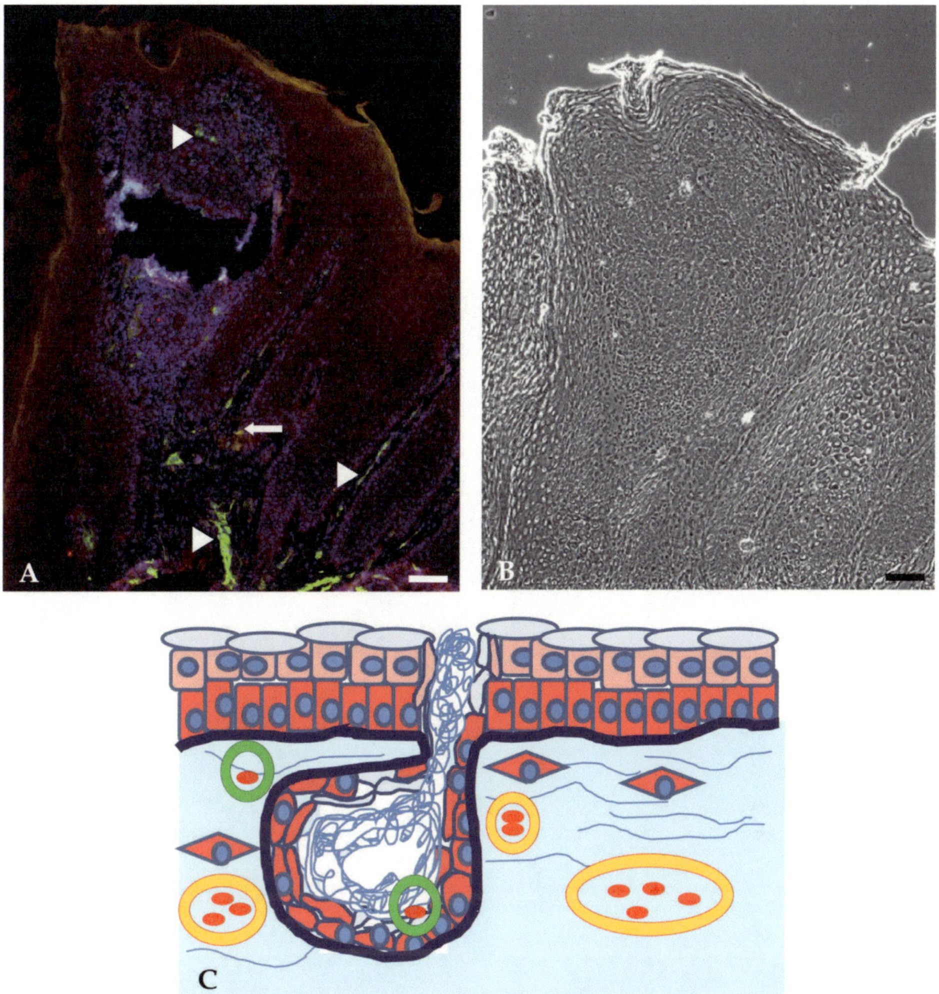

Fig. 4. Double immunofluorescent staining of keratoacanthoma at the stage of growth with antibodies against T-cadherin (red) and vWF (green) (A). Nuclei were counterstained with DAPI (blue). Figure B depicts phase contrast image of the parallel section. T-cadherin expression was verified in all keratinocytes. Part of the blood vessels showed no T-cadherin expression, at the same time some of the blood vessels were found among keratinizing squamous cells at the site of the future pearl (A). Colocalization of T-cadherin and vWF is shown by the arrow, blood vessels which do not express T-cadherin are marked by arrowheads. Bars, 100 μm. The diagram shows strong (red) and moderate (pink) T-cadherin expression in keratinocytes. Blood vessels expressing T-cadherin and vWF are shown in yellow, blood vessels with no T-cadherin expression are shown in green.

However, abnormal or premature keratin production (dyskeratosis) is observed resulting in individually keratizing cells or formation of keratin pearls (Fig.5). The stroma is vascular and infiltrated (Fig.4 and Fig.5). In KA T-cadherin expression was verified in all keratinocyte layers (Fig.4 and Fig.5). At stabilization stage of KA, T-cadherin expression was detected in all the surrounding blood vessels as verified by immunofluorescent staining with antibody against T-cadherin, endothelial marker vWF and mural cell marker - α–actin (Fig.5). However, part of the blood vessels in KA at the growth stage did not express T-cadherin (Fig.4). Noteworthy, is the abnormal location of blood vessels within the epidermal hypertrophied layer and among keratinizing squamous cells at the site of the future pearl (Fig.4). The abnormal vessel location and down-regulated T-cadherin expression in KA at the growth stage most probably reflects the rapid and locally aggressive behavior of the tumor, while at stabilization stage, T-cadherin expression in keratinocytes and blood vessels resembles their expression in the normal skin samples.

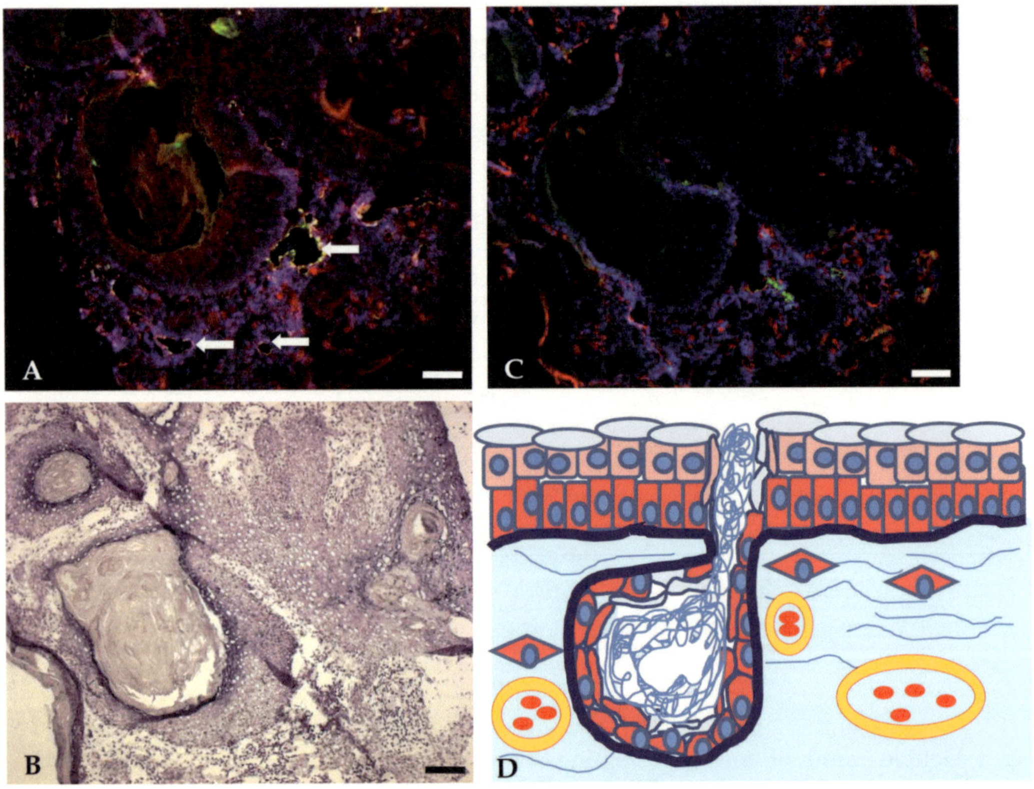

Fig. 5. Double immunofluorescent staining of keratoacanthoma at stabilization stage with antibodies against T-cadherin (red) and vWF (green) (A) or vWF (green) and α–actin (red) (C). Nuclei were counterstained with DAPI (blue). Figure B represents hematoxylin staining of the parallel section. T-cadherin expression was verified in all keratinocytes. Most of the blood vessels showed colocalization of vWF and T-cadherin expression, as shown by the arrows (A). Stabilized vessels were located in derma and were double positive for vWF and α–actin. Bars, 100 μm. The diagram shows strong (red) and moderate (pink) T-cadherin expression in keratinocytes. Blood vessels expressing T-cadherin and vWF are shown in yellow.

6.1.5 Basal Cell Carcinoma (BCC)

BCC is the most common malignant tumor of the skin composed of cells originating from the basal cell layer of the epidermis and its appendages, namely BCCs arise from the hair follicle bulge stem cell or from the interfollicular epidermis (Quinn & Perkins, 2010; Wang et al., 2011). The typical BCC progresses slowly and rarely metastases. The early tumors are usually small, translucent or pearly and covered by thin epidermis. The more advanced tumors show a variety of forms. Some tumors grow at a very slow rate and they are in practical terms benign. This is true for many superficial lesions and some of the nodular types of BCCs (Quinn & Perkins, 2010). BCCs are truly invasive in only a small proportion of cases. Then the tumors show no tendency to grow as rounded masses, have no palisade or organized stroma, and penetrate the dermis and deeper structures, destroying them as they grow. Such tumors are almost always ulcerated, usually from an early stage (Quinn & Perkins, 2010).

In the present study we examined T-cadherin expression in superficial, nodular and infiltrative samples of BBC. In superficial BCC, expression of T-cadherin was prominent in tumor cells and in the surrounding stroma. The majority of vessels around the tumor aggregates coexpressed markers of endothelial cells vWF and T-cadherin, however, blood vessels with no expression of T-cadherin were also noted (Fig. 6).

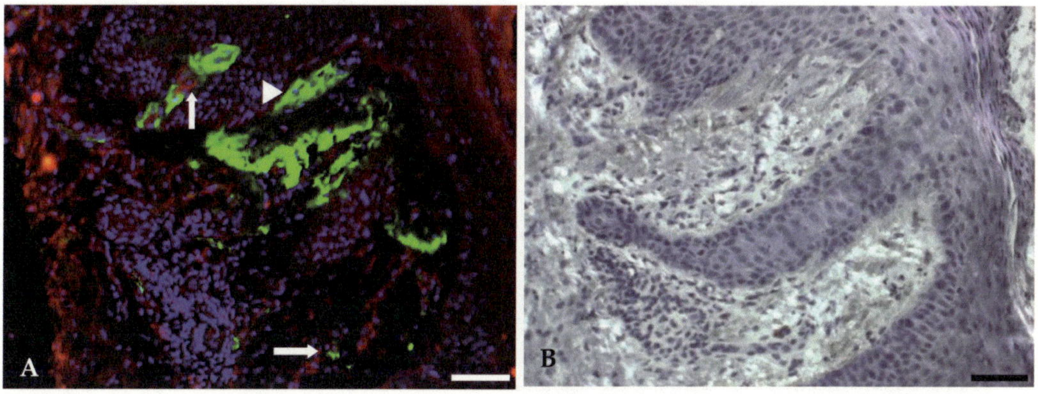

Fig. 6. Double immunofluorescent staining of superficial BCC with antibodies against T-cadherin (red) and vWF (green) (A). Nuclei were counterstained with DAPI (blue). Figure B shows hematoxylin staining of the parallel section. T-cadherin expression was observed in tumor cells and in the surrounding stroma. Not all blood vessels as detected by vWF staining were positive for T-cadherin. Colocalization of T-cadherin and vWF is shown by the arrows, blood vessels which do not express T-cadherin - by arrowhead. Bars, 100 μm.

The nodular BCC samples demonstrated "classic" features of basalioma, including large tumor nests with a smooth palisaded border and stromal retraction. In nodular BCC the expression of T-cadherin was heterogeneous: some tumor nests were strongly positive for T-cadherin expression (Fig. 7), while weak or undetectable expression of T-cadherin occurred in some tumor nests or individual cells within these nests (Fig. 7). These results coincide with the results obtained by other authors (Buechner et al., 2009), but are in contrast to data obtained by Takeuchi and colleagues (Takeuchi et al., 2002). Most of the blood vessels coexpressed endothelial cells marker vWF and T-cadherin. However, in some samples of nodular BCC, the aberrant expression of vessel markers and T-cadherin was revealed: in part of vWF-positive vessels T-cadherin expression was lost; while structures, morphologically resembling

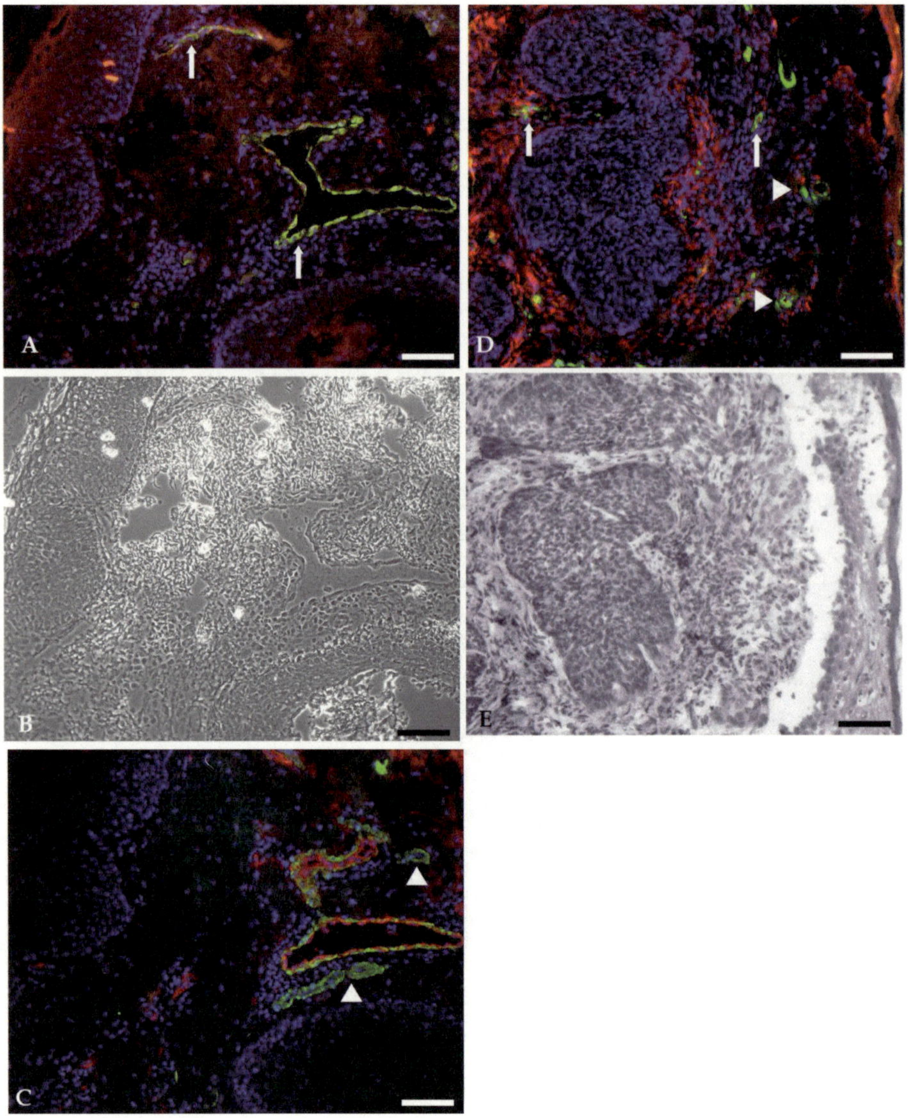

Fig. 7. Double immunofluorescent staining of nodular BCCs with antibodies against T-cadherin (red) and vWF (green) (A, D) or vWF (red) and α–actin (green) (C). Nuclei were counterstained with DAPI (blue). Figure E shows hematoxylin staining the parallel section of the same sample shown in Figure D; Figure B reflects phase contrast image of the parallel section of the same sample shown in Figures A and C. Some tumor nests were T-cadherin positive (A), while other nodules or individual cells within them demonstrated weak T-cadherin expression (D). Most of the blood vessels coexpressed endothelial cells marker vWF and T-cadherin as shown by the arrows in A and D. However, in some samples, the aberrant expression of vessel markers and T-cadherin was revealed: in part of vWF-positive vessels T-cadherin expression was lost (arrowhead pointing to the vessels in A and D); while some samples structures, morphologically resembling blood vessels and expressing α–actin but vWF-negative were observed (arrowhead in C). Bars, 100 μm.

blood vessels and expressing α–actin were vWF-negative (Fig. 7). In samples of infiltrating BCC, nests of variable size with irregular borders were detected. There was frequently little palisading and sometimes no stromal retraction. Tumor cells and cells of the surrounding stroma expressed T-cadherin, while in the blood vessels located among the stromal cells, aberrant vessel markers and T-cadherin was marked: in part of vWF-positive vessels T-cadherin expression was lost (Fig. 8). While T-cadherin expression was present in keratinocytes in 90% of the samples, in the vessels surrounding BCC nests, its expression was lost in part of the blood vessels.

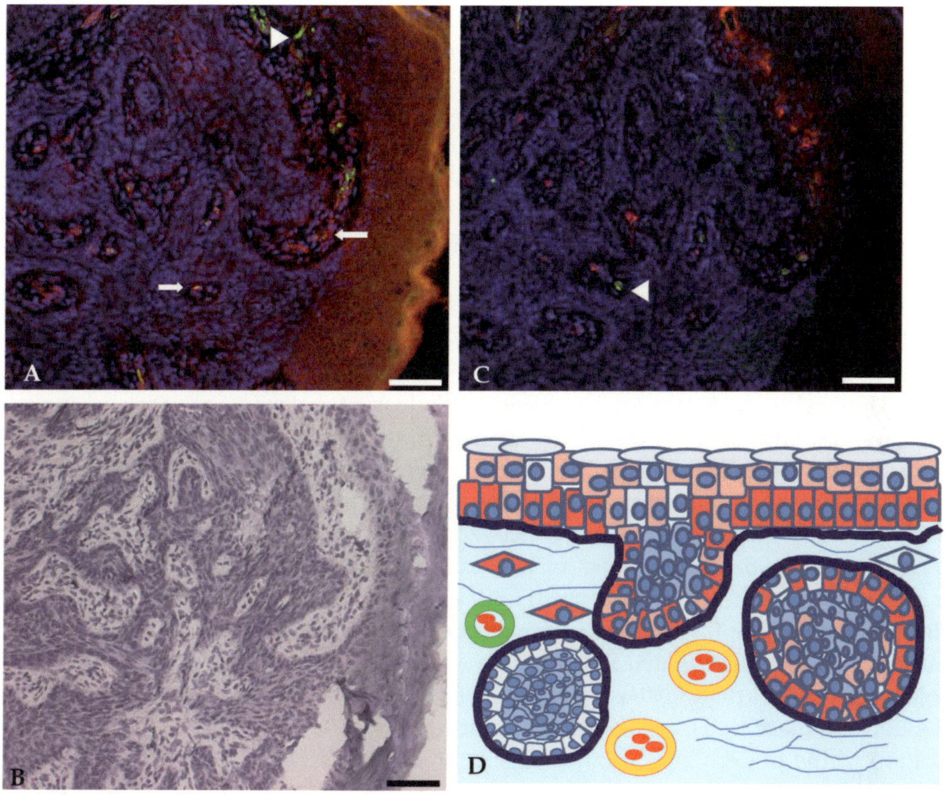

Fig. 8. Double immunofluorescent staining of infiltrating BCC sample with antibodies against T-cadherin (red) and vWF (green) (A) or vWF (red) and α–actin (green) (C). Nuclei were counterstained with DAPI (blue). Figure B shows hematoxylin staining of the parallel section. T-cadherin expression was observed in tumor cells and in the surrounding stroma. In part of vWF-positive blood vessels located among the stromal cells T-cadherin expression was noted (arrows in A). However, in some vessel-like structures aberrant expression of vessel markers and T-cadherin was observed: in part of vWF-positive vessels T-cadherin expression was not detected (arrowheads in A); while in some samples, structures, morphologically resembling blood vessels and expressing α–actin were demonstrated to be vWF-negative (arrowheads in C). Bars, 100 μm. The diagram shows strong T-cadherin expression in red and moderate - in pink. Some of the tumor cells in BCC nests retain T-cadherin expression, while in the others T-cadherin is lost. Blood vessels expressing T-cadherin and vWF are shown in yellow, blood vessels with no T-cadherin expression are shown in green.

6.1.6 Squamous Cell Carcinoma (SCC)

A SCC of the skin is a malignant neoplasm of epidermal keratinocytes and its appendages. Cutaneous SCCs include many subtypes with different clinical behaviors, ranging from indolent to aggressive tumors with significant metastatic potential (Cassarino et al., 2006a; Cassarino et al., 2006b). Various classifications of SCC were proposed basing upon the malignant potential of SCC variants with low, intermediate or high metastatic rate (Cassarino et al., 2006a; Cassarino et al., 2006b; Yanofsky et al., 2011). According to the latest classification, histopathologically SCC can be divided into three separate categories including: actinic or solar keratoses (AKs) and SCC *in situ* (Bowen's disease), - common precursors of SCC arising from excessive sun exposure; invasive SCC (SCCI), clear-cell SCC, spindle cell (sarcomatoid) SCC, and SCC with single cell infiltrates - tumor subtypes emerging from invasive progression of AKs and SCC *in situ; de novo* SCC, lymphoepithelioma-like carcinoma of the skin (LELCS), and verrucous carcinoma (VC) - very rare variants of SCC with no direct correlation to sun exposure or actinic neoplasms (Yanofsky et al., 2011).

SCCIs are often referred to as conventional SCCs. SCCI are subdivided into three histological grades based on their associated degree of nuclear atypia and keratinization (well-differentiated, moderate and poorly-differentiated SCCI). The majority of SCCI's arising from AKs, are well-differentiated tumors, containing slightly enlarged cells with hyperchromatic nuclei, which produce large amounts of keratin, resulting in the formation of keratin pearls. These tumors are associated with a very low malignant potential. The histological and cytopathological changes seen in the individual cells of AK and SCCI are identical. Both show atypical keratinocytes with loss of polarity, nuclear pleomorphism, disordered maturation and increased numbers of mitotic figures; many of them atypical and pleomorphic. In contrast to AK, SCCI are characterized by the presence of infiltrative cells passing through the basement membrane into the dermis. This infiltrate can be difficult to detect at the early stages of invasion, however, additional indicators such as full thickness epidermal atypia or the involvement of hair follicles can be used to facilitate the diagnosis. Later stages of invasion are characterized by the formation of nests of atypical tumor cells in the dermis often with inflammatory infiltrate (Yanofsky et al., 2011).

In contrast to well-differentiated SCCI, in poor-differentiated tumors, cells are characterized by enlarged, pleomorphic nuclei with high degree of atypia and frequent mitosis. Keratin production in these cells is markedly reduced. Poorly-differentiated SCCI show deep infiltration of the underlying dermis and subcutaneous tissues. These SCCI demonstrate a much more aggressive clinical behavior, with an increased rate of metastasis and recurrence. A third, moderately-differentiated subtype of SCCI shares the features of both well-differentiated and poor-differentiated tumors (Yanofsky et al., 2011). It is thought that poorly differentiated tumors have a higher rate of metastasis (Dinehart et al., 1997; Dinehart & Pollack, 1989; Lund et al., 1984). Another essential component in assessing the malignant potential of a tumor is the presence of perineural and perivascular spread. Invasion of capillaries and nerves reflects a more aggressive tumor behavior and correlates with an increased rate of metastases, local recurrence and disease-specific death (Yanofsky et al., 2011). The accurate microscopy diagnostics between these variants is critically important for prognosis and the treatment of SCCI (Yanofsky et al., 2011).

In our study in moderate-to-poorly-differentiated SCCI samples tumor cells deeply invaded the underlying dermis (Fig.9). Occasionally, some atypical cells in isolated tumor nests and stromal cells exhibited week T-cadherin staining. However, in basaloid cells of most of the tumor nests T-cadherin expression was down-regulated. The activated stroma expressed α–actin.

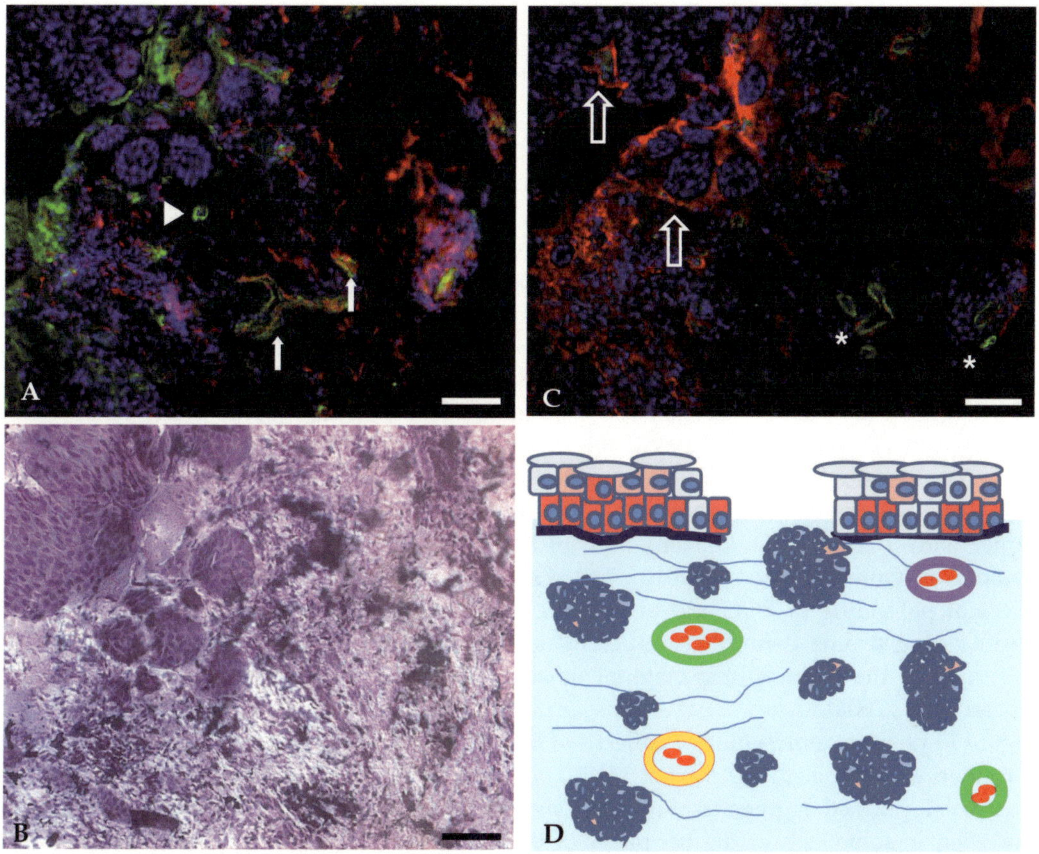

Fig. 9. Double immunofluorescent staining of moderate-to-poorly-differentiated SCCI sample with antibodies against T-cadherin (red) and vWF (green) (A) or CD31 (red) and α–actin (green) (C). Nuclei were counterstained with DAPI (blue). Figure B shows hematoxylin staining of the parallel section. Some atypical cells in isolated tumor nests and stromal cells exhibited T-cadherin staining (A), however, basaloid cells in most of the tumor nests show no T-cadherin expression (A). Vessel-like structures, which do not express CD31 but exhibit α–actin are noted (asterisk in C), moreover, CD31-positive areas, morphologically different from vessels are also present (empty arrows in C). Bars, 100 μm. The diagram marks strong T-cadherin expression in red, and moderate - in pink. In most tumor cells growing in small aggregates T-cadherin expression is absent. Blood vessels expressing T-cadherin and vWF are shown in yellow, blood vessels with no T-cadherin expression are shown in green. Vessel-like structures expressing α–actin are shown in violet.

This data correlate with results obtained by other authors (Mykoyama et al., 2005; Pfaff et al., 2010; Takeuchi et al., 2002b; Zhou et al., 2003) and indicate that T-cadherin loss due to aberrant methylation of the T-cadherin gene or its deletion correlates with SCC invasive phenotype and potentially more aggressive tumor behavior.
However, our results demonstrated that in SCCI not only T-cadherin expression was lost in atypical keratinocytes. Among other abnormalities the aberrant expression of vessel markers and T-cadherin was noted: in part of vWF-positive vessels T-cadherin expression was lost; at

the same time, we observed vessel-like structures, which did not express vWF but bear T-cadherin or α–actin. Strikingly, CD31/vWF-positive areas, morphologically different from vessels were also noted (Fig.9).

6.1.7 Basosquamous Cell Carcinoma (BSCC) or metatypical basal cell carcinoma

The term basosquamous cell carcinoma is used for tumors that exhibit the features of both BCC and SCC (Garcia et al., 2009). BSCC is not widely discussed in the literature and little attention has been paid to this subtype in recent comprehensive reviews of cutaneous SCC (Cassarino et al., 2006a; Cassarino et al., 2006b). The importance of diagnostics of these tumors is based on the fact that BSCC pathological pattern is associated with a more aggressive behavior and a significantly higher incidence of metastasis than BCC or SCC (Banks et al., 1992; Farmer & Helwig, 1980; Smith & Irons, 1983; Winzenburg et al., 1998). The diagnosis of BSCC is currently based on histological criteria, initially proposed by Wain and coauthors (Wain et al., 1986). BSCCs are characterized by exaggerated nuclear to cytoplasmic ratio of the tumor nests which results in their basaloid appearance. Atypical mitotic figures can be readily visualized (Zbären et al., 2004; Boyd et al., 2011). The cells are larger with a larger paler nucleus than in the classic BCC and have a more eosinophilic cytoplasm (Quinn & Perkins, 2010). The BSCC is characterized by cell aggregates lacking classical palisading of BCC and embedded in a dense and profound fibrous stroma. The surrounding stroma is fibrotic with occasional deposits of hyaline basement membrane in the form of the extracellular material adjacent to tumor aggregates (Sarbia et al., 1997; Zbären et al., 2004).

Figure 10 presents representative patterns of immunostaining of BSCC with antibodies against T-cadherin, endothelial cell marker vWF and smooth muscle/pericyte cell marker α–actin. Tumor cells formed aggregates of different size, which generally lacked T-cadherin expression; however, in some cells at the periphery of these aggregates T-cadherin expression was still observed (Fig. 10). Tumor masses were surrounded by stroma expressing T-cadherin (Fig.10). The majority of vessels around the tumors aggregates coexpressed markers of endothelial cells - vWF and T-cadherin or vWF and α–actin (Fig. 10), thus resembling capillaries and stable blood vessels of the normal skin (Fig. 10). However, structures morphologically resembling blood vessels and expressing T-cadherin or α–actin, but lacking expression of classical endothelial marker vWF was noted (Fig. 10). Alternatively, vWF-positive vessels with no expression of T-cadherin were observed (data not shown).

To summarize, the obtained data confirm the fact that the initially occasional loss of T-cadherin expression in keratinocytes and blood vessels of pre-malignant lesions but subsequently progressive down-regulation of T-cadherin expression in tumor cells, appearance of blood vessels aberrantly expressing T-cadherin and endothelial/mural cell markers of more aggressive tumors correlate with the malignant transformation of the skin neoplasms.

7. Conclusion

The presented data support the statement that the loss of T-cadherin expression in epidermal keratinocytes is biologically relevant to malignant transformation of normal epidermal cells into cancer and correlates with the literature data. It has been proposed that T-cadherin expression may contribute to maintenance of tissue integrity in resting

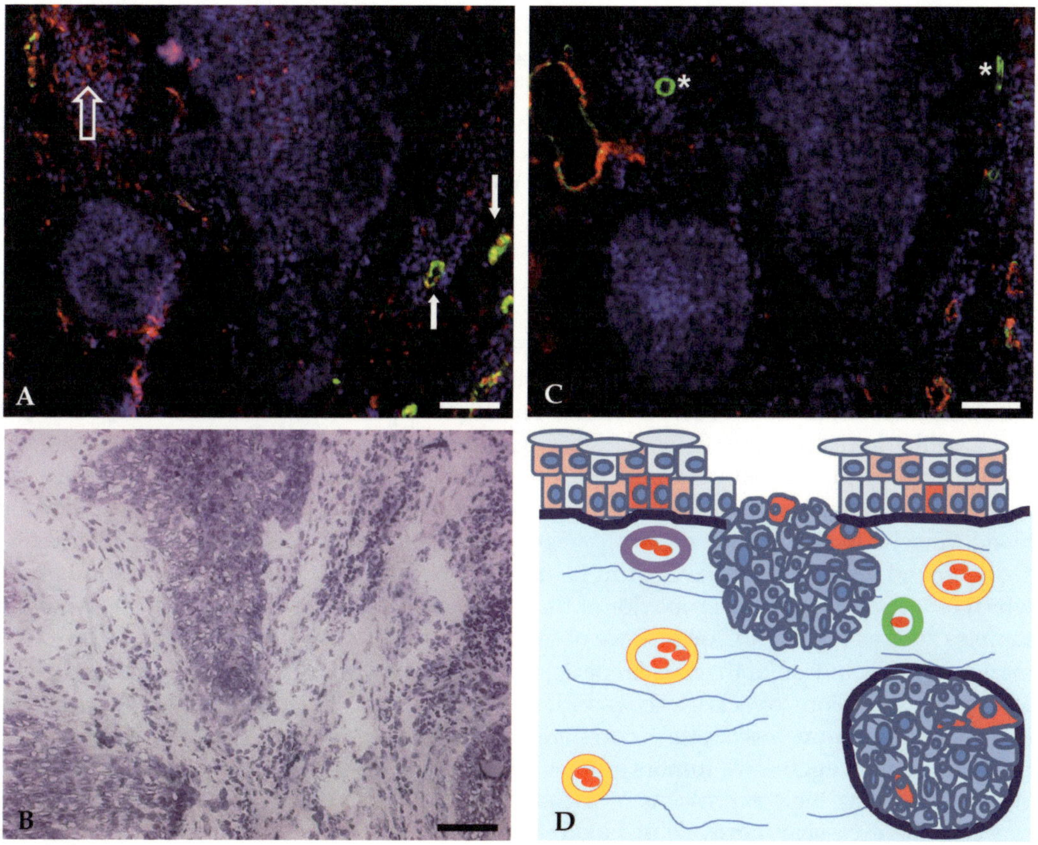

Fig. 10. Double immunofluorescent staining of BSCCs sample with antibodies against T-cadherin (red) and vWF (green) (A) or CD31 (red) and α–actin (green) (C). Nuclei were counterstained with DAPI (blue). Figure B shows hematoxylin staining of the parallel section. Tumor cells formed aggregates of different size, which generally lacked T-cadherin expression, however, in some tumor nests or in cells at the periphery of tumor aggregates T-cadherin expression is still observed (A). The majority of vessels around the tumor aggregates coexpressed markers of endothelial cells - vWF and T-cadherin (arrows in A) or vWF and α–actin (C). However, aberrant expression of vessel markers and T-cadherin could be seen: vessel-like T-cadherin positive structures with no expression of vWF are marked by empty arrow in B and α–actin vessel-like structures with no expression of CD31 by asterisk in C. The diagram marks strong T-cadherin expression in red, and moderate - in pink. In most tumor cells growing in small aggregates T-cadherin expression is absent. Blood vessels expressing T-cadherin and vWF are shown in yellow, blood vessels with no T-cadherin expression are shown in green. Vessel-like structures expressing α–actin are shown in violet.

conditions by preventing cell dislocation (Ivanov et al, 2003), that's why T-cadherin expression is well marked in the basal layer of keratinocytes attached to the basal membrane and bordering with underlying derma.

In the normal skin proliferation takes place in the basal layer of keratinocytes which correlates with the maximal T-cadherin expression in these cells. Interestingly, upon maturation epidermal keratinocyte are moved from the basal cell layer towards skin surface not crossing the layer with the maximal T-cadherin expression. In pre-malignant skin lesions such as KA at stabilization stage, psoriasis, AK and superficial basalioma, which demonstrate slow or controlled growth and, in most cases, where keratinocytes maintain interactions with the basal membrane, the pattern of T-cadherin expression partly resembles that in the normal skin. Upon tumorigenesis in some BSCCs, SCCs, and in some cases of BCC, when tumors are characterized by a higher proliferative, invasive and metastatic potential, keratinocytes tend to grow in smaller cell aggregates and down-regulate T-cadherin expression. It is tempting to speculate that T-cadherin acts as a tumor suppressor in the normal skin and pre-malignant lesions by restricting keratinocyte proliferation and migration and by enhancing their homophilic interactions within the cell layer. In cancer, aggressive behavior of tumor cells correlates with the loss of T-cadherin expression.

In normal skin samples and in pre-malignant lesions such as psoriasis, KA at stabilization stage and superficial BCC all blood vessels uniformly express endothelial cells marker vWF and T-cadherin. Although AK in some papers is regarded as premalignant skin lesion, we revealed that in AK not all vWF-positive blood vessels expressed T-cadherin. This puts AK in line with malignant skin lesions such as SCC where T-cadherin is partly lost from the blood vessels. In KA at the growing stage part of the blood vessels do not express T-cadherin and grow into the layer of hypertrophied and rapidly proliferating keratinocytes, which reflects the aggressive behavior of this tumor at the stage of the fast growth. In cancer samples such as BSCC, BCC or SCC we observed heterogeneity in the expression of vascular markers (vWF and smooth muscle/pericyte cell marker α–actin) and T-cadherin. Thus, aberrant expression of classical vascular markers and heterogeneity in T-cadherin expression in tumor vasculature correlates with the histological features and invasive behavior of more aggressive tumors such as BSCC, BCC or SCC.

We propose that high expression of T-cadherin in normal tissue and in benign tumors prevents the excessive ingrowth of blood vessels that also express T-cadherin. During the tumor transformation, expression of T-cadherin on vascular endothelial cells is disturbed, and this causes abnormality in vascularization of tumor nodules and surrounding stroma.

8. References

Ackerman, A.B. & Mones, J.M. (2006). Solar (actinic) keratosis is squamous cell carcinoma. *British Journal of Dermatology*, Vol.155, No.1, (July 2006), pp. 9–22, ISSN 0007-0963

Adachi, Y.; Takeuchi, T.; Nagayama, T; Ohtsuki, Y. & Furihata, M. (2009). Zeb1-mediated T-cadherin repression increases the invasive potential of gallbladder cancer. *FEBS Letters*, Vol.583, No.2, (January 2009), pp. 430-436, ISSN 0014-5793

Adachi, Y.; Takeuchi, T.; Sonobe, H. & Ohtsuki, Y. (2006). An adiponectin receptor, T-cadherin, was selectively expressed in intratumoral capillary endothelial cells in hepatocellular carcinoma: possible cross talk between T-cadherin and FGF-2 pathways. *Virchows Archiv*, Vol.448, No.3, (March 2006), pp. 311-318, ISSN 0945-6317

Adams, R.H.; Wilkinson, G.A.; Weiss, C.; Diella, F.; Gale, N.W.; Deutsch, U.; Risau, W. & Klein, R. (1999). Roles of ephrinB ligands and EphB receptors in cardiovascular development: demarcation of arterial/venous domains, vascular morphogenesis, and sprouting angiogenesis. *Genes & Development*, Vol.13, No.3, (February 1999), pp. 295-306, ISSN 0890-9369

Andreeva, A.V.; Han, J.; Kutuzov, M.A.; Profirovic, J.; Tkachuk, V.A. & Voyno-Yasenetskaya, T.A. (2010). T-cadherin modulates endothelial barrier function. *Journal of Cellular Physiology*, Vol.223, No.1, (April 2010), pp. 94–102, ISSN 0021-9541

Andreeva, A.V. & Kutuzov, M.A. (2010). Cadherin 13 in cancer. *Genes, Chromosomes and Cancer*, Vol.49, No.9, (September 2010), pp. 775-790, ISSN 1045-2257

Andreeva, A.V.; Kutuzov, M.A.; Tkachuk, V.A. & Voyno-Yasenetskaya, T.A. (2009). T-cadherin is located in the nucleus and centrosomes in endothelial cells. *American Journal of Physiology Cell Physiology*, Vol.297, No.5, (November 2009), pp. C1168–C1177, ISSN 0363-6143

Banks, E.R.; Frierson, H.F.Jr.; Mills, S.E.; George, E.; Zarbo, R.J. & Swanson, P.E. (1992). Basaloid squamous cell carcinoma of the head and neck. A clinicopathologic and immunohistochemical study of 40 cases. *American Journal of Surgical Pathology*, Vol.16, No.10, (October 1992), pp. 939–946, ISSN 0147-5185

Bauer, E.A.; Uitto, J.; Walters, R.C. & Eisen, A.Z. (1979). Enhanced collagenase production by fibroblasts derived from human basal cell carcinomas. *Cancer Research*, Vol.39, No.11, (November 1979), pp. 4594–4599, ISSN 0008-5472

Beckermann, B.M.; Kallifatidis, G.; Groth, A.; Frommhold, D.; Apel, A.; Mattern, J.; Salnikov, A.V.; Moldenhauer, G.; Wagner, W.; Diehlmann, A.; Saffrich, R.; Schubert, M.; Ho, A.D.; Giese, N.; Büchler, M.W.; Friess, H.; Büchler, P. & Herr I. (2008). VEGF expression by mesenchymal stem cells contributes to angiogenesis in pancreatic carcinoma. *British Journal of Cancer*, Vol.99, No.4, (August 2008), pp. 622–631, ISSN 0007-0920

Berx, G. & van Roy, F. (2009). Involvement of members of the cadherin superfamily in cancer. *Cold Spring Harbor Perspectives in Biology*, Vol.1, No.6, (December 2009), pp. 1-27, ISSN 1943-0264

Boyd, A.S.; Stasko, T.S. & Tang, Y.W. (2010). Basaloid squamous cell carcinoma of the skin. *Journal of the American Academy of Dermatology*, Vol.64, No.1, (January 2011), pp. 144-151, ISSN 0190-9622

Brown, D.A. & London, E. (2000). Structure and function of sphingolipid- and cholesterol-rich membrane rafts. *The Journal of Biological Chemistry*, Vol.275, No.23, (June 2000), pp. 17221–17224, ISSN 0021-9258

Buechner, S.A.; Philippova M.; Erne P.; Mathys T. & Resink T.J. (2009) High T-cadherin expression is a feature of basal cell carcinoma. *British Journal of Dermatology*. Vol.161, No.1, (July 2009), pp. 199–202, ISSN 0007-0963

Carmeliet, P. (2000). Mechanisms of angiogenesis and arteriogenesis. *Nature Medicine*, Vol.6, No.4, (April 2000), pp. 389-395, ISSN 1061-4036

Cassarino, D.S.; Derienzo, D.P. & Barr, R.J. (2006a). Cutaneous squamous cell carcinoma: a comprehensive clinicopathologic classification. Part one. *Journal of Cutaneous Pathology*, Vol.33, No.3, (March 2006), pp. 191-206, ISSN 0303-6987

Cassarino, D.S.; Derienzo, D.P. & Barr R.J. (2006b). Cutaneous squamous cell carcinoma: a comprehensive clinicopathologic classification. Part two. *Journal of Cutaneous Pathology*, Vol.33, No.4, (April 2006), pp. 261-279, ISSN 0303-6987

Cavallaro, U.; Liebner, S. & Dejana, E. (2006). Endothelial cadherins and tumor angiogenesis. *Experimental Cell Research*, Vol.312, No.5, (March 2006), pp. 659 - 667, ISSN 0014-4827

Chan, D.W.; Lee, J.M.; Chan, P.C. & Ng, I.O. (2008). Genetic and epigenetic inactivation of T-cadherin in human hepatocellular carcinoma cells. *International Journal of Cancer,* Vol.123, No.5, (September 2008), pp. 1043–1052, ISSN 0020-7136

Chaplin, D.J.; Pettit, G.R. & Hill, S.A. (1999). Antivascular approaches to solid tumour therapy: evaluation of combretastatin A4 phosphate. *Anticancer Research,* Vol.19, No.1A, (February 1999), pp. 189–195, ISSN 0250-7005

Chaplin, D.J.; Pettit, G.R.; Parkins, C.S. & Hill, S.A. (1996). Antivascular approaches to solid tumour therapy: evaluation of tubulin binding agents. *British Journal of Cancer,* Vol.27, (July 1996), pp. S86–S88, ISSN 0007-0920

Denekamp, J. (1993). Review article: angiogenesis, neovascular proliferation and vascular pathophysiology as targets for cancer therapy. *British Journal of Radiology,* Vol.66, No.783, (March 1993), pp. 181–196, ISSN 0007-1285

Dinehart, S. M.; Nelson-Adesokan, P.; Cockerell, C.; Russell, S. & Brown, R. (1997). Metastatic cutaneous squamous cell carcinoma derived from actinic keratosis. *Cancer,* Vol.79, No.5, (March 1997), pp. 920–923, ISSN 1097-0142

Dinehart, S.M. & Pollack, S.V. (1989). Metastases from squamous cell carcinoma of the skin and lip. An analysis of twenty - seven cases. *Journal of the American Academy of Dermatology,* Vol.21, No.2 Pt. 1, (August 1989), pp. 241–248, ISSN 0190-9622

Efimenko, A.Iu.; Starostina, E.E.; Rubina, K.A.; Kalinina, N.I. & Parfenova, E.V. (2010). Viability and angiogenic activity of mesenchymal stromal cells from adipose tissue and bone marrow in hypoxia and inflammation in vitro. *Tsitologiia,* Vol.52, No.2, (February 2010), pp. 144-154, ISSN 0041-3771

Epstein, E. (2004). Quantifying actinic keratosis: assessing the evidence. *American Journal of Clinical Dermatology,* Vol.5, No.3, (2004), pp. 141–144, ISSN 1175-0561

Farmer, E.R. & Helwig, E.B. (1980). Metastatic basal cell carcinoma: a clinicopathologic study of seventeen cases. *Cancer,* Vol.46, No.4, (August 1980), pp. 748–757, ISSN 1097-0142

Folkman J. Tumor Angiogenesis: from Bench to Bedside (2008). *Tumor Angiogenesis. Basic Mechanisms and Cancer Therapy, pp. 3-28,* ISBN 978-3-540-33176-6

Folkman, J. (1995). Angiogenesis in cancer, vascular, rheumatoid and other diseases. *Nature Medicine,* Vol.1, No.1, (January 1995), pp. 37–31, ISSN 1061-4036

Fredette, B.J.; Miller, J. & Ranscht, B. (1996). Inhibition of motor axon growth by T-cadherin substrata. *Development,* Vol.122, No.10, (October 1996), pp. 3163-3171, ISSN 1011-6370

Freeman, R.G.; Barr, R.J. & Elder, D.E. (1984). What is the boundary that separates a thick actinic keratosis from a thin squamous-cell carcinoma? *The American Journal of Dermatopathology,* Vol.6, (1984), pp. 301–306, ISSN 0193-1091

Garcia, C.; Poletti, E. & Crowson, A.N. (2009). Basosquamous carcinoma. *Journal of the American Academy of Dermatology,* Vol.60, No.1, (January 2009), pp. 137-143, ISSN 0190-9622

Ghosh, S.; Joshi, M.B.; Ivanov, D.; Feder-Mengus, C.; Spagnoli, G.C.; Martin, I.; Erne, P. & Resink, T.J. (2007). Use of multicellular tumor spheroids to dissect endothelial cell-tumor cell interactions: a role for T-cadherin in tumor angiogenesis. *FEBS Letters,* Vol.581, No.23, (September 2007), pp. 4523-4528, ISSN 0014-5793

Gloushankova, N.A. (2008). Changes in regulation of cell-cell adhesion during tumor transformation. *Biochemistry (Moscow)*, Vol.73, No.7, (July 2008), pp. 742-750, ISSN 0006-2979

Godic, A. (2004). New approaches to psoriasis treatment. A review. *Acta Dermatovenerologica. ALPINA*, Vol.13, No.2, (2004), pp. 50-57, ISSN 1318-4458

Gumbiner, B.M. (2005). Regulation of cadherin-mediated adhesion in morphogenesis. *Nature Reviews Molecular Cell Biology*, Vol.6, No.8, (August 2005), pp. 622-634, ISSN 1471-0072

Gutmann, D.H.; Wu, Y.L.; Hedrick, N.M.; Zhu, Y.; Guha, A. & Parada, L.F. (2001). Heterozygosity for the neurofibromatosis 1 (NF1) tumor suppressor results in abnormalities in cell attachment, spreading and motility in astrocytes. *Human Molecular Genetics*, Vol.10, No.26, (December 2001), pp. 3009-3016, ISSN 0964-6906

Hanahan, D. & Folkman, J. (1996). Patterns and emerging mechanisms of the angiogenic switch during tumorigenesis. *Cell*, Vol.86, No.3, (August 1996), pp. 353–364, ISSN 0092-8674

Hasan, J.; Byers, R. & Jayson, G.C. (2002). Intra-tumoural microvessel density in human solid tumours. *British Journal of Cancer*, Vol.86, No.10, (May 2002) pp. 1566-1577, ISSN 0007-0920

Hebbard, L.W.; Garlatti, M.; Young, L.J.; Cardiff, R.D.; Oshima, R.G. & Ranscht, B. (2008). T-cadherin supports angiogenesis and adiponectin association with the vasculature in a mouse mammary tumor model. *Cancer Research*, Vol.68, No.5, (March 2008), pp. 1407-1416, ISSN 0008-5472

Holmgren, L.; O'Reilly, M.S. & Folkman, J. (1995). Dormancy of micrometastases: balanced proliferation and apoptosis in the presence of angiogenesis suppression. *Nature Medicine*, Vol.1, No.2, (February 1995), pp. 149-153, ISSN 1061-4036

Huang, Z.Y.; Wu, Y.; Hedrick, N. & Gutmann, D.H. (2003). T-cadherin-mediated cell growth regulation involves G_2 phase arrest and requires p21 (CIP1/WAF1) expression. *Molecular and Cellular Biology*, Vol.23, No.2, (January 2003), pp. 566-578, ISSN 0270-7306

Ivanov, D.; Philippova, M.; Allenspach, R.; Erne, P. & Resink, T. (2004). T-cadherin upregulation correlates with cell-cycle progression and promotes proliferation of vascular cells. *Cardiovascular Research*, Vol.64, No.1, (October 2004), pp. 132–143, ISSN 0008-6363

Ivanov, D.; Philippova, M.; Antropova, J.; Gubaeva, F.; Iljinskaya, O.; Tararak, E.; Bochkov, V.; Erne, P.; Resink, T. & Tkachuk, V. (2001). Expression of cell adhesion molecule T-cadherin in the human vasculature. *Histochemistry and Cell Biology*, Vol.115, No.3, (March 2001), pp. 231- 242, ISSN 0948-6143

Ivanov, D.; Philippova, M.; Tkachuk, V.; Erne, P. & Resink, T. (2003). Cell adhesion molecule T-cadherin regulates vascular cell adhesion, phenotype and motility. *Experimental Cell Research*, Vol.293, No.2, (February 2004), pp. 207-218, ISSN 0014-4827

Jain, R.K. & Carmeliet, P.F. (2001). Vessels of death or life. *Scientific American*, Vol.285, No.6, (December 2001), pp. 38-45, ISSN 0036-8733

Jorizzo, J.L.; Carney, P.S.; Ko, W.T.; Robins, P.; Weinkle, S.H. & Werschler, W.P. (2004). Treatment options in the management of actinic keratosis. *Cutis*, Vol.74, No.6 Suppl, (December 2004), pp. 9–17, ISSN 0011-4162

Joshi, M.B.; Philippova, M.; Ivanov, D.; Allenspach, R.; Erne P. & Resink, T.J. (2005). T-cadherin protects endothelial cells from oxidative stress0induced apoptosis. *FASEB Journal*, Vol.19. No.12, (October 2005), pp. 1737-1739, ISSN 0892-6638

Keehn, C.A.; Smoller, B.R. & Morgan, M.B. (2004). Ets-1 immunohistochemical expression in non-melanoma skin carcinoma. *Journal of Cutaneous Pathology*, Vol.31, No.1, (January 2004), pp. 8-13, ISSN 0303-6987

Kinnaird, T.; Stabile, E.; Burnett, M.S.; Lee, C.W.; Barr, S.; Fuchs, S. & Epstein, S.E. (2004). Marrow-derived stromal cells express genes encoding a broad spectrum of arteriogenic cytokines and promote in vitro and in vivo arteriogenesis through paracrine mechanisms. *Circulation Research*, Vol.94, No.5, (March 2004), pp. 678–685, ISSN 0009-7330

Kipmen-Korgun, D.; Osibow, K.; Zoratti, C.; Schraml, E.; Greilberger, J.; Kostner, G.M.; Jürgens, G. & Graier, W.F. (2005). T-cadherin mediates low-density lipoprotein-initiated cell proliferation via the Ca(2+)-tyrosine kinase-Erk1/2 pathway. *Journal of Cardiovascular Pharmacology*, Vol.45, No.5, (May 2005), pp. 418-430, ISSN 0160-2446

Klopp, A.H.; Gupta, A.; Spaeth, E.; Andreeff, M. & Marini, F. (2011). Concise Review: Dissecting a Discrepancy in the Literature: Do Mesenchymal Stem Cells Support or Suppress Tumor Growth? *Stem Cells*, Vol.29, No.1, (January 2011), pp. 11–19, ISSN 1066-5099

Knudson, W.; Biswas, C. & Toole, B.P. (1984). Interactions between human tumor cells and fibroblasts stimulate hyaluronate synthesis. *Proceedings of the National Academy of Sciences of the United States of America*, Vol.81, No.21, (November 1984), pp. 6767–6771, ISSN 0027-8424

Kossard, S; Epstein, E.H. & Cerio, R. (2006). Basal cell carcinoma, In: *World Health Organization Classification of Tumours. Pathology and Genetics: Skin Tumours*, LeBoit P.E., Burg G., Weedon D., Sarasin A., pp. 13-19, IARC Press, ISBN 92-832-2417-5, Lyon, France

Kuphal, S.; Martyn, A.C.; Pedley, J.; Crowther, L.M.; Bonazzi, V.F.; Parsons, P.G.; Bosserhoff, A.K.; Hayward, N.K. & Boyle, G.M. (2009). H-cadherin expression reduces invasion of malignant melanoma. *Pigment Cell and Melanoma Research*, Vol.22, No.3, (June 2009), pp. 296-306, ISSN 1755-1471

Kurzen, H.; Münzing, I. & Hartschuh, W. (2003). Expression of desmosomal proteins in squamous cell carcinomas of the skin. *Journal of Cutaneous Pathology*, Vol.30, No.10, (November 2003), pp. 621-630, ISSN 0303-6987

Laskin, W.B. & Miettinen, M. (2003). Epithelioid sarcoma: new insights based on an extended immunohistochemical analysis. *Archives of Pathology & Laboratory Medicine*, Vol.127, No.9, (September 2003), pp. 1161-1168, ISSN 0003-9985

Lebwohl, M.; Dinehart, S.; Whiting, D.; Lee, P.K.; Tawfik, N.; Jorizzo, J.; Lee, J.H. & Fox, T.L. (2004). Imiquimod 5% cream for the treatment of actinic keratosis: results from two phase III, randomized, double-blind, parallel-group, vehicle-controlled trials. *Journal of the American Academy of Dermatology*, Vol.50, No.5, (May 2004), pp. 714–721, ISSN 0190-9622

Lee, S.W. (1996). H-cadherin, a novel cadherin with growth inhibitory functions and diminished expression in human breast cancer. *Nature Medicine*, Vol.2, No.7, (July 1996), pp. 776-782, ISSN 1061-4036

Lee, S.W.; Reimer, C.L.; Campbell, D.B.; Cheresh, P.; Duda, R.B. & Kocher, O. (1998). H-cadherin expression inhibits in vitro invasiveness and tumor formation in vivo. *Carcinogenesis*, Vol.19, No.6, (June 1998), pp. 1157-1159, ISSN 0143-3334

Lund, H.Z. (1984). Metastasis from sun-induced squamous-cell carcinoma of the skin: an uncommon event. *The Journal of Dermatologic Surgery and Oncology*, Vol.10, No.3, (March 1984), pp. 169–170, ISSN 0148-0812

Maloney, M.E. (1995). Histology of Basal Cell Carcinoma. *Clinics in Dermatology*, Vol.13, No.6, (November-December 1995), pp. 545-549, ISSN 0738-081X

Maxfield, F.R. (2002). Plasma membrane microdomains. *Current Opinion in Cell Biology*, Vol.14, No.4, (August 2002), pp. 483–487, ISSN 0955-0674

Mishra, P.J.; Humeniuk, R.; Medina, D.J.; Alexe, G.; Mesirov, J.P.; Ganesan, S.; Glod, J.W. & Banerjee, D. (2008). Carcinoma-associated fibroblast-like differentiation of human mesenchymal stem cells. *Cancer Research*, Vol.68, No.11, (June 2008), pp. 4331–4339, ISSN 0008-5472

Mukoyama, Y.; Zhou, S.; Miyachi, Y. & Matsuyoshi, N. (2005). T-cadherin negatively regulates the proliferation of cutaneous squamous carcinoma cells. *The Journal of Investigative Dermatology*, Vol.124, No.4, (April 2005), pp. 833-888, ISSN 0022-202X

Offersen, B.V.; Borre, M.; Sørensen, F.B. & Overgaard, J. (2002). Comparison of methods of microvascular staining and quantification in prostate carcinoma: relevance to prognosis. *APMIS*, Vol.110, No.2, (February 2002), pp. 177-185, ISSN 0903-4641

Ogawa, K.; Pasqualini, R.; Lindberg, R.A.; Kain, R.; Freeman, A.L. & Pasquale, E.B. (2000). The ephrin-A1 ligand and its receptor, EphA2, are expressed during tumor neovascularization. *Oncogene*, Vol.19, No.52, (December 2000), pp. 6043-6052, ISSN 0950-9232

Oh, C.W. & Penneys, N. (2004). p27 and mib1 expression in actinic keratosis, Bowen disease, and squamous cell carcinoma. *The American Journal of Dermatopathology*, Vol.26, No.1, (February 2004), pp. 22-26, ISSN 0193-1091

Olumi, A.F.; Grossfeld, G.D.; Hayward, S.W.; Carroll, P.R.; Tlsty, T.D. & Cunha, G.R. (1999). Carcinoma-associated fibroblasts direct tumor progression of initiated human prostatic epithelium. *Cancer Research*, Vol.59, No.19, (October 1999), pp. 5002–5011, ISSN 0008-5472

Orimo, A.; Gupta, P.B.; Sgroi, D.C.; Arenzana-Seisdedos, F.; Delaunay, T.; Naeem, R.; Carey, V.J.; Richardson, A.L. & Weinberg, R.A. (2005). Stromal fibroblasts present in invasive human breast carcinomas promote tumor growth and angiogenesis through elevated SDF-1/CXCL12 secretion. *Cell*, Vol.121, No.3, (May 2005), pp. 335–348, ISSN 0092-8674

Parangi, S.; O'Reilly, M.; Christofori, G.; Holmgren, L.; Grosfeld, J.; Folkman, J. & Hanahan, D. (1996). Antiangiogenic therapy of transgenic mice impairs de novo tumor growth. *Proceedings of the National Academy of Sciences of the United States of America*, Vol.93, No.5, (March 1996), pp. 2002-2007, ISSN 0027-8424

Pfaff, D.; Philippova, M.; Buechner, S.A.; Maslova, K.; Mathys, T.; Erne, P. & Resink, T.J. (2010). T-cadherin loss induces an invasive phenotype in human keratinocytes and squamous cell carcinoma (SCC) cells in vitro and is associated with malignant transformation of cutaneous SCC in vivo. *British Journal of Dermatology*, V.163, No.2, (August 2010), pp. 353-363, ISSN 0007-0963

Philippova, M.P.; Bochkov, V.N.; Stambolsky, D.V.; Tkachuk, V.A. & Resink, T.J. (1998). T-cadherin and signal-transducing molecules co-localize in caveolin-rich membrane domain of vascular smooth muscle cells. *FEBS Letters*, Vol.429, No.2, (June 1998), pp. 207-210, ISSN 0014-5793

Philippova, M.; Ivanov, D.; Allenspach, R.; Takuwa, Y.; Erne, P. & Resink, T. (2005). RhoA and Rac mediate endothelial cell polarization and detachment induced by T-cadherin. *FASEB Journal*, Vol.19, No.6, (April 2005), pp. 588-590, ISSN 0892-6638

Philippova, M.; Ivanov, D.; Joshi, M.B.; Kyriakakis, E.; Rupp, K.; Afonyushkin, T.; Bochkov, V.; Erne, P. & Resink, T.J. (2008). Identification of proteins associating with glycosylphosphatidylinositol-anchored T-cadherin on the surface of vascular endothelial cells: role for Grp78/BiP in T-cadherin-dependent cell survival. *Molecular and Cellular Biology*, Vol.28, No.12, (June 2008), pp. 4004-4017, ISSN 0270-7306

Philippova, M.; Ivanov, D.; Tkachuk, V.; Erne, P. & Resink, T.J. (2003). Polarisation of T-cadherin to the leading edge of migrating vascular cells in vitro: a function in vascular cell motility? *Histochemistry and Cell Biology*, Vol.120, No.5, (November 2003), pp. 353-360, ISSN 0948-6143

Philippova, M.; Joshi, M.B.; Kyriakakis, E.; Pfaff, D.; Erne, P. & Resink, T.J. (2009). A guide and guard: the many faces of T-cadherin. *Cellular Signalling*, Vol.21, No.7, (July 2009), pp. 1035–1044, ISSN 0898-6568

Pinkus, H.; Jallad, M. & Mehregan, A.H. (1963). The inflammatory infiltrate of precancerous skin lesions. *The Journal of Investigative Dermatology*, Vol.41, (November 1963), pp. 247–248, ISSN 0022-202X

Potapova, I.A.; Gaudette, G.R.; Brink, P.R.; Robinson, R.B.; Rosen, M.R.; Cohen, I.S. & Doronin, S.V. (2007). Mesenchymal stem cells support migration, extracellular matrix invasion, proliferation, and survival of endothelial cells in vitro. *Stem Cells*, Vol.25, No.7, (July 2007), pp. 1761–1768, ISSN 1066-5099

Quinn, A.G. & Perkins, W. (2010). Non-melanoma skin cancer and other epidermal skin tumors, In: *Rook's Textbook of Dermatology*, Burns, T., Breathnach, S., Cox, N. & Griffiths, C, Blackwell Publishing Ltd, ISBN 978-1-405-16169-5, Chichester, United Kingdom

Ranscht, B. & Dours-Zimmermann, M.T. (1991). T-cadherin, a novel cadherin cell adhesion molecule in the nervous system lacks the conserved cytoplasmic region. *Neuron*, Vol.7, No.3, (September 1991), pp. 391-402, ISSN 0896-6273

Rasmussen, A.A. & Cullen, K.J. (1998). Paracrine/autocrine regulation of breast cancer by the insulin-like growth factors. *Breast Cancer Research and Treatment*, Vol.47, No.3, (February 1998), pp. 219–233, ISSN 0167-6806

Riener, M.O.; Nikolopoulos, E.; Herr, A.; Wild, P.J.; Hausmann, M.; Wiech, T.; Orlowska-Volk, M.; Lassmann, S.; Walch, A. & Werner, M. (2008). Microarray comparative genomic hybridization analysis of tubular breast carcinoma shows recurrent loss of the CDH13 locus on 16q. *Human Pathology*, Vol.39, No.11, (November 2008), pp. 1621-1629, ISSN 0046-8177

Riou, P.; Saffroy, R.; Chenailler, C.; Franc, B.; Gentile, C.; Rubinstein, E.; Resink, T.; Debuire, B.; Piatier-Tonneau, D. & Lemoine, A. (2006). Expression of T-cadherin in tumor cells influences invasive potential of human hepatocellular carcinoma. *FASEB Journal*, Vol.20, No.13, (November 2006), pp. 2291-2301, ISSN 0892-6638

Rippey, J.J. (1998). Why classify basal cell carcinomas? *Histopathology*, Vol.32, No.5, (May 1998), pp. 393-398, ISSN 0309-0167

Risau, W. (1997). Mechanisms of angiogenesis. *Nature*, Vol.386, No.6626, (April 1997), pp. 671–674, ISSN 0028-0836

Röwert-Huber, J.; Patel, M.J.; Forschner, T.; Ulrich, C.; Eberle, J.; Kerl, H.; Sterry, W. & Stockfleth, E. (2007). Actinic keratosis is an early in situ squamous cell carcinoma: a proposal for reclassification. *British Journal of Dermatology*, Vol.156, No.Suppl. 3, (May 2007), pp. 8–12, ISSN 0007-0963

Rubin, M.A.; Buyyounouski, M.; Bagiella, E.; Sharir, S.; Neugut, A.; Benson, M.; de la Taille, A.; Katz, A.E.; Olsson, C.A. & Ennis, R.D. (1999). Microvessel density in prostate cancer: lack of correlation with tumor grade, pathologic stage, and clinical outcome. *Urology*, Vol.53, No.3, (March 1999), pp. 542-547, ISSN 0090-4295

Rubina, K.A; Kalinina, N.I.; Bochkov, V.N.; Parfyonova, Ye.V. & Tkachuk, V.A. (2005a). T-cadherin as an antiadhesive and guidance molecule interacting with low density lipoproteins. *Annals EAS*, pp. 1-14, ISSN 1784-0686

Rubina, K.; Kalinina, N.; Efimenko, A.; Lopatina, T.; Melikhova, V.; Tsokolaeva, Z.; Sysoeva, V.; Tkachuk, V. & Parfyonova, Y. (2009). Adipose stromal cells stimulate angiogenesis via promoting progenitor cell differentiation, secretion of angiogenic factors and enhancing vessel maturation. *Tissue Engineering. Part A*, Vol.15, No.8, (August 2009), pp. 2039-2050, ISSN 1937-3341

Rubina, K.; Kalinina, N.; Potekhina, A.; Efimenko, A.; Semina, E.; Poliakov, A.; Wilkinson, D.G.; Parfyonova, Y. & Tkachuk, V. (2007). T-cadherin suppresses angiogenesis in vivo by inhibiting migration of endothelial cells. *Angiogenesis*, Vol.10, No.3, (May 2007), pp. 83-195, ISSN 0969-6970

Rubina, K.; Talovskaya, E.; Cherenkov, V.; Ivanov, D.; Stambolsky, D.; Storozhevikh, T.; Pinelis, V.; Shevelev, A.; Parfyonova, Y.; Resink, T.; Erne, P. & Tkachuk, V. (2005b). LDL induces intracellular signaling and cell migration via atypical LDL-binding protein T-cadherin. *Molecular and Cellular Biochemistry*, Vol.273, No.1-2, (May 2005), pp. 33-41, ISSN 0300-8177

Rubina, K.A. & Tkachuk, V.A. (2004). Antiadhesive molecule T-cadherin is an atypical low-density lipoprotein receptor in vascular cells. *Rossiiskii Fiziologicheskii Zhurnal Imeni I. M. Sechenova*, Vol.90, No.8, (August 2004), pp. 968-986, ISSN 0869-8139

Sarbia, M.; Verreet, P.; Bittinger, F.; Dutkowski, P.; Heep, H.; Willers, R. & Gabbert, H.E. (1997). Basaloid squamous cell carcinoma of the esophagus: diagnosis and prognosis. *Cancer*, Vol.79, No.10, (May 1997), pp. 1871-1878, ISSN 1097-0142

Sasano, H.; Ohashi, Y.; Suzuki, T. & Nagura, H. (1998). Vascularity in human adrenal cortex. *Modern Pathology*, Vol.11, No.4, (April 1998), pp. 329-33, ISSN 0893-3952

Sato, M.; Mori, Y.; Sakurada, A.; Fujimura, S. & Horii, A. (1998). The H-cadherin (CDH13) gene is inactivated in human lung cancer. *Human Genetics*, Vol.103, No.1, (July 1998), pp. 96-101, ISSN 0340-6717

Semina, E.V.; Rubina, K.A.; Rutkevich, P.N.; Voyno-Yasenetskaya, T.A.; Parfyonova, Y.V. & Tkachuk, V.A. (2009). T-cadherin activates Rac1 and Cdc42 and changes endothelial permeability. *Biochemistry (Moscow)*, Vol.74, No.4. (April 2009), pp. 362-370, ISSN 0006-2979

Smith, J.M. & Irons, G.B. (1983). Metastatic basal cell carcinoma: review of the literature and report of three cases. *Annals of Plastic Surgery*, Vol.11, No.6, (December 1983), pp. 551–553, ISSN 0148-7043

Spaeth, E.L.; Dembinski, J.L.; Sasser, A.K.; Watson, K.; Klopp, A.; Hall, B.; Andreeff, M. & Marini, F. (2009). Mesenchymal stem cell transition to tumor-associated fibroblasts contributes to fibrovascular network expansion and tumor progression. *PLoS One*, Vol.4, No.4, (April 2009), pp. e4992, ISSN 1932-6203

Spaeth, E.; Klopp, A.; Dembinski, J.; Andreeff, M. & Marini, F. (2008). Inflammation and tumor microenvironments: defining the migratory itinerary of mesenchymal stem cells. *Gene Therapy*, Vol.15, No.10, (May 2008), pp. 730–738, ISSN 0969-7128

Suehiro, Y.; Okada, T.; Anno, K.; Okayama, N.; Ueno, K.; Hiura, M.; Nakamura, M.; Kondo, T.; Oga, A.; Kawauchi, S.; Hirabayashi, K.; Numa, F.; Ito, T.; Saito, T.; Sasaki, K. & Hinoda, Y. (2008). Aneuploidy predicts outcome in patients with endometrial carcinoma and is related to lack of CDH13 hypermethylation. *Clinical Cancer Research*, Vol.14, No.11, (June 2008), pp. 3354-3361, ISSN 1078-0432

Takeuchi, T.; Liang, S.B.; Matsuyoshi, N.; Zhou, S.; Miyachi, Y.; Sonobe, H. & Ohtsuki, Y. (2002a). Loss of T-cadherin (CDH13, H-cadherin) expression in cutaneous squamous cell carcinoma. *Laboratory Investigation*, Vol.82, No.8, (August 2002), pp. 1023-1029, ISSN 0023-6837

Takeuchi, T.; Liang, S.B. & Ohtsuki, Y. (2002b). Downregulation of expression of a novel cadherin molecule, T-cadherin, in basal cell carcinoma of the skin. *Molecular Carcinogenesis*, Vol.35, No.4, (December 2002), pp. 173-179, ISSN 0899-1987

Takeuchi, T.; Misaki, A.; Liang, S.B.; Tachibana, A.; Hayashi, N.; Sonobe, H. & Ohtsuki, Y. (2000). Expression of T-cadherin (CDH13, H-cadherin) in human brain and its characteristics as a negative growth regulator of epidermal growth factor in neuroblastoma cells. *Journal of Neurochemistry*, Vol.74, No.4, (April 2000), pp. 1489-1497, ISSN 0022-3042

Takeuchi, T. & Ohtsuki, Y. (2001). Recent progress in T-cadherin (CDH13, H-cadherin) research. *Histology and Histopathology*, Vol.16, No.4, (October 2001), pp. 1287-1293, ISSN 0213-3911

Tlsty, T.D. & Coussens, L.V. (2006). Tumor stroma and regulation of cancer development. *Annual Review of Pathology*, Vol.1, (February 2006), pp. 119–50, ISSN 1553-4006

van den Hooff, A. (1988). Stromal involvement in malignant growth. *Advances in Cancer Research*, Vol.50, (1988), pp. 159–196, ISSN 0065-230X

Verdolini, R.; Amerio, P.; Goteri, G.; Bugatti, L.; Lucarini, G.; Mannello, B.; Filosa, G.; Offidani, A.; Brancorsini, D.; Biagini, G. & Giangiacomi, M. (2001). Cutaneous carcinomas and preinvasive neoplastic lesions. Role of MMP-2 and MMP-9 metalloproteinases in neoplastic invasion and their relationship with proliferative activity and p53 expression. *Journal of Cutaneous Pathology*, Vol.28, No.3, (March 2001), pp. 120-126, ISSN 0303-6987

Vieira, S.C.; Zeferino, L.C.; Da Silva, B.B.; Aparecida Pinto, G.; Vassallo, J.; Carasan, G.A. & De Moraes, N.G. (2004). Quantification of angiogenesis in cervical cancer: a comparison among three endothelial cell markers. *Gynecologic Oncology*, Vol.93, No.1, (April 2004), pp. 121-124, ISSN 0090-8258

Wain, S.L.; Kier, R.; Vollmer, R.T. & Bossen, E.H. (1986). Basaloid-squamous carcinoma of the tongue, hypopharynx, and larynx: report of 10 cases. *Human Pathology*, Vol.17, No.11, (November 1986), pp. 1158–1166, ISSN 0046-8177

Wang, G.Y.; Wang, J.; Mancianti, M.L. & Epstein, E.H.Jr. (2011). Basal cell carcinomas arise from hair follicle stem cells in Ptch1(+/-) mice. *Cancer Cell*, Vol.19, No.1, (January 2011), pp. 114-124, ISSN 1535-6108

Weigelt, B.; Peterse, J.L. & van 't Veer, L.J. (2005). Breast cancer metastasis: markers and models. *Nature Reviews Cancer*, Vol.5, No.8, (August 2005), pp. 591-602, ISSN 1474-175X

Weinstein, B.M. (2005). Vessels and nerves: matching to the same tune. *Cell*, Vol.120, No.3, (February 2005), pp. 299-302, ISSN 0092-8674

Widschwendter, A.; Ivarsson, L.; Blassnig, A.; Müller, H.M.; Fiegl, H.; Wiedemair, A.; Müller-Holzner, E.; Goebel, G.; Marth, C. & Widschwendter, M. (2004). CDH1 and CDH13 methylation in serum is an independent prognostic marker in cervical cancer patients. *International Journal of Cancer*, Vol.109, No.2, (March 2004), pp. 163-166, ISSN 0020-7136

Winzenburg, S.M.; Niehans, G.A.; George, E.; Daly, K. & Adams, G.L. (1998). Basaloid squamous carcinoma: a clinical comparison of two histological types with poorly differentiated squamous cell carcinoma. *Otolaryngology – Head and Neck Surgery*, Vol.119, No.5, (November 1998), pp. 471–475, ISSN 0194-5998

Wyder, L.; Vitality, A.; Schneider, H.; Hebbard, L.W.; Moritz, D.R.; Wittmer, M.; Ajmo, M. & Klemenz, R. (2000). Increased expression of H/T-cadherin in tumor-penetrating blood vessels. *Cancer Research*, Vol.60, No.17, (September 2000), pp. 4682-4688, ISSN 0008-5472

Yancopoulos, G.D.; Davis, S.; Gale, N.W.; Rudge, J.S.; Wiegand, S.J. & Holash, J. (2000). Vascular-specific growth factors and blood vessel formation. *Nature*, Vol.407, No.6801, (September 2000), pp. 242-248, ISSN 0028-0836

Yanofsky, V.R.; Mercer, S.E. & Phelps, R.G. (2011). Histopathological variants of cutaneous squamous cell carcinoma: a review. *Journal of Skin Cancer*, Vol.2011, (December 2010), pp. 1-13, ISSN 2090-2905

Yu, T.C.; Rahman, Z. & Ross, B.S. (2003). Actinic keratosis – surgical and physical therapeutic modalities. *Cutis*, Vol.71, No.5, (May 2003), pp. 381–384, ISSN 0011-4162

Yurlova, E.I.; Rubina, K.A.; Sysoeva, V.Yu.; Sharonov, G.V.; Semina, E.V.; Parfenova, Ye.V. & Tkachuk, V.A. (2010). T-cadherin suppresses the cell proliferation of mouse melanoma B16F10 and tumor angiogenesis in the model of chorioallantoic membrane. *Ontogenez*, Vol.41, No.4, (July-August 2010), pp. 261-270, ISSN 0475-1450

Zalaudek, I.; Bonifazi, E.; Ferrara, G. & Argenziano, G. (2009). Keratoacanthomas and spitz tumors: are they both 'self-limiting' variants of malignant cutaneous neoplasms? *Dermatology*, Vol.219, No.1, (April 2009), pp. 3–6, ISSN 1018-8665

Zbären, P.; Nuyens, M. & Stauffer, E. (2004). Basaloid squamous cell carcinoma of the head and neck. *Current Opinion in Otolaryngology and Head and Neck Surgery*, Vol.12, No.2, (April 2004), pp. 116-121, ISSN 1068-9508

Zhou, S.; Matsuyoshi, N.; Liang, S.B.; Takeuchi, T.; Ohtsuki, Y. & Miyachi, Y. (2002). Expression of T-cadherin in basal keratinocytes of skin. *The Journal of Investigative Dermatology*. Vol.118, No.6, (June 2002), pp. 1080–1084, ISSN 0022-202X

Zhou, S.; Matsuyoshi, N.; Takeuchi, T.; Ohtsuki, Y. & Miyachi, Y. (2003). Reciprocal altered expression of T-cadherin and P-cadherin in psoriasis vulgaris. *British Journal of Dermatology*, Vol.149, No.2, (August 2003), pp. 268-273, ISSN 0007-0963

Zucchini, C.; Bianchini, M.; Valvassori, L.; Perdichizzi, S.; Benini, S.; Manara, M.C.; Solmi, R.; Strippoli, P.; Picci, P.; Carinci, P. & Scotlandi, K. (2004). Identification of candidate genes involved in the reversal of malignant phenotype of osteosarcoma cells transfected with the liver/bone/kidney alkaline phosphatase gene. *Bone*, Vol.34, No.4, (April 2004), pp. 672-679, ISSN 8756-3282

7

Modeling Tumor Angiogenesis in Zebrafish

Massimo M. Santoro
Molecular Biotechnology Center,
University of Torino, Torino,
Italy

1. Introduction

The process of angiogenesis is essential for tumor progression and metastasis. New pathways have been identified to play a critical role in promoting and regulating blood vessel formation both in embryogenesis and in pathophysiological conditions. These pathways provide potential molecular targets for anti-angiogenic therapies to treat cancer and other vascular diseases. The critical cellular targets of these therapies are vascular endothelial cells (ECs) and supporting mural cells or pericytes (MCs) that are recruited from surrounding healthy tissue to form new vessels in the growing tumor. A challenging task has always been to visualize these biological processes in vivo as well as to screen for drugs affecting these pathological pathways. In this context, the zebrafish model represents an emerging vertebrate system to study the tumor angiogenesis process and to better understand the modification of tumor microenvironment by anti-angiogenesis therapy. Can a small tropical fish help to better understand the tumor angiogenesis process and identify new therapies for tumor angiogenesis ? In this chapter we illustrate how the zebrafish has emerged as a novel in vivo cancer model to study tumor-induced neovascularization and metastases. In the transparent zebrafish embryos, invasion and migration of tumor cells, their circulation in the vascular system, as well as the formation tumor-induced neovascularization can all be followed with high resolution in real time. Importantly, these zebrafish models allow to quantitate both metastatic behavior of transplanted tumor cells and tumor-cell induced neovascularization. The zebrafish model has the advantage of being a vertebrate equipped with easy and powerful genetic and imaging tools to investigate the mechanisms of tumor development and progression. In particular the transparency of embryos and lately also adult are transforming this model system in the leading in vivo model for cancer biology and tumor angiogenesis.

2. The zebrafish model

The zebrafish (*Danio rerio*) system has emerged in the past years as an ideal vertebrate model organism in which to study a wide variety of biological processes (Thisse and Zon, 2002). Zebrafish is a small, freshwater teleost native of Ganges river in South-East India. Some of the advantages of the zebrafish animal model system, together with its small size and low cost, include fecundity, with each female capable of laying 200-300 eggs per week, external fertilization that permits manipulation of embryos ex utero, and rapid development of optically clear embryos, which allows the direct observation of developing internal organs and tissues in vivo (Thisse and Zon, 2002). These attributes have led to the emergence of the zebrafish as a preeminent embryological model. The zebrafish has proven to be a powerful vertebrate model system for the genetic analysis of developmental pathways and has just started to be exploited as a model for human disease and clinical research (Lieschke and Currie, 2007; Skromne and Prince, 2008). If in the past 20 years zebrafish has served as an excellent model for understanding normal development using its powerful genetics and embryology, now is becoming a unique opportunity to uncover novel insights into the molecular genetics of human diseases.

2.1 Zebrafish and angiogenesis

The zebrafish system possesses many advantages for vascular studies. By 24 h after fertilization the zebrafish embryo has already developed a functional cardiovascular system (beating heart, aorta, cardinal vein and blood). Since the zebrafish embryo is relatively small and aquatic, zebrafish embryos are not completely dependent on a functional vascular system to continue to survive and develop. This happens because embryos receive enough oxygen by passive diffusion, thereby allowing a detailed analysis of animals with severe vascular defects (Stainier, 2001). Embryos without cardiac contraction or blood thus develop normally until their size outstrips diffusive oxygenation. This allows the consequences of genetic manipulation on cardiovascular development to be observed for longer than would be possible in mammals, in which abnormal heart or vascular development is fatal very early in development. By contrast avian and mammalian embryos die rapidly in the absence of a functional cardiovascular system and are not easy visualized internally without fixation and staining.

Until 5 days post fertilization, the embryos are nearly transparent, allowing in vivo visualization of any tissue without instrumentation or manipulation other than microscopy. This feature allows observation of the heart and blood vessels during development even at single cell resolution. The availability of the fertilized egg for injection with genetic constructs greatly facilitates the generation of tissue-specific transgenics (Kawakami, 2007). Such transgenesis usually uses a native tissue-specific promoter to drive expression of a fluorescent reporter protein, such as green fluorescent protein (GFP). Examples of cardiovascular transgenic lines include Fli1:GFP (expresses GFP in endothelial cells and some neural crest-derived cells) (Lawson and Weinstein, 2002), kdrl:GFP (expresses GFP localized to endothelial cell) (Jin et al., 2005), GATA1:dsRED (expresses dsRED in erythrocytes) (Traver et al., 2003), CD41:GFP (expresses GFP in thrombocytes) (Lin et al., 2005) and cmlc2:GFP (expresses GFP in cardiomyocytes) (Burns et al., 2005) and TGNL-Cherry (expresses cherry in smooth muscle cells)(Gays and Santoro, personal communication).

Coupled with the embryo's optical clarity, these transgenic lines allow observation of in vivo cellular behavior in a manner impossible in other models. The striking transparency of the embryos facilitates morphological observation of internal organs in vivo under a simple stereomicroscope, and at the single-cell level using confocal and single plan microscopy. Transparent zebrafish embryos are also well suited for in vivo time-lapse imaging. The fast acquisition speed of spinning disk and 2-photon confocal microscopy reduces the recording times significantly when millimeter-sized embryos need to be imaged at high resolution and at short time intervals. Light Sheet Fluorescence Microscopy could also be very useful in zebrafish (Keller et al., 2008). These attributes, that have led to the emergence of the zebrafish as a preeminent embryological model, including its capacity for gain- and loss-

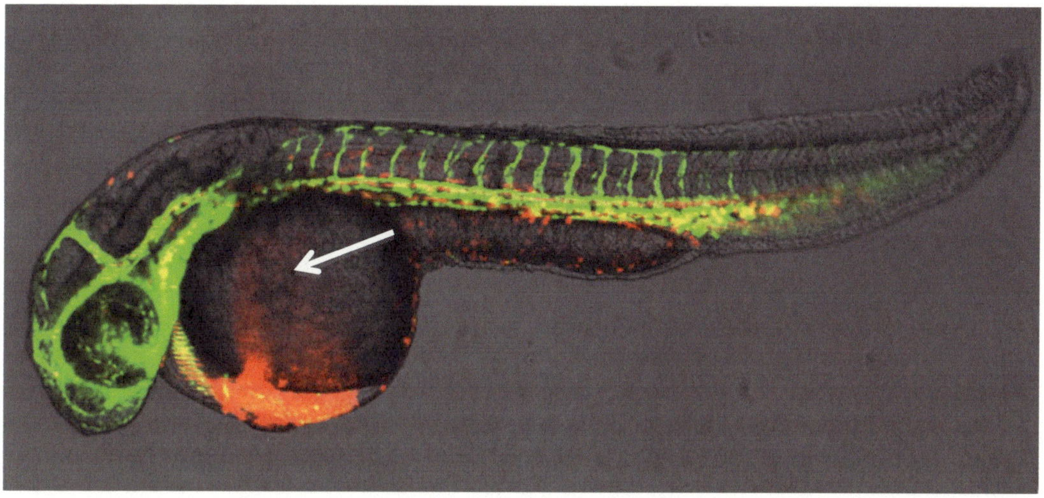

Fig. 1. Representative images of 30hpf transgenic Tg(kdrl:GFP^{s843},gata1:deRed^{sd2}) zebrafish embryos. Green fluorescent blood vessels and red fluorescent erythrocytes and macrophages are evident in all embryo. Arrow indicates point of tumor cells injections.

of-function studies, provides a unique opportunity to uncover novel insights into the molecular genetics of development and diseases. The zebrafish system also offers the opportunity to carry out forward genetic analysis to identify as yet unidentified loci/genes affecting vascular development (Patton and Zon, 2001). Different techniques exist to generate point mutations, deletions and mutagenic insertions, which can be bred to homozygosis in order to determine their phenotypic consequences. Zebrafish also allows the powerful combination of loss-of-function and gain-of-function analyses (Zon and Peterson, 2005). Altogether these data suggest the zebrafish system as an optimal model to study angiogenesis not only during development but also in pathological conditions such as tumor angiogenesis.

2.2 Zebrafish and cancer

The zebrafish (*Danio rerio*) has proven to be a powerful vertebrate model system for the genetic analysis of developmental pathways and is only beginning to be exploited as a model for human disease and clinical research. More recently, research with zebrafish has extended to model human diseases and to analyze the formation and functions of cell populations within organs (Dooley and Zon, 2000). This work has generated new human disease models and has begun to establish therapeutic possibilities, including genes that modify disease states and chemicals that rescue organs from disease. Zebrafish has recently entered the stage as a promising model system to study human cancer. This is largely due to the development of zebrafish transgenic lines expressing oncogenes and their amenability to genetic and pharmacological testing. Cancer progression in these animals recapitulates many aspects of human disease and opens the door for studies to identify genetic and chemical modifiers of cancer. The zebrafish is amenable to transgenic and genetic strategies that can be used to identify or generate zebrafish models of different types of cancer and may also present significant advantages for the discovery of tumor suppressor genes that promote tumorigenesis when inactivated by mutations (Amatruda et al., 2002). Importantly, the transparency and accessibility of the zebrafish embryo and adult allows the unprecedented direct analysis of pathologic processes in vivo, in particular tumor angiogenesis (Moshal et al., 2010; Nicoli and Presta, 2007; Stoletov and Klemke, 2008). The attention has been further fueled by the development of xenograft models that allow the propagation and visualization of human cancer cells engrafted in optically transparent. The integration of zebrafish genetics with the large tool chest of reagents available to study human cancer cells provides a powerful new vertebrate model to visualize and dissect the mechanisms that drive cancer formation, angiogenesis and metastasis. Finally, zebrafish have many attributes that cancer researchers find attractive. Compared to mice, zebrafish require minimal care and are cost effective to maintain in the laboratory. A pair of adult fish produces several hundred fertilized eggs a week. The embryos develop externally and are transparent up to 1 month of age. Adult, casper mutant (noy$^{-/-}$; nacre$^{-/-}$) animals are also available that remain transparent throughout life and are amenable to in vivo transplantation studies (White et al., 2008). The remarkable transparency of zebrafish tissues allows direct imaging of cancer progression including cell invasion, intravasation, extravasation and angiogenesis (Rouhi et al., 2010b; Stoletov et al., 2007).

Ultimately, high-throughput modifier screens based on zebrafish cancer models can lead to the identification of chemicals or genes involved in the suppression or prevention of the malignant phenotype (Lieschke and Currie, 2007). The identification of small molecules or gene products through such screens will serve as ideal entry points for novel drug development for cancer treatment. Here we focus on the current technology that takes advantage of the zebrafish model system to advance our understanding of the genetic basis of tumor angiogenesis and its treatment.

2.3 Molecular mechanisms involved in angiogenesis

The vascular system is the first organ to form and function during embryogenesis. Vascular development begins with the organization of endothelial cells (ECs) into a primitive vascular plexus that becomes progressively remodeled to ultimately form a complex vascular network, a process called angiogenesis (Carmeliet, 2003; Cleaver and Melton, 2003; Red-Horse et al., 2007). Afterwards, the developing vessels differentiate and mature by generating extracellular matrices, by expressing specific cell-cell molecules, and by recruiting mural cells (MCs)(pericytes and vascular smooth muscle cells) in a process called vascular maturation. MCs are recruited to the endothelial vasculature and sheathe it, providing support and contractility to the mature vascular system (Bergers and Song, 2005; Carmeliet, 2005). Formation and stabilization of the vascular system is essential for proper development of vertebrate embryos, as well as for the survival of adults. Mature vessels continue to provide metabolic homeostasis by supplying oxygen and nutrients and removing metabolic wastes. Several molecular mechanisms are involved during the vascular maturation process, including signaling pathways (e.g. PDGF, Angiopoietins, TGFb1, DlGF, S1P-EDG1), cell-cell and cell-matrix interactions (e.g. cadherins, connexins, integrins, MMPs, PAI1). Formation of new blood vessels is desirable for regenerative purposes, such as during tissue healing or transplantation, but can be pathological, as in diabetic retinopathy and cancer.

Several studies in zebrafish have identified new mechanism involved in angiogenesis. It has been demonstrated that numerous angiogenic factors not only induce angiogenesis but also function as EC survival factors. Using genetic studies in zebrafish, we previously discovered that Birc2/cIap1, an inhibitor of apoptosis (IAP), is critical for the survival of endothelial cells, which line the inner portion of blood vessels (Santoro et al., 2007). Apart from the relevance of these findings for improving understanding of vascular development, they may create new opportunities for further development of anti- angiogenic drug therapies. In fact, several reports demonstrate that IAP antagonist potentiate apoptosis in cancer cells by promoting induction of auto-ubiquitination and degradation of cIAPs, which culminates in TNFα-mediated cell death suggesting an important role of this pathway in tumor angiogenesis (Wu et al., 2005).

Non-coding RNAs called microRNAs also modulate the response of the vascular endothelium to angiogenic stimuli. Recently different microRNA (e.g. miRNA126, and miRNA296 have been found to be associated with angiogenesis in zebrafish (Fish and Srivastava, 2009). However, many other mechanisms remain to be discovered.

2.4 Tumor angiogenesis

A tumor consists of a population of rapidly dividing and growing cancer cells. Cancer cells have lost their ability to divide in a controlled fashion as a consequence tumor cells rapidly accumulate mutations that allow cancer cells (or sub-populations of cancer cells within a tumor) to grow more (Carmeliet, 2003; Folkman, 2007). Tumors cannot grow beyond a certain size, generally 1–2 mm^3 due to a lack of oxygen and other essential nutrients. Tumors cells have then have acquired a specific feature that is to induce blood vessel growth (a process called tumor angiogenesis) by secreting various endothelial growth factors. Endothelial specific growth factors such as bFGF and VEGF-A can induce capillary growth into the tumor that in turn allow tumor expansion. Tumor angiogenesis is a necessary and required step for transition from a small harmless cluster of cells to a large tumor. Angiogenesis is also required for the spread of a tumor, or metastasis. Single cancer cells can break away from an established solid tumor, enter the blood vessel, and be carried to a distant site, where they can implant and begin the growth of a secondary tumor. Evidence now suggests the blood vessel in a given solid tumor may, in fact, be mosaic vessels, composed of endothelial cells, mural cells and neoplastic cells. The subsequent growth of such metastases will also require a supply of nutrients and oxygen and a waste disposal pathway.

Endothelial cells have long been considered genetically more stable than cancer cells. This genomic stability confers an advantage to targeting endothelial cells using antiangiogenic therapy, compared to chemotherapy directed at cancer cells, which rapidly mutate and acquire 'drug resistance' to treatment. For this reason, endothelial cells are thought to be an ideal target for therapies directed against them (Folkman, 2007). Tumor blood vessels have perivascular detachment, vessel dilation, and irregular shape. It is believed that tumor blood vessels are not smooth like normal tissues, and are not ordered sufficiently to give oxygen to all of the tissues. Endothelial precursor cells are organized from bone marrow, which are then integrated into the growing blood vessels. Afterwards endothelial cells differentiate and migrate into perivascular space, providing nutrients that allow neoplastic cells to growth the tumor mass. In this process VEGF-A plays a crucial role since it is important for *denovo* formation of new blood vessels at sites of tumor formation allowing cancer cell to growth (Bergers and Hanahan, 2008).

Tumor angiogenesis is one of the most prominent mechanisms driving tumor development and progression. Tumor angiogenesis research is a cutting-edge field in cancer research and recent evidence also suggests traditional therapies, such as radiation therapy, may actually work in part by targeting the genomic stable endothelial cell compartment, rather than the genomic unstable tumor cell compartment. New blood vessel formation is a relatively fragile process, subject to disruptive interference at several levels. In short, the therapy is the selection agent that is being used to kill a cell compartment. Tumor cells evolve resistance rapidly due to rapid generation time (days) and genomic instability (variation), whereas endothelial cells are a good target because of a long generation time (months) and genomic stability (low variation). As a consequence crucial targets for therapeutic intervention have been identified and validated. Based on these efforts and achievements, targeted drug development programs have been implemented to interfere with tumor angiogenesis as an attractive strategy in cancer treatment. As a promising result the first targeted anti-angiogenic drugs have been approved for a variety of solid metastasizing cancers. The first generation of these molecules targets the two most prominent regulatory components of tumor angiogenesis: the vascular endothelial growth factor (VEGF-A), produced by tumor cells, and the VEGF-A receptor tyrosine kinase, which is expressed on vascular endothelial cells. Beyond the VEGF receptor system, additional tumor-angiogenic systems are presented as new potential targets for anti-angiogenic therapy (Bergers and Benjamin, 2003).

Over the last decades studies of tumor angiogenesis have concentrated mainly on the endothelial cells component, while the interest for mural cells has lagged behind (Bergers and Hanahan, 2008). Mural cells (MCs)(aka pericytes or vascular smooth muscle cells) are perivascular cells that wrap around blood capillaries. They communicate with endothelial cells by direct physical contact through a jointly synthesized basement membrane and reciprocal paracrine signalling. MCs and endothelial cells are thereby interdependent and, as such, defects in either endothelial cells or pericytes can affect the vascular system. Mural cells have various demonstrable functions in different physiological contexts, including stabilization and homeostatic regulation of mature blood vessels; facilitation of vessel maturation in the context of neovascularization; provision by their intimate association of endothelial cell survival signals; and limitation of cell transit across the vascular wall. The functional significance of mural cells in development is underscored by genetic depletion or disruption of mural cells association with the developing vasculature, which results in blood vessel dilation, widespread microvascular leakage and subsequent lethality during late gestation (Bergers and Song, 2005; Conway et al., 2001; Red-Horse et al., 2007). In tumors, MCs are typically less abundant and more loosely attached to blood vessels than in normal tissues, but their association is still important, as shown in a growing body of experimental evidence which indicates that pericytes help to maintain the integrity and functionality of the tumor vasculature (Armulik et al., 2005; Majesky, 2007). Interestingly, a growing body of evidence indicates that MCs, the periendothelial support cells of the microvasculature, are also important cell constituents of the aberrant tumor vasculature. When therapies impair neovascularization and/or elicit vascular regression, some tumors evidently rely on pericytes to help keep a core of pre-existing blood vessels alive and functional. This concept has evolved from the observation by several groups that, although inhibition of VEGF signalling can lead to substantial reduction in tumor vascularization, distinctive functional vessels remain that are slim and tightly covered with pericytes. These observations suggest that endothelial cells can induce MCs recruitment to protect themselves from death consequent to the lack of the crucial tumor-derived survival signals conveyed by VEGF-A. This hypothesis is supported by the findings that tumor vessels lacking adequate MCs coverage are more vulnerable to VEGF-A inhibition and that tumor MCs, which are juxtacrine to endothelial cells, express appreciable levels of VEGF-A and potentially other factors that support endothelial cell survival. The understanding of these mechanisms represents an important first step to elucidate pathways leading to many vascular-associated disorders, including tumor angiogenesis. The integration of zebrafish transgenic technology with human cancer biology may aid in the development of cancer models that target specific organs, tissues, or cell types within the tumors. Zebrafish could also provide a cost-effective means for the rapid development of therapeutic agents directed at blocking human cancer progression and tumor-induced angiogenesis (Amatruda et al., 2002).

2.5 Zebrafish as a model to study tumor angiogenesis

It has already been shown that blood vessels can grow by positional cues as well as secreted factors from other tissues. During pathological states, solid tumors use molecular mechanisms that are involved during normal angiogenesis to promote the disease state and establish a microenvironment to render normally quiescent endothelial cells to proliferate. In this respect, tumor tissue secretes angiogenic factors that can regulate blood vessel development (Bergers and Benjamin, 2003). However, not much is known about the cellular signals that initiate or establish cross talk between the tumor and the stromal cells. The study of the cellular interaction of tumor cells with its surrounding endothelial cells is expected to aid in the discovery of genes/pathways involved in the process of blood vessel formation in vivo. The microenvironment of a host-tumor interface has a profound influence on disease progression and has the potential for cancer therapy. Despite the importance of tumor-stromal interactions, there is a limited understanding of signaling cross talk between the tumor and the host microenvironment. Much of the information regarding the signaling networks comes from cell culture studies; however, the main drawback of this approach is the difficulty in extrapolating these findings to the whole organism. Thus, there is a need to develop suitable whole animal models to study the host- tumor interface.

In this respect, the zebrafish xenotransplantation system represents a novel model for defining tumor angiogenesis by the means of high-throughput manipulation of host environment, via morpholino knockdown of genetic pathways and treatment with small molecule inhibitors (Haldi et al., 2006; Nicoli et al., 2007; Rouhi et al., 2010a; Stoletov et al., 2007). Although embryonic and tumor vasculatures have morphological differences, they are mechanistically similar in the process of angiogenesis; therefore, studying the zebrafish xeno-transplantation model will allow us to better understand the impact of manipulation of the host microenvironment on tumor angiogenesis.

2.6 The xenotranplant experiments

The xenotransplantation studies conducted in mice and humans are limited by difficulties for direct observation in real time of cellular and signaling events in the context of the whole organism. Therefore, the future challenge will be to analyze the functional role of signaling interaction in modulating tumor angiogenesis by the host environment and determining its relationship with the inflammatory response and tumor cell metastasis using zebrafish as a transparent and tractable whole animal model system. In this regard, the use of transparent adult zebrafish casper mutant with fluorescently tagged blood vessels and myeloid-specific transgenic zebrafish will be advantageous to study cellular responses in real time (White et al., 2008). The other advantages include the speed of analysis for tumor angiogenesis (24-48 hours) and the ability to perform whole- mount in situ gene expression analyses in heterologous tumor cells vs the tumor-induced gene expression in the surrounding host environment leading to the attractiveness and appropriateness of the zebrafish model to study tumor angiogenesis. Various groups have shown that human cancer cells when grafted in early zebrafish embryos (1/2-day-old) may promote neoangiogenesis from embryos vessels and spread of metastasis in all embryos, thereby validating the xenotransplantation procedure to study tumor angiogenic and metastatic processes in zebrafish (Haldi et al., 2006; Nicoli et al., 2007; Stoletov et al., 2007) (Topczewska et al., 2006; Marques et al., 2009). The major advantage of the xenotransplantation in early embryos is the immature immune system that permits cancer cell engraftment without rejection. The studies by Haldi and collaborators demonstrated the feasibility of using 2 days postfertilization (dpf) zebrafish for xeno-transplantation where the fluorescently labeled human carcinoma was grafted into the yolk sac and observed until 7 days postinjection for cancer cell proliferation, migration, infiltration of tumor masses by endothelial cells, vessel remodeling, and stimulation of angiogenesis (Haldi et al., 2006). This technique represents a promising vertebrate model to study tumor-host microenvironment and to screen for antiangiogenic compounds. Later on, Presta and collaborators have refined the xenotransplantation process by transplanting tumor cells directly into the perivitelline space between the periderm and the yolk syncytial layer of the zebrafish embryos at 48 hours postfertilization and observed the neoangiogenic response originating from the subintestinal vessel plexus (Nicoli et al., 2007). Using the early zebrafish xenotransplantation model, Cao and collaborators monitored the dissemination of single-tumor cells from the primary sites and recapitulated early stages of clinical metastasis (Rouhi et al., 2010b). They concluded that hypoxia and VEGF-A-induced neovascularization promoted tumor invasion and metastasis by increasing dissemination of tumor cells into the circulation. Using the zebrafish xenotransplantation, Vlecken and Bagowski documented the significance of LIM domain kinases 1 and 2 signal molecules in tumor metastasis and angiogenesis of human pancreatic cancer cell lines and suggested that simultaneous targeting of both LIM domain kinases could inhibit tumor progression and metastasis (Vlecken and Bagowski, 2009). Hence, zebrafish early xenotransplantation may represent a powerful tool to understand how the angiogenic phenotype of the cancer culminates in metastatic spread of tumor and will be beneficial to study the molecular mechanism of antiangiogenesis therapy.

Later on, Stoletov and colleques successfully transplanted human cancer cells in a 30-day-old transparent zebrafish and studied the dynamics of microtumor formation and angiogenesis, thereby making this an excellent model appropriate to study the basics of vessel remodeling and alteration in subcellular compartments during tumorigenesis (Stoletov et al., 2007). It is not fully understood whether the new vessels triggered by human cancer cells are the result of redirection of the preexisting vessels and/or recruiting from the circulating endothelial cells. Therefore, using this late zebrafish xenotransplantation model will be better suited to investigate the origin of these endothelial cells in the transparent zebrafish host in which the vasculature has already established. The other advantages of using late xenotransplantation include easy interpretation of tumor-induced vascular effects, since the major organs in the juvenile fish including the vasculature have fully formed including smooth muscle cells and pericytes that can play a key role in tumor angiogenesis and it eliminates the concern related to the developmental defects due to embryologic manipulation. On the other hand, a limitation for this late model is the requirement of chemical suppression of the host immune function for successful grafting of the cancer cells. Recently, the generation of homozygous diploid clonal zebrafish lines by heat shock method made it possible to perform transplantation of hepatic tumor from one fish to another without rejection of the graft and without compromised by immunosuppression or sublethal γ-irradiation (Mizgireuv and Revskoy, 2006). However, clonal zebrafish model is suitable for studying various cancer types of zebrafish origin; it cannot be used as a host for transplanting human cancer cells without immunosuppression. To date, the early events that trigger vascular remodeling and tumor angiogenesis during tumor formation are not known. In addition, micrometastasis is a major cause of deaths in cancer patients. In this regard, a 30-day-old zebrafish xenotransplantation might also represent an adequate model to dissect the molecular and cellular mechanisms leading to micro-tumor formation.

2.7 Tumor angiogenesis-associated molecular mechanisms in zebrafish

Novel function of important genes associated with the process of tumor angiogenesis has been identified recently using the zebrafish model, including galectin-1 (Thijssen et al., 2006), Chemokine receptor 7 (Miao et al., 2007), LIM domain kinase 1 and 2 (Vlecken and Bagowski, 2009), angiomodulin (Hooper et al., 2009), Hypoxia inducible factor (Lee et al., 2009). In the past we identified a new molecule, Birc2/cIAP, important for endothelial survival in normal and pathological conditions (Gyrd-Hansen et al., 2008; Santoro et al., 2007). This study has implications for future design of antiangiogenic therapy. Available antiangiogenic agents (all VEGF inhibitors) induce endothelial cell apoptosis in existing vessels. Hence, additional antiangiogenic agents with complementary mechanisms are required. Because Birc2 has enzymatic activity, it might become an attractive target for drug development. We are currently testing a specific cIAP antogonists (BV6 and derivates) in endothelial cells in zebrafish (Varfolomeev et al., 2007). These small molecules potentiate apoptosis in cancer cells by promoting caspases activation. We will test these compounds and its derivates on out xenograft model of tumor angiogenesis in zebrafish. During the last years we also worked on characterization of mural cells (pericytes and vascular smooth muscle cells) (Santoro et al., 2009). Identify the molecular mechanisms involved in mural cell differentiation is very important to target tumor angiogenesis because it is known that tumor endothelial cells required pericytes/mural cells to survive (von Tell et al., 2006). Better understanding of the molecular genetic of mural cells may lead to the identification of new important targets for tumor angiogenesis and help to design anti-angiogenic drugs.

Nicoli et al., showed that morpholino knockdown of VE-cadherin expression selectively prevented tumor cell-induced angiogenesis by FGF2, but not normal vessel development including formation of the intersegmental and subintestinal vessels (Nicoli et al., 2007). These findings are surprising in light of the fact that VE-cadherin null mice display several vascular defects in vessel assembly that cause embryonic lethality at day 9.5 (Carmeliet et al., 1999). The apparent discrepancy in these studies may be due to differences in the vascular programs utilized by fish and mammals. It is also possible that tumor-induced vessel formation in zebrafish may be uniquely sensitive to perturbation of VE-cadherin expression or that the same programs that drive tumor-induced angiogenesis are different from those that drive developmental vasculogenesis.

Recently, Stoletov and Klemke demonstrate that highly invasive human cancer cell lines such as HT1080 or Hep3 are also invasive in zebrafish host while low invasive human cells as MDA-435 do not disseminate in the host zebrafish tissue (Stoletov and Klemke, 2008). Human cancer cells overexpressing RhoC or src display increased cell dissemination when transplanted in zebrafish demonstrating that the molecules (ECM, growth factors, MMPs) and mechanisms playing a role in cancer cell-host tissue interaction are highly conserved between human and zebrafish.

3. Conclusions

Zebrafish recently entered the stage as a promising model system to study human cancer. This has been largely due to the development of transgenic and xenograft models of cancer, and their amenability to genetic and pharmacological testing. Cancer progression in these animals recapitulates many aspects of human disease and opens the door for studies to identify genetic and chemical modifiers of cancer. There are general advantages and limitations of using zebrafish as an in vivo model to study tumor angiogenesis. These include:

Advantages

- Zebrafish husbandry: inexpensive to obtain and maintain large number of adult and embryo zebrafish.
- Generation of larvae with deletion or overexpression of specific genes can be easily accomplished using available tools (e.g. morpholinos, RNA, mimics).
- Genetically manipulated zebrafish strains that are defective or have acquired functions of certain gene products are available (e.g. zinc-fingers, ENU, tilling).
- Transgenic zebrafish lines that express reporter genes in particular cell types are also available in the scientific community.
- Addition of active chemical stimulators or inhibitors to the water enables analysis of intervention of these compounds on physiological and pathological processes.
- Turnover time for experiments is relatively short.
- Optical clarity of zebrafish embryos allows visualization of vascular and hematopoietic cells as well as tumor cell dissemination in living animals.
- Zebrafish embryos allows implantation of mammalian tumor cells, including human and mouse tumor cells, due to the absence of a functional immune system at this stage

Limitations

- Few antibodies against zebrafish proteins are available so far. For this reason it is difficult to perform immunofluorescence analyses in zebrafish samples.
- Due relative small size of zebrafish larvae, you need skillful and careful trainees to perform experiments.
- As most mammalian tumors grow at 37 °C, it is difficult to study the process of xenograft tumor growth at the optimal temperature.
- Microinjection of tumor cells into the perivitelline space of a large number of zebrafish embryos is a tedious procedure and requires highly skillful micro-operations.

These models are already being utilized by academia and industry to search for genetic and chemical modifiers of cancer with success. The attention has been further stimulated by the amenability of zebrafish to pharmacological testing and the superior imaging properties of fish tissues that allow visualization of cancer progression and angiogenesis in live animals.

Here we have described how the zebrafish/tumor xenograft model is becoming an emerging vertebrate system to study tumor angiogenesis. In particular this model become very interesting to analyze the molecular and cellular mechanisms of tumor angiogenesis in real time. Within the past several years, zebrafish has shown great promise to become a powerful animal model to study cancer progression and several laboratories have focused on zebrafish and tumor biology. However, despite a significant progress, more work is required to fully explore how closely these processes in zebrafish may parallel mammalian cancer mechanisms and how well they might be translated to human disease. This improvement will require more specific comparative studies among transgenic and xenograft zebrafish and mouse/mammalian models of cancer/tumor angiogenesis and their relevance to the disease. When all these studies and analyses will be performed the zebrafish model will have the full potential to be used and embraced by the cancer research community.

4. Acknowledgment

I apologize to the many researchers whose work was not cited in this review due to space limitations. We would like to thank all members of Santoro laboratory for support and discussion as well as Ellen Jane Corcoran. Work in Santoro 's laboratory is supported by grants from HFSP, Marie Curie IRG, Telethon and AIRC.

5. References

Amatruda, J. F., Shepard, J. L., Stern, H. M. and Zon, L. I. (2002). Zebrafish as a cancer model system. *Cancer Cell* 1, 229-31.

Armulik, A., Abramsson, A. and Betsholtz, C. (2005). Endothelial/pericyte interactions. *Circ Res* 97, 512-23.

Bergers, G. and Benjamin, L. E. (2003). Tumorigenesis and the angiogenic switch. *Nat Rev Cancer* 3, 401-10.

Bergers, G. and Hanahan, D. (2008). Modes of resistance to anti-angiogenic therapy. *Nat Rev Cancer* 8, 592-603.

Bergers, G. and Song, S. (2005). The role of pericytes in blood-vessel formation and maintenance. *Neuro Oncol* 7, 452-64.

Burns, C. G., Milan, D. J., Grande, E. J., Rottbauer, W., MacRae, C. A. and Fishman, M. C. (2005). High-throughput assay for small molecules that modulate zebrafish embryonic heart rate. *Nat Chem Biol* 1, 263-4.

Carmeliet, P. (2003). Angiogenesis in health and disease. *Nat Med* 9, 653-60.

Carmeliet, P. (2005). Angiogenesis in life, disease and medicine. *Nature* 438, 932-6.

Cleaver, O. and Melton, D. A. (2003). Endothelial signaling during development. *Nat Med* 9, 661-8.

Conway, E. M., Collen, D. and Carmeliet, P. (2001). Molecular mechanisms of blood vessel growth. *Cardiovasc Res* 49, 507-21.

Coultas, L., Chawengsaksophak, K. and Rossant, J. (2005). Endothelial cells and VEGF in vascular development. *Nature* 438, 937-45.

Dooley, K. and Zon, L. I. (2000). Zebrafish: a model system for the study of human disease. *Curr Opin Genet Dev* 10, 252-6.

Duval, H., Harris, M., Li, J., Johnson, N. and Print, C. (2003). New insights into the function and regulation of endothelial cell apoptosis. *Angiogenesis* 6, 171-83.

Duval, H., Johnson, N., Li, J., Evans, A., Chen, S., Licence, D., Skepper, J., Charnock-Jones, D. S., Smith, S. and Print, C. (2007). Vascular development is disrupted by endothelial cell-specific expression of the anti-apoptotic protein Bcl-2. *Angiogenesis* 10, 55-68.

Eimon, P. M., Kratz, E., Varfolomeev, E., Hymowitz, S. G., Stern, H., Zha, J. and Ashkenazi, A. (2006). Delineation of the cell-extrinsic apoptosis pathway in the zebrafish. *Cell Death Differ* 13, 1619-30.

Fish, J. E. and Srivastava, D. (2009). MicroRNAs: opening a new vein in angiogenesis research. *Sci Signal* 2, pe1.

Folkman, J. (2007). Angiogenesis: an organizing principle for drug discovery? *Nat Rev Drug Discov* 6, 273-86.

Gyrd-Hansen, M., Darding, M., Miasari, M., Santoro, M. M., Zender, L., Xue, W., Tenev, T., da Fonseca, P. C., Zvelebil, M., Bujnicki, J. M. et al. (2008). IAPs contain an evolutionarily conserved ubiquitin-binding domain that regulates NF-kappaB as well as cell survival and oncogenesis. *Nat Cell Biol* 10, 1309-17.

Haldi, M., Ton, C., Seng, W. L. and McGrath, P. (2006). Human melanoma cells transplanted into zebrafish proliferate, migrate, produce melanin, form masses and stimulate angiogenesis in zebrafish. *Angiogenesis* 9, 139-51.

Hooper, A. T., Shmelkov, S. V., Gupta, S., Milde, T., Bambino, K., Gillen, K., Goetz, M., Chavala, S., Baljevic, M., Murphy, A. J. et al. (2009). Angiomodulin is a specific marker of vasculature and regulates vascular endothelial growth factor-A-dependent neoangiogenesis. *Circ Res* 105, 201-8.

Jin, S. W., Beis, D., Mitchell, T., Chen, J. N. and Stainier, D. Y. (2005). Cellular and molecular analyses of vascular tube and lumen formation in zebrafish. *Development* 132, 5199-209.

Kawakami, K. (2007). Tol2: a versatile gene transfer vector in vertebrates. *Genome Biol* 8 Suppl 1, S7.

Keller, P. J., Schmidt, A. D., Wittbrodt, J. and Stelzer, E. H. (2008). Reconstruction of zebrafish early embryonic development by scanned light sheet microscopy. *Science* 322, 1065-9.

Lawson, N. D. and Weinstein, B. M. (2002). In vivo imaging of embryonic vascular development using transgenic zebrafish. *Dev Biol* 248, 307-18.

Lee, B. W., Chae, H. Y., Tuyen, T. T., Kang, D., Kim, H. A., Lee, M. and Ihm, S. H. (2009). A comparison of non-viral vectors for gene delivery to pancreatic beta-cells: delivering a hypoxia-inducible vascular endothelial growth factor gene to rat islets. *Int J Mol Med* 23, 757-62.

Lieschke, G. J. and Currie, P. D. (2007). Animal models of human disease: zebrafish swim into view. *Nat Rev Genet* 8, 353-67.

Lin, H. F., Traver, D., Zhu, H., Dooley, K., Paw, B. H., Zon, L. I. and Handin, R. I. (2005). Analysis of thrombocyte development in CD41-GFP transgenic zebrafish. *Blood* 106, 3803-10.

Majesky, M. W. (2007). Developmental basis of vascular smooth muscle diversity. *Arterioscler Thromb Vasc Biol* 27, 1248-58.

Marques, I. J., Weiss, F. U., Vlecken, D. H., Nitsche, C., Bakkers, J., Lagendijk, A. K., Partecke, L. I., Heidecke, C. D., Lerch, M. M. and Bagowski, C. P. (2009). Metastatic behaviour of primary human tumours in a zebrafish xenotransplantation model. *BMC Cancer* 9, 128.

Mazzone, M., Ruiz de Almodovar, C. and Carmeliet, P. (2007). Building in resistance to endothelial cell death. *Nat Genet* 39, 1308-9.

Miao, Z., Luker, K. E., Summers, B. C., Berahovich, R., Bhojani, M. S., Rehemtulla, A., Kleer, C. G., Essner, J. J., Nasevicius, A., Luker, G. D. et al. (2007). CXCR7 (RDC1) promotes breast and lung tumor growth in vivo and is expressed on tumor-associated vasculature. *Proc Natl Acad Sci U S A* 104, 15735-40.

Micheau, O. and Tschopp, J. (2003). Induction of TNF receptor I-mediated apoptosis via two sequential signaling complexes. *Cell* 114, 181-90.

Mizgireuv, I. V. and Revskoy, S. Y. (2006). Transplantable tumor lines generated in clonal zebrafish. *Cancer Res* 66, 3120-5.

Moshal, K. S., Ferri-Lagneau, K. F. and Leung, T. (2010). Zebrafish model: worth considering in defining tumor angiogenesis. *Trends Cardiovasc Med* 20, 114-9.

Nicoli, S. and Presta, M. (2007). The zebrafish/tumor xenograft angiogenesis assay. *Nat Protoc* 2, 2918-23.

Nicoli, S., Ribatti, D., Cotelli, F. and Presta, M. (2007). Mammalian tumor xenografts induce neovascularization in zebrafish embryos. *Cancer Res* 67, 2927-31.

Patton, E. E. and Zon, L. I. (2001). The art and design of genetic screens: zebrafish. *Nat Rev Genet* 2, 956-66.

Red-Horse, K., Crawford, Y., Shojaei, F. and Ferrara, N. (2007). Endothelium-microenvironment interactions in the developing embryo and in the adult. *Dev Cell* 12, 181-94.

Rouhi, P., Jensen, L. D., Cao, Z., Hosaka, K., Lanne, T., Wahlberg, E., Steffensen, J. F. and Cao, Y. (2010a). Hypoxia-induced metastasis model in embryonic zebrafish. *Nat Protoc* 5, 1911-8.

Rouhi, P., Lee, S. L., Cao, Z., Hedlund, E. M., Jensen, L. D. and Cao, Y. (2010b). Pathological angiogenesis facilitates tumor cell dissemination and metastasis. *Cell Cycle* 9, 913-7.

Sakamaki, K. (2004). Regulation of endothelial cell death and its role in angiogenesis and vascular regression. *Curr Neurovasc Res* 1, 305-15.

Santoro, M. M., Pesce, G. and Stainier, D. Y. (2009). Characterization of vascular mural cells during zebrafish development. *Mech Dev* 126, 638-49.

Santoro, M. M., Samuel, T., Mitchell, T., Reed, J. C. and Stainier, D. Y. (2007). Birc2 (cIap1) regulates endothelial cell integrity and blood vessel homeostasis. *Nat Genet.*

Skromne, I. and Prince, V. E. (2008). Current perspectives in zebrafish reverse genetics: moving forward. *Dev Dyn* 237, 861-82.

Stainier, D. Y. (2001). Zebrafish genetics and vertebrate heart formation. *Nat Rev Genet* 2, 39-48.

Stoletov, K. and Klemke, R. (2008). Catch of the day: zebrafish as a human cancer model. *Oncogene* 27, 4509-20.

Stoletov, K., Montel, V., Lester, R. D., Gonias, S. L. and Klemke, R. (2007). High-resolution imaging of the dynamic tumor cell vascular interface in transparent zebrafish. *Proc Natl Acad Sci U S A* 104, 17406-11.

Thijssen, V. L., Postel, R., Brandwijk, R. J., Dings, R. P., Nesmelova, I., Satijn, S., Verhofstad, N., Nakabeppu, Y., Baum, L. G., Bakkers, J. et al. (2006). Galectin-1 is essential in tumor angiogenesis and is a target for antiangiogenesis therapy. *Proc Natl Acad Sci U S A* 103, 15975-80.

Thisse, C. and Zon, L. I. (2002). Organogenesis--heart and blood formation from the zebrafish point of view. *Science* 295, 457-62.

Topczewska, J. M., Postovit, L. M., Margaryan, N. V., Sam, A., Hess, A. R., Wheaton, W. W., Nickoloff, B. J., Topczewski, J. and Hendrix, M. J. (2006). Embryonic and tumorigenic pathways converge via Nodal signaling: role in melanoma aggressiveness. *Nat Med* 12, 925-32.

Traver, D., Paw, B. H., Poss, K. D., Penberthy, W. T., Lin, S. and Zon, L. I. (2003). Transplantation and in vivo imaging of multilineage engraftment in zebrafish bloodless mutants. *Nat Immunol* 4, 1238-46.

Varfolomeev, E., Blankenship, J. W., Wayson, S. M., Fedorova, A. V., Kayagaki, N., Garg, P., Zobel, K., Dynek, J. N., Elliott, L. O., Wallweber, H. J. et al. (2007). IAP antagonists induce autoubiquitination of c-IAPs, NF-kappaB activation, and TNFalpha-dependent apoptosis. *Cell* 131, 669-81.

Varfolomeev, E. E., Schuchmann, M., Luria, V., Chiannilkulchai, N., Beckmann, J. S., Mett, I. L., Rebrikov, D., Brodianski, V. M., Kemper, O. C., Kollet, O. et al. (1998). Targeted disruption of the mouse Caspase 8 gene ablates cell death induction by the TNF receptors, Fas/Apo1, and DR3 and is lethal prenatally. *Immunity* 9, 267-76.

Vlecken, D. H. and Bagowski, C. P. (2009). LIMK1 and LIMK2 are important for metastatic behavior and tumor cell-induced angiogenesis of pancreatic cancer cells. *Zebrafish* 6, 433-9.

von Tell, D., Armulik, A. and Betsholtz, C. (2006). Pericytes and vascular stability. *Exp Cell Res* 312, 623-9.

White, R. M., Sessa, A., Burke, C., Bowman, T., LeBlanc, J., Ceol, C., Bourque, C., Dovey, M., Goessling, W., Burns, C. E. et al. (2008). Transparent adult zebrafish as a tool for in vivo transplantation analysis. *Cell Stem Cell* 2, 183-9.

Wu, C. J., Conze, D. B., Li, X., Ying, S. X., Hanover, J. A. and Ashwell, J. D. (2005). TNF-alpha induced c-IAP1/TRAF2 complex translocation to a Ubc6-containing compartment and TRAF2 ubiquitination. *Embo J* 24, 1886-98.

Zon, L. I. and Peterson, R. T. (2005). In vivo drug discovery in the zebrafish. *Nat Rev Drug Discov* 4, 35-44.

8

The Role of VEGF in the Process of Neovasculogenesis

Aleksandra Sobczyńska-Rak
Department of Veterinary Surgery, Faculty of Veterinary Medicine, Lublin University of Life Sciences, Lublin, Poland

1. Introduction

Neovasculogenesis is a multi-stage process of blood vessel formation which plays a vital role in neoplasia. The formation of blood vessels in tumours is closely related to invasive cancerous growth.

The process of angiogenesis is closely regulated by the system of cooperating stimulants and inhibitors. Factors stimulating neovasculogenesis are characterised by a fairly broad spectrum of activity. Three key attributes of proangiogenic factors have been identified as:

1. The specific effect on endothelial cells, i.e. the given factor's presence induces angiogenesis.
2. The presence of specific receptors in endothelial cells.
3. Neutralisation of the factor inhibits angiogenesis (Grunstein et al., 1999; McMahon, 2000; Szala & Radzikowski, 1997).

There are a number of proteins that have been referred to as pro-angiogenic factors that actively participate in the formation of capillaries. VEGF meets all key requirements of being classified as a pro-angiogenic factor: it specifically affects vascular epithelial cells, it is present only during angiogenesis, it does not occur in adults unless new vessels are being formed. Its overexpression is connected to the formation of capillaries and its neutralisation inhibits the process (Grunstein et al., 1999; McMahon, 2000).

2. VEGF - Vascular Endothelial Growth Factor

The two main biological activities of VEGF - mitogenic activity and vascular permeability inducing activity - were described, purified and designated independently as VPF (vascular permeability factor) and VEGF (vascular endothelial growth factor).

The release of a vascular permeability-increasing agent by guinea pig hepatocarcinoma cells was reported in 1979 (Dvorak et al., 1979). Vascular leakage was subsequently used to monitor purification of VEGF from the supernatant of this (Senger et al., 1983; Senger et al., 1986) and of the human histiocytic lymphoma cell line U-937 (Connolly et al., 1989b). Therefore, the factor was later designated as vascular permeability factor –VPF (Senger et al., 1983) or vasculotropin (Plouët et al., 1989).

The mitogenic activity of this agent towards vascular endothelial cells was used to monitor its purification, and on the basis of its target cell selectivity the purified agent was designated VEGF (Ferrara & Henzel, 1989; Gospodarowicz et al., 1989).

VEGF is a strong and specific mitogen for endothelial vascular cells of the circulatory and lymphatic systems (Baillie et al., 2001; Barańska et al., 2005; Chhieng et al., 2003). It is secreted by a number of cell types: T lymphocytes, monocytes, macrophages, activated platelets, fibroblasts, smooth muscle cells, and most importantly neoplastic cells (Namiecińska et al., 2005; Restucci et al., 2002; Rosen, 2002; Szala & Radzikowski, 1997). The factor is characterised by mitogenic activity towards endothelial cells, which causes their increased proliferation, migration and formation of new vessels from endothelial cells (Baillie et al., 2001; Bałan, 2000; Breier & Risau, 1996; Conti, 2002; Dvorak, 2002; Epstein et al., 2001; Gawrychowski et al., 1997; Nicosia, 1998; Restucci et al., 2002; Rofstad & Halsor, 2000; Terman & Stoletov, 2001). The newly formed blood vessels serve not only to provide neoplastic cells with nutrients and oxygen, but are also responsible for the neoplastic cells permeating to the circulatory system, thus facilitating tumour dissemination and metastasis (Litwiniuk et al., 2007).

VEGF is also a 50 times stronger inductor of blood vessel permeability than histamine, it allows the permeation of plasma proteins as well as neoplastic cells into the extravascular space, allowing for their hyperplasia into the new location (Epstein et al, 2001; Kondo et al., 2000; Łojko & Komarnicki, 2004; Szala & Radzikowski, 1997).

VEGF is the main proangiogenic factor responsible for the formation of blood vessels in neoplastic tumours (Fang et al., 2001; Papetti & Herman, 2002).

It was demonstrated that the increase of VEGF-A expression is one of the mechanisms greatly enhances a tumour's resistance to chemotherapy (Volk et al., 2008). VEGF-A protects tumor cells from apoptosis through autocrine activation of VEGF-A receptors expressed on tumour cells (Volk et al., 2011).

2.1 VEGF–A isoforms

VEGF is a glycosilated homodimer whose molecular mass is 46-48 kDa (Barańska et al., 2005, Chhieng et al., 2003; Clifford et al., 2001; Kondo et al., 2000; Nicosia, 1998; Papetti & Herman, 2002; Ranieri et al., 2004). The gene for VEGF-A is located on chromosone 6 at band 21.3, and comprises 8 exons separated by 7 introns (Ferrara, 1999; Gruchlik et al., 2007). Through alternative mRNA maturation, isoforms of VEGF are formed comprising respectively 121, 145, 148, 162, 165, 183, 189, or 206 amino acids ($VEGF_{121}$, $VEGF_{145}$, $VEGF_{148}$, $VEGF_{183}$, $VEGF_{165}$, $VEGF_{189}$, $VEGF_{206}$). The shortest isoform, $VEGF_{121}$, is encoded by exons 1-5 and 8, VEGF165 includes additionally exon 7. $VEGF_{189}$ and $VEGF_{206}$ mRNAs contain all 8 exons, and the usage of a variable 5'-splice donor site within exon 6 creates the difference between the VEGF189 and $VEGF_{206}$ mRNA .The particular isoforms vary in terms of biochemical and biological qualities (Bałan, 2000; Barańska et al., 2005; Ferrara, 1999; Ferrara & Davis-Smyth 1997; Łojko & Komarnicki, 2004; Łukasik et al., 2003; Namiecińska et al., 2005; Nicosia, 1998; Oshika et al., 1998; Papetti & Herman, 2002; Webb et al., 1998; Yu et al., 2002). Additionally, a form of $VEGF_{110}$ also exists as a product of $VEGF_{165}$ and $VEGF_{189}$ proteolysis.

The most common form, synthesised by a wide range of both healthy and altered cells, which is at the same time the most active biologically, is $VEGF_{165}$ and $VEGF_{121}$ (Gruchlik et al., 2007). Other commonly observed isoforms are $VEGF_{121}$, $VEGF_{165}$, $VEGF_{189}$, while

$VEGF_{145}$, $VEGF_{183}$ and $VEGF_{206}$ are rarely observed *in vivo*, e.g. the longest of the forms is found exclusively in embryonic tissues (Barańska et al., 2005). $VEGF_{121}$ and $VEGF_{165}$ are soluble proteins observed extracellularly. $VEGF_{121}$ is a weak acidic polypeptide that does not bind to heparin due to the lack of the heparin-binding domain encoded by exons 6 and 7. In contrast, $VEGF_{165}$ is basic and binds to heparin. $VEGF_{189}$ and $VEGF_{206}$ are even more basic and bind to heparin with greater affinity. The differences in affinity for heparin affect the fate of the VEGF isoforms (Houck et al., 1992). $VEGF_{121}$ is secreted and is freely diffusible in the medium of transfected cells. $VEGF_{165}$ is also secreted but a significant fraction remains bound to heparin-containing proteoglycans. A part of $VEGF_{165}$ remains anchored to the cell membrane and the extracellular matrix. $VEGF_{189}$ and $VEGF_{206}$ are alkaline and are found almost exclusively as proteins anchored to the extracellular matrix. They display stronger mitogenic activity than the shorter isoforms (Barańska et al., 2005; Gruchlik et al., 2007; Łojko & Komarnicki, 2004; Łukasik et al., 2003). They may take the soluble form after binding with heparin as well as under the effect of heparinase, metaloproteases or other extracellular proteases. The mRNA molecule for all the isoforms comprises exons 1-5 carrying information necessary to recognise the specific receptors - VEGFR-1 or VEGFR-2. Discrepancies in this respect are observed only in terms of presence or absence of exons 6, 6', 7 or 8. (Michalski et al., 2003)

2.2 The VEGF protein family

Purified VEGF (VEGF-A) was first obtained by Gospodarowicz et al. and Ferrara and Hanzel in 1989 (Ferrara & Henzel, 1989; Gospodarowicz et al., 1989). It is one of the most thoroughly studied factors partaking in all stages of angiogenesis.

In normal tissues, the highest levels of VEGF-A mRNA are found in adult lung, kidney, heart, and adrenal gland. Lower, but still readily detectable, quantities of VEGF-A transcript levels occur in liver, spleen, and gastric mucosa (Hoeban et al., 2004)

VEGF-A displays a variety of qualities, one of the most important of which is the increase of vascular permeability. The same allows blood proteins, e.g. plasminogen, fibrinogen, macrophages and platelets to permeate into the extravascular space.

Plasmitogen is transformed into plasmin which, through proteolytic action, activates metalloproteases destroying the basement membranes of the existing vessels. Fibrinogen is transformed into fibrin which provides a form of scaffold for the precipitating endothelial cells. Macrophages and platelets in turn stimulate angiogenesis by secreting cytokines and VEGF.

VEGF-A is the key mitogenic factor but it also displays strong protective action. It was observed that it can induce the expression of proteins which prevent apoptosis in blood vascular endothelial cells and increase the probability of the cells' survival (Hoeban et al., 2004; Bałan & Słowiński, 2008)

It was demonstrated that overexpression VEGF may inhibit differentiation and maturation of dendritic cells and thus weaken the host immunological response against a tumour (Swidzińska et al., 2006).

Furthermore, VEGF stimulates the expression of the tissue factor (TF) in ECs and monocytes, which facilitates the activation of blood coagulation (Wojtkiewicz & Sierko, 2009).

At a molecular level, VEGF-A reprograms endothelial cell gene expression, leading to increased expression of a number of different proteins, including the procoagulant tissue factor, proteins associated with the fibrinolytic pathway, matrix metalloproteases, the GLUT-1 glucose transporter, nitric oxide synthase, numerous mitogens, and a number of antiapoptotic factors (e.g. bcl-2, A1, survivin, XIAP)(Bałan & Słotwiński 2008).

VEGF-A is a cytokine which plays a key role in postnatal angiogenesis, both pathological, i.e. the formation of undesirable vessels (in tumours, retinopathy), and physiological (healing).

VEGF-A is over expressed not only by invasive cancer cells, but also by at least some premalignant lesions (eg, precursor lesions of breast, cervix, and colon cancers);furthermore, expression levels increased in parallel with malignant progression (Bałan & Słotwiński 2008).

The VEGF group also includes other structurally related, yet varying in terms of biological activity, proteins VEGF-B, VEGF-C, VEGF-D and VEGF-E as well as the placental growth factor (PIGF) (Barańska et al., 2005; Łojko & Komarnicki, 2004; Namiecińska et al., 2005; Papetti & Herman, 2002; Ranieri et al., 2004; Terman & Stoletov, 2001).

Cytokine VEGF-B was discovered in 1996 (Grimmond et al., 1996; Olofsson et al., 1996). Its gene is located in the region of the 11q13 chromosome and contains 7 exons.

It is observed in two forms formed through alternative splicing of mRNA contained in molecule 167 or 186 of amino acids. VEGF-B is a VEGFR-1 ligand, and after the formation of the heterodimer from VEGF-A it can also react with the VEGF-2 receptor (Olofsson et al., 1998) The two splice isoforms, VEGF-B_{167} and VEGF-B_{186}, differ in their C-terminal amino acid sequences and show different diffusion properties and receptor-binding affinities. Both isoforms are expressed in adult tissues, with the highest expression in the myocardium, brown adipose tissue (BAT), skeletal muscle and pancreas. The expression of VEGF-B is not induced by hypoxia, in contrast to all the other VEGF-ligands (Li et al., 2001)

VEGF –B_{167} has a heparyn-binding domain so that upon secretion, VEGF –B_{167} binds to cell-surface heparyn sulphate proteoglycans. VRGF-B_{186} does not contain the heparin-binding domain and there-fore is more soluble (Li, 2010)

Several studies have shown that VEGF-B gene or protein transfer into different types of organs did not induce angiogenesis under most conditions (Li et al., 2009)

VEGF-B is not necessary in the process of angiogenesis, however, recent studies have shown that the factor is needed for vessel survival. In fact many researchers have suggested changing the VEGF-B functional denotation to "survival" rather than an "angiogenic" factor.

We recently found that VEGF-B is a survival factor for multiple types of vascular cells, including vascular endothelial cells (EC), pericytes (PC) and smooth muscle cells (SMC) (Zhang et al., 2009).

VGF-B186 delivery to the heart upregulated the expression of many antiapoptotic genes in cardiomyocytes, and inhibited cardiac myocyte apoptosis, demonstrating a survival effect of VEGF-B_{186} on them (Lahteenvuo et al., 2009).

Certain researchers claim VEGF-B to be necessary in adults to ensure proper functioning, however, it is not required in the development of the cardiovascular system and angiogenesis (Roskoski, 2007)

Moreover, Dr Eriksson's group showed that VEGF-B is a critical regulator of energy metabolism by regulating fatty acid uptake (Hagberg et al., 2010)

It has also been observed that the protein can regulate the FATP (Fatty Acid Transport Proteins) level in vascular walls.

The human VEGF-C gene was first cloned in 1996, while VEGF-D in 1997 (Joukov V et al. 1996; Yamada Y 1997).

Both factors are synthesised as inactive, multi-molecular pre-pro-proteins comprising end pro-peptides NH_2- and COOH - and the central homological VEGF domain. The domain contains receptor binding sites (Achen et al., 1998; Joukov et al., 1996; Stacker et al.,1999; Yamada 1997; Kuuk et al., 1996).

The active VEGF-C and VEGF-D forms are formed through inter- and extra-cellular proteolysis of –C and –N ends (Achen et al., 1998; Joukov et al., 1996).

The precursor forms of the growth factor interact mainly with the VEGFR-3 receptor while active forms display strong affinity for VEGFR-2 (Joukov et al., 1997; Stacker et al., 1999).

The functions of VEGF-C and VEGF-D are mainly determined by the receptor they bind with and its location. When either of the factors interacts with the VEGFR-3 receptor located in the lymphatic epithelium, they induce the development and restructuring of lymphatic vessels. In turn, when the active forms of the growth factor bind with the VEGFR-2 receptor in blood vessel epithelium, they influence angiogenesis.

In the course of research conducted on embryos and transgenic animals, it was observed that VEGF-C and the VEGFR-3 receptor play a vital role in the embryonic development of the lymphoid system. Homozygous mice VEGF-C$^{-/-}$ with inactive VEGF-C gene died due to undeveloped lymphoid system. Heterozygous mice VEGF-C $^{-/+}$ displayed significant malformation in terms of this system.

In adult humans, high levels of VEGF-C mRNA have been observed in a number of organs, i.e.: the heart, lungs, skeletal muscles, large intestine, small intestine, and thyroid. Relatively small amounts of VEGF-C are known to be produced in the kidneys, pancreas, prostate, and spleen (Roskoski 2007).

VEGF-C overexpression has been observed in a number of tumours in humans, including: breast cancer, colorectal cancer, stomach cancer, thyroid neoplasm, and prostate cancer. High levels of the factor indicate a negative prognosis (Sucha & Ganesan 2008)

Structural similarities between VEGF-C and VEGF-D as well as their affinity for the VEGFR-2 and VEGFR-3 receptors would suggest similar biological qualities of the two. However, VEGF-D does not play as significant a role in the embryonic development of the lymphoid system (Karkkainen et al., 2004). It has been observed that apart from mitogenic activity on endothelial cells, it also stimulates fibroblast division.

High VEGF-D levels are observed in humans mainly in the heart, lungs, skeletal muscles, and small intestine. VEGF-D overexpression is observed in a number of tumours as well, i.e.: breast cancer, colorectal cancer, stomach cancer, thyroid neoplasm, and cervical cancer. Furthermore, the VEGF-D expression level has proved to be an independent prognostic factor in respect to ovarian cancer (Yokoyama et al 2003).

To sum up, VEGF-C and VEGF-D play important roles in lymphangiogenesis and angiogenesis, they also facilitate lymphatic metastasis in lymph nodes.

VEGF-E was identified in the genome of the orf virus (parapoxvirus) which is pathogenic in goats, sheep and sporadically in humans. It is in homological sequence with other proteins of the VEGF family, which may suggest that the gene of the virus VEGF originated from mammal hosts and underwent a genetic drift. It displays proangiogenic activity (Barańska et al., 2005).

PIGF - occurs in homodimer form. Increased concentrations of this factor have been observed in cases of myocardial infarction, retinopathy and neoplastic disease. It is responsible for stimulating the growth of endothelial cells and smooth muscles. Through action synergistic with VEGF-B, it influences the diversification and activation of monocytes (Clauss, 2000; Namiecińska et al., 2005).

The VEGF family also includes sv-VEGF proteins isolated from snake venom. Due to their homology similar to the VEGF found in mammals, they are often referred to as "VEGF-like" proteins. One such protein has been isolated from the venom of a Bothrops insularis snake (Barańska et al., 2005).

2.3 VEGF receptors

VEGF binds to at least three different types of receptors: VEGFR-1 (Flt-1- fms-like tyrosine kinase-1), VEGFR-2 (KDR- kinase domain region in humans and Flk-1- fetal liver kinase-1 in mice), and VEGFR-3 (Flt-4 - fetal liver kinase 4) which belong to a family of receptors containing a tyrosine-kinase domain (Bałan, 2000; Barańska et al, 2005; Breier & Risau, 1996; Ferrara & Davis-Smyth, 1997; Namiecińska et al., 2005; Papetti, 2002; Ranieri et al., 2004; Szala & Radzikowski, 1997; Webb et al., 1998).

VEGFR-1 is found in the epithelium, as well as on the surface of macrophages and monocytes. The receptor is characterised by the highest affinity for the ligand (Kd-10-20 pM). Its expression remains constant in dividing as well as latent cells. It has been observed that the absence of said receptor results in disorders in terms of the structure and morphology of the formed vessels. The same is due to the increase in the number of hemangioblasts accumulating inside the forming vessels and closing them off (Barańska et al., 2005).

In homozygous mice, the receptor's insufficiency leads to vessel hypertrophy and premature death of foetuses in mid pregnancy (Hucz & Szala, 2006).

VEGFR-1 displays significant affinity for bonding VEGF-A as well as PIGF and VEGF-B (Barańska et al., 2005).

VEGFR-2 is expressed in epithelium cells, retinal stem cells, as well as platelets and hematopoietic cells, mainly during foetal life when the processes of angiogenesis and vasculogenesis are particularly intensive (Bałan, 2000). The amount of mRNA for VEFGR-2 is reduced in the cells of an adult organism. Embryos deprived of the VEGFR-2 receptor do not develop vascularisation and die in early embryogenesis (Shibuya & Claesson-Welsh 2006) The receptor's affinity for the ligand is lower than in the case of VEGFR-1 (Barańska et al., 2005).

The Flt-1 and KDR/Flk-1 receptors vary in terms of signal transduction mechanisms. Stimulation of the KDR/Flk-1 receptor results in a violent reaction while stimulation of the Flt-1 receptor induces a significantly weaker response. The above suggests that Flt-1 may negatively regulate the process of angiogenesis (Ferrara, 1999), whereas activation of the KDR/Flk-1 receptor increases the proliferational activity of endothelium cells while at the same time inhibiting the process of apoptosis and increasing blood vessel permeability. It has been observed that mouse embryos deprived of the VEGFR-2 receptor will be non-vascularised and will die in the early stage of embryogenesis (Thielemann et al., 2010). The receptor reacts to VEGF-C and VEGF D.

Two distinct receptor tyrosine kinases have been identified for VEGF-A on endothelial cells: VEGFR-1 and VEGFR-2 (Olsson et al., 2006; Shibuya & Claesson-Welsh, 2006). The affinity of VEGF-A for VEGFR-1 is 10-fold stronger than its affinity for VEGFR-2; nonetheless, most VEGF-A–mediated downstream signaling events associated with angiogenesis require VEGFR-2 activation (Waltenberger et al., 1994, Zachary 2003, Szala 2009). Binding of VEGFR-2 to VEGF induces dimerization and consequent phosphorylation of a subset of intracellular tyrosine residues (Rydén et al., 2003, Chen et al., 2010).

VEGFR-3 has been detected in embryonic epithelial cells. In mature tissue it is present almost exclusively in the lymphatic vessel epithelium cells, which indicates its participation in lymphangiogenesis. The receptor does not recognise VEGF-A but does bind with VEGF-C and VEGF-D (Barańska et al., 2005; Namiecińska et al., 2005).

In the 1990s, soluble forms of sVEGFR-1, unanchored in the cell membrane, were discovered. The particulars of the biochemical structure of sVEGFR-1 remain to be determined, but we know that by binding with each isoform of VEGF they serve as negative angiogenesis regulators and inhibit the formation of blood vessels in neoplastic tumours (Thielemann et al., 2010).

2.4 Regulation of VEGF expression

VEGF expression is regulated by a number of mechanisms, the most important of which is hypoxia. In conditions of lowered oxygen partial pressure, a sudden increase can be observed in terms of the presence of hypoxia inducible factor - HIF-1α - which activates the VEGF gene promoter - HRE (hypoxia response element), thus intensifying VEGF expression (Breier & Risau, 1996; Fang et al., 2001; Ferrara, 1999; Namiecińska et al., 2005; Papetti & Herman, 2002; Rosen, 2002).

The gene's stimulation independent of HIF-1 has also been observed as a result of hypoxia. Due to low oxygen pressure, accumulation of adenosine may occur activating its receptor A2 and causing an increase of cAMP concentration, which in turn leads to elevated levels of mRNA for VEGF. Stimulation of VEGF expression can also be due to the influence of cytokines: EGF, TGF-β, KGF, PGF_2, IGF-1, interleukin - IL-1, IL -5, IL-6, IL-9, IL-13, or due to a mutation of certain oncogenes leading to a neoplastic transformation (Barańska et al., 2005; Breier & Risau, 1996; Gruchlik et al., 2007, Xue et al., 2009). An example of the latter case may be the mutation of gene p-53, which stimulates VEGF expression.

3. VEGF expression in tumours

3.1 VEGF expression profiles in human tumours

The opinion prevalent in literature is that increased vascular density may result from overexpression of proangiogenic factors, particularly VEGF (Han et al., 2001).

The induction of vessel growth is a process closely regulated by positive and negative angiogenesis regulators. In a mature organism, the two balance each other out, thus preventing vessel carcinogenesis. Any distortion of the balance results in the increased production and action of one or more proangiogenic factors, which leads to the stimulation of angiogenesis (Jośko et al., 2000; Conti, 2002).

It has been suggested by a number of researchers that VEGF is a mitogen of epithelium cells and a strong factor inducing increased vessel permeability. It plays a vital role in the process of neovascularisation, tumour growth and metastasis (Baillie et al., 2001; Barańska et al., 2005; Chhieng et al., 2003; Dvorak, 2002; Grunstein et al., 1999; Hicklin & Ellis, 2005; Kraft et al., 1999; Litwiniu et al., 2007; Poon et al., 2003; Zheng et al., 2003). Chechlińska also observes that it can activate specific types of integrins on neoplastic cells, which increases invasiveness by allowing tumour cells to anchor to degraded elements of the extracellular matrix (Chechlińska, 2003).

There are a number of publications pertaining to the assessment of immunohistochemical expression of VEGF receptors in cancerous tissues. In the research, anti-VEGF antibodies were used to show receptors in endothelial cells. Takahashi observed elevated expression of the KDR/Flk-1 receptor for VEGF in metastased malignant colorectal cancers, as compared to non-metastased cancers (Takahashi et al., 1995).

Research has also been conducted on patients suffering from lung cancer (Oshika et al., 1998; Yuan et al., 2001) and women diagnosed with malignant breast cancer (Adams et al., 2000; Lewis et al., 2000; Terman & Stoletov, 2001). Overexpression of the vascular endothelial growth factor correlated with tumour growth, development of new vessels, and early relapse of the neoplastic disease.

With the use of the real-time PCR exam, the presence of VEGF mRNA can be determined in tumour cells. The highest VEGF mRNA levels have been observed in malignant tumour tissue contiguous with necrotic areas (Ferrara & Davis-Smyth 1997; Restucci et al., 2002).

Increased VEGF expression, both in terms of mRNA in neoplastic tissues and the protein itself in blood plasma, serum and urine, has been observed in numerous types of neoplastic disease in humans (Ferrara & Davis-Smyth, 1997; Łojko & Komarnicki, 2004). Elevated VEGF concentrations in blood plasma have been noted in patients diagnosed with colorectal cancer, lung cancer, and breast cancer in women. It typically constituted a bad prognosis and indicated the presence of distant metastases (Chhieng et al., 2003; Ferrara & Davis-smyth, 1997; Han et al., 2001; Litwiniuk et al., 2007; Zheng et al., 2003; Kopczyńska et al., 2008; Wójcik et al., 2010).

Overproduction of VEGF has also been observed in neoplastic cells of aberrant ovaries. The growth factor was identified in the peritoneal effusions from female patients diagnosed with malignant neoplastic growths, which suggests its secretion by cancerous cells (Gawrychowski et al., 1997).

Elevated VEGF levels have also been noted in hematologic hyperplasia. In myeloid leukaemia, elevated VEGF levels correlated with shorter survivability and lower probability of full remission (Łojko & Komarnicki, 2004).

Kozaczka et al. observed significantly higher levels of serum VEGF in patients diagnosed with surgical colorectal andenocarcinoma, when compared to the control population. They concluded that the level of vascular endothelial growth factor was the only statistically significant parameter of prognostic value (Kozaczka et al., 2004).

Elevated levels of VEGF expression, related to bad prognoses and high likelihood of metastasis, have been observed in various types of malignant tumours in humans (Epstein et al., 2001; Poon et al., 2003; Yu et al., 2002; Yuan et al., 2001). A correlation has also been observed between the VEGF value and the level of malignancy in tumours of: lungs, breasts, thyroids, stomachs, intestines, kidneys, bladders, ovaries, oral cavities, as well as angiosarcomas, and nervous system neoplasms (Chao et al., 2001; Han et al., 2001; Nicosia, 1998; Yuan et al., 2001).

Research has also been conducted into the expression of serum VEGF in patients suffering from melanoma. Elevated VEGF levels in the serum were observed in patients with advanced neoplastic process. It indicated significantly shorter periods of remission and, as suggested by the author, was of prognostic value (Ascierto et al., 2004;Yu et al., 2002).

Available literature devotes significant attention to the correlation between the vessel density in cancerous tissue and the expression of VEGF in blood serum or tumour cells (Adams et al., 2000; Ferrara, 1999; Kondo et al., 2000; Loggini et al., 2003; Takahashi et al., 1995; Zheng et al., 2003).

Said correlation has been observed in squamous skin carcinomas in humans. Some researchers suggest that the correlation between the number of vessels and the increased expression of vascular endothelial growth factor mRNA can prove valuable in determining the malignancy level of such cancers (Loggini et al., 2003). The development of vessels accompanied by increased concentrations of VEGF mRNA as well as of the protein itself in tumour tissues has also been observed in cases of colorectal adenoma (Kondo et al., 2000; Takahashi et al., 1995) and breast cancer (Adams et al., 2000) in humans, where it indicated unfavourable prognoses.

It is assumed that the negative correlation between the number of vessels in a tumour and the level of VEGF as the main proangiogenic factor may be due to the process known as vascular mimicry. It is a process in which angioid channels are formed outside the epithelium. Literature indicates that said phenomenon can be observed in the case of malignant melanomas (Folberg et al., 2000; McDonald et al., 2000).

3.2 VEGF expression profiles in dog tumours

Comparative studies have been performed in respect to human and animal VEGF structure. It was demonstrated that all main isoforms of the vascular endothelial growth factor are present in dogs, and that amino acid sequences in the areas responsible for binding with receptors are identical in humans and animals. Furthermore, it has been observed that canine VEGF activates human endothelial cells to the same extent as the human growth factor. In dogs, it occurs in tumours at similar volumetric ratios to those observed in human malignant tumours (Mohammed et al., 2002; Scheidegger et al., 1999).

The immunohistochemiacal reaction of VEGF expression has also been studied in squamous carcinomas and skin basaliomas in dogs (Maiolino et al., 2004). The presence of the growth factor was observed in all squamous cancers, particularly those located in the vicinity of toes, while it was not detected in the studied basaliomas. Similar results were obtained in the course of research on human squamous carcinoma (Loggini et al., 2003; Oshika et al., 1998). It is believed that the presence of VEGF in squamous cancers may serve as a viable, additional criterion in determining the malignancy and growth capacity of tumours in both dogs and humans.

The growth factor has been determined in the blood serum of dogs diagnosed with angiosarcoma. It was observed that elevated VEGF levels in dog blood serum occurred in dogs suffering from cancer. It did not, however, correlate with the advancement stage of the disease or the size of the tumour (Clifford et al., 2001). Similar results were obtained by Wergin and Kaser-Hotz. They observed that in healthy dogs the level of VEGF was indiscernible, while in dogs suffering from the neoplastic disease it was high and the obtained results were statistically significant (Wergin & Kaser-Hotz, 2004; Wergin et al., 2004).

Elevated VEGF levels have also been observed in the urine of dogs diagnosed with malignant bladder cancer (Mohammed et al., 2002).

Our own research indicated statistically significant VEGF values in the blood serum of dogs suffering from malignant skin neoplasms. An analysis of own research results as well as data available in literature suggests that the blood serum levels of VEGF may indeed constitute a valuable prognostic criterion and be a viable indicator in early diagnoses of carcinomas. Overexpression of the vascular endothelial growth factor observed in malignant tumours, confronted with the clinical picture of the neoplasia, may influence the choice of treatment and facilitate the prognosis of its therapeutic effect (Sobczyńska-Rak, 2009).

A study on vascular density in mammary carcinomas in dogs yielded similar results to those obtained in humans. The correlation between the number of capillaries and elevated VEGF levels was again observed (Restucci et al., 2002).

In the course of own research, a correlation was observed between vessel density and serum VEGF levels in benign and malignant skin cancers in dogs. A negative correlation was indicated in the case of oral cancer, while no correlation was observed in the case of

mammary cancer. The results indicate that both angiogenesis and the growth factor have significant prognostic value in terms of determining the malignancy level of skin cancer. The potential value of the same in respect to oral cancer and mammary cancer remains to be determined (Sobczyńska-Rak, 2009).
Research by other authors conducted on dogs suffering from mammary cancer indicates that VEGF stimulates the proliferation and migration of endothelial cells and therefore influences angiogenesis. However, for a functional vessel to be formed other growth factors are required (Restucci et al. 2002; Troy et al., 2006).
To sum up, overexpression of VEGF in blood serum, bodily fluids, or neoplastic tissue often correlates with angiogenesis, growth and metastasis in both human and animal cancers. The observed close relations suggest the notion of treating neoplastic disease through inhibiting the formation of blood vessels in cancerous tissues. A particularly promising treatment approach may prove to be the use of VEGF antibodies (Gruchlik et al., 2007; Stępień-Wyrobiec et al., 2007, Hashizume et al., 2010) and clinical research into the matter is currently being conducted worldwide. In recent years, intensive research has been underway into anti-neoplasmic treatments with the use of cytostatic agents in combination with agents inhibiting VEGF expression or blocking its receptors. The results so far show considerable promise and may constitute a significant breakthhrough in the fight against neoplastic disease (Volk et al., 2011)

4. References

Achen M.G., Jeltsch M., Kukk E., Makinen T., Vitali A., Wilks A.F., Alitalo K., Stacker S.A. 1998. Vascular endothelial growth factor D (VEGF-D) is a ligand for the tyrosine kinases VEGF receptor 2 (Flk1) and VEGF receptor 3 (Flt4). Proc. Natl. Acad. Sci. 95, 548-53

Adams J., Carder P. J., Downey S., Forbes M. A., MacLennan K., Allgar V., Kaufman S., Hallam S., Bicknell R., Walker J. J., Cairnduff F., Selby P. J., Perren T. J., Lansdown M., Banks R. E. 2000. Vascular Endothelial Growth Factor (VEGF) in breast cancer: comparison of plasma, serum, and tissue VEGF and microvessel density and effects of Tamoxifen. Cancer Res. 60, 2898-2905.

Ascierto P. A., Leonardi E., Ottaiano A., Napolitano M., Scala S., Castello G. 2004. Prognostic volue of serum VEGF in melanoma patients: a pilot study. Anticancer Res. 24, 4255-4258.

Baillie R., Carlile J., Pendleton N., Schor A. M. 2001. Prognostic value of vascularity and vascular endothelial growth factor expression in non-small cell lung cancer. J. Clin. Pathol. 54, 116-120.

Bałan B. J. 2000. Angiogenesis – problem of XXI century. Nowa Medycyna 4, 8-14.

Bałan B. J., Słotwiński R. 2008. VEGF and tumor angiogenesis. Centr. Eur. J Immunol. 33, 232-236.

Barańska P., Jerczyńska H., Pawłowska Z. 2005. Vascular endothelial growth factor-structure and functions. Postępy Biochem. 51, 13-21.

Biedka M., Makarewicz R., Lebioda A., Kardymowicz H., Goralewska A. 2010. Vascular endothelial growth factor C as a predictive factor In cervical cancer? Współczesna Onkologia, 14, 87-92.

Breier G., Risau W. 1996. The role of vascular endothelial growth factor in blood vessel formation. Cell Biol. 6, 454-456.

Chao C., Al-Saleem T., Brooks J. J., Rogatko A., Kraybill W. G., Eisenberg B. 2001. Vascular Endothelial Growth Factor and soft tissue sarcomas: tumor expression correlates with grade. Ann. Surg. Oncol. 8, 260-267.

Chechlińska M. 2003. The role of cytokines in carcinogenesis. Nowotwory 6, 648-659.

Chen T. T., Luque A., Lee S., Anderson S. M., Segura T., Iruela-Arispe M. L. 2010. Anchorage of VEGF to the extracellular matrix conveys differential signaling responses to endothelial cells. J. Cell Biol. 188, 595–609

Chhieng D. C., Tabbara S. O., Marley E. F., Talley L. I., Frost A. R. 2003. Microvassel density and Vascular Endothelil Growth Factor expression in infiltrating lobular mammary carcinoma. Breast J. 9, 200-207.

Clauss M. 2000. Molecular biology of the VEGF and VEGF receptor family. Semin. Tromb. Hemost. 26, 561-569.

Clifford C. A., Hughes D., Beal M. W., Mackin A. J., Henry C. J., Shofer F. S., Sorenmo K. U. 2001. Plasma vascular endothelial growth factor concentrations in healthy dogs and dogs with hemangiosarcoma. J. Vet. Intern. Med. 15, 131-135.

Connolly, D. T., Olander, J. V., Heuvelman, D., Nelson, R., Monsell, R., Siegel, N., Haymore, B. L., Leimgruber, R., and Feder, J. 1989. Human vascular permeability factor. Isolation from U937 cells. J. Biol. Chem. 264, 20017-24.

Conti C. J. 2002. Vascular endothelial growth factor: regulation in the mouse skin carcinogenesis model and use in antiangiogenesis cancer therapy. Oncologist. 7, 4-11.

Dvorak H. F., Orenstein, N. S., Carvalho A. C., Churchill, W. H., Dvorak A. M., Galli S. J., Feder J., Bitzer A. M., Rypysc J., Giovinco P. 1979. Induction of a fibrin-gel investment: an early event in line 10 hepatocarcinoma growth mediated by tumor-secreted products. J. Immunol. 122, 166-174.

Dvorak H. F. 2002. Vascular permeability factor/ Vascular Endothelial Growth Factor: a critical cytokine in tumor angiogenesis and a potential target for diagnosis and therapy. J. Clin. Oncol. 20, 4368-4380.

Epstein S. E., Kornowski R., Fuchs S., Dworak H. F. 2001. Angiogenesis therapy. Circulation 104, 115.

Fang J., Yan L., Shing Y., Moses M. A. 2001. HIF-1α-mediated up-regulation of Vascular Endothelial Growth Factor, independent of Basic Fibroblast Growth Factor, is important in the switch to the angiogenic phenotype during early tumorigenesis. Cancer Res. 61, 5731-5735.

Ferrara N. 1999. Molecular and biological properties of Vascular Endothelial Growth Factor. J. Mol. Med. 77, 527-543.

Ferrara N., Davis-Smyth T. 1997. The biology of vascular endothelial growth factor. Endocr. Rev. 18, 4-25.

Ferrara N., Henzel W. J. 1989. Pituitary follicular cells secrete a novel heparin-binding growth factor specific for vascular endothelial cells. Biochem. Biophys. Res. Commun. 161, 851-858.

Folberg R., Hendrix M. J. C., Maniotis A. J. 2000. Vasculogenic mimicry and tumors angiogenesis. Am. J. Pathol. 156, 361-381.

Gawrychowski K., Barcz E., Kamiński P. 1997 Angiogenesis in the ovarian cancer. Nowotwory 47, 775-784.

Gospodarowicz D., Abraham J. A., Schilling J. 1989. Isolation and characterization of a vascular endothelial cell mitogen produced by pituitary-derived folliculo stellate cells. Proc. Natl. Acad. Sci. USA 86, 7311-7315.

Grimmond S., Lagercrantz J., Drinkwater C., Silins G., Townson S., Pollock P., Gotley D., Carson E., Rakar S., Nordenskjold M., Ward L., Hayward N., Weber G. 1996. Cloning and characterization of a novel human gene related to vascular endothelial growth factor. Genome Res. 6, 124–13.

Gruchlik A., Chodurek E., Domal-Kwiatkowska D., Dzierżewicz Z. 2007. VEGF-A-target of antiangiogenic cancer therapy. Postępy Biol. Kom. 3, 557-580.

Grunstein J., Roberts W. G., Mathieu- Castello O., Hanahan D., Johnson R. S. 1999. Tumor-derived expression of vascular endothelial growth factor is a critical factor in tumor expansion and vascular function. Cancer Res. 59, 1592-1598.

Han H., Silverman J. F., Santucci T. S., Macherey R. S., dAmato T. A., Tung M. Y., Weyant R. J., Landreneau R. J. 2001. Vascular Endothelial Growth Factor expression in stage I non-small cell lung cancer correlates with neoangiogenesis and a poor prognosis. Ann. Surg. Oncol. 8, 72-79.

Hargberg C. E., Falkevall A., Wang X., Larsson E., Huusko J., Nilsson I., van Meeteren L. A., Samen E., Lu L., Vanwildemeersch M., Klar J., Genove G., Pietras K., Stone-Elander S., Claesson-Welsh L., Ylä-Herttuala S., Lindahl P., Eriksson U. 2010. Vascular endothelial growth factor B controls endothelial fatty acid uptake. Nature 464, 917-921.

Hashizume H., Falcón B. L., Kuroda T., Baluk P., Coxon A., Yu D., Bready J.V., Oliner J.D., McDonald D.M. 2010. Complementary actions of inhibitors of angiopoietin-2 and VEGF on tumor angiogenesis and growth Cancer Res. 70, 2213-2223.

Hicklin D. J., Ellis L. M. 2005. Role of Vascular Endothelial Growth factor pathway in tumor growth and angiogenesis. J. Clin. Oncol. 23, 1011-1027.

Hoeben A., Landuyt B., Highley M. S., Wildiers H., Van Osterom A. T., De Bruijn E. A. 2004. Vascular Endothelial Growth Factor and Angiogenesis. Pharmacol. Rev. 56, 549-580

Houck K. A., Leung D. W., Rowland A. M., Winer J., Ferrara N. 1992. Dual regulation of vascular endothelial growth factor bioavailability by genetic and proteolytic mechanisms. J. Biol. Chem. 267, 26031-26037.

Hucz J., Szala S. 2006. VEGFR-2 receptor - target for anticancer therapy. Współczesna Onkologia 10, 506-514.

Jośko J., Gwóźdź B., Jędrzejowska-Szypułka H., Henryk S. 2000. Vascular endothelial growth factor (VEGF) and its effect on angiogenesis. Med. Sci. Monit. 6, 1047-1052.

Joukov V., Pajusola K., Kaipainen A., Chilov D., Lahtinen I., Kukk E., Saksela O., Kalkkinen N., Alitalo K. 1996. A novel vascular endothelial growth factor, VEGF-C, is a ligand for the Flt4 (VEGFR-3) and KDR (VEGFR-2) receptor tyrosine kinases. EMBO J. 15, 290-298.

Joukov V., Pajusola K., Kaipainen A., Chilov D., Lahtinen I., Kukk E., Saksela O., Kalkkinen N., Alitalo K. 1996. A novel vascular endothelial growth factor, VEGF-C, is a ligand for the Flt4 (VEGFR-3) and KDR (VEGFR-2) receptor tyrosine kinases. EMBO J. 15, 290-298.

Karkkainen M.J., Haiko P., Sainio K., Partanen J., Taipale J., Petrova T.V., Jeltsch M., Jackson D.G., Talikka M., Rauvala H., Betsholtz C., Alitalo K. 2004. Vascular endothelial growth factor C is required for sprouting of the first lymphatic vessels from embryonic veins. Nat. Immunol. 5, 74-80.

Kondo Y., Arii Sh., Mori A., Furutani M., Chiba T., Imamura M. 2000. Enhancement of angiogenesis, tumor growth, and metastasis by transfection of Vascular Endothelial Growth Factor into LoVo human colon cancer cell line. Cancer Res. 6, 622-630.

Kopczyńska E., Dancewicz M., Kowalewski J., Tyrakowski T. 2008. The comparison of prognostic value of VEGF and MMP-9 in non-small cell lung cancer during three-year observation after anti-tumour treatment Współcz. Onkol. 12, 370-373.

Kozaczka A., Najda J., Waszczyk D. 2004: Angiogenesis controlling mechanisms and their clinical application in advanced cases of colorectal cancer. Współcz. Onkol. 8, 373-378.

Kraft A., Weindel K., Ochs A., Marth C., Zmija J., Schumacher P., Unger C., Marme D., Gastl G. 1999. Vascular endothelial growth factor in the sera and effusion of patients with malignant and nonmalignant disease. Cancer 85, 178-187.

Kukk E, Lymboussaki A, Taira S, Jeltsch M, Joukov V, Alitalo K. 1996. VEGF-C receptor binding and pattern of expression with VEGFR-3 suggests a role in lymphatic vascular development. Development 122, 3829-3837

Lahteenvuo J. E., Lahteenvuo M. T., Kivela A., Rosenlew C., Falkevall A, Klar J, Heikura T., Rissanen T. T., Vähäkangas E., Korpisalo P., Enholm B., Carmeliet P., Alitalo K., Eriksson U., Ylä-Herttuala S. 2009. Vascular endothelial growth factor-B induces myocardium-specific angiogenesis and arteriogenesis via vascular endothelial growth factor receptor-1- and neuropilin receptor-1-dependent mechanisms. Circulation 119, 845–856.

Lewis J. S., Landers R. J., Underwood J. C., Harris A. L., Lewis C. E. 2000. Expession of vascular endothelial growth factor by macrophages is upregulated in poorly vascularized areas of breast carcinomas. J. Pathol. 192, 150-158.

Li X., Aase K., Li H., Von Euler G., Eriksson U. 2001. Isoform-specific expression of VEGF-B in normal tissues and tumors. Growth Factors 19, 49-59

Li X., Lee Ch., Tang Z., Zhang F., Arjunan P., Li Y., Hou X., Kumar A., Dong L. 2009 VEGF-B a survival or angiogenic factor? Cell Adh. Migr. 3, 322-327

Li X. 2010.VEGF-B: a thing of beauty. Cell Res. 20, 741-744.

Litwiniuk M., Łojko A., Thielemann A., Kopczyński Z. 2007. Vascular endothelial growth factor (VEGF) and selected clinicopathological parameters in breast carcinoma. Współcz Onkol. 11, 300-304.

Loggini B., Boldrini L., Gisfredi S., Ursino S., Camacci T., De Jeso K., Cervadoro G., Pingitore R., Barachini P., Leocata P., Fontanini G. 2003. C34 microvessel density and VEGF expression in basal and squqmous cell carcinoma. Pathol. Res. Pract. 199, 705-712.

Łojko A., Komarnicki M. 2004. Vascular endothelial growth factor In tumor angiogenesis. Współ. Onkol. 8, 1-4.

Łukasik A., Fila A., Michalski B., Pordzik P., Poręba R., Wilczok T., Mazurek U. 2003. Estimation of risk progression in low grade squamous intraepithelial lesions in aspect of occurrence of alternative splice mRNA VEGF forms -$VEGF_{121}$, $VEGF_{145}$, $VEGF_{165}$, $VEGF_{183}$, $VEGF_{189}$, $VEGF_{206}$. Współcz. Onkol. 7, 286-293.

Maiolino P, De Vico G, Restucci B. 2000. Expression of vascular endothelial growth factor in basal cell tumours and in squamous cell carcinomas of canine skin. J Comp. Pathol. 123, 141-145.

McDonald D. M., Munn L., Jain R. K. 2000. Vasculogenic mimicry: how convinicing, how novel and how sifnificant? Am. J. Pathol. 156, 383-388.

McMahon G. 2000. VEGF receptor signaling in tumor angiogenesis. Oncologist. 5, 3-10.

Mohammed S. I, Bennett P. F, Craig B. A, Glickman N. W., Mutsaers A. J., Snyder P. W., Widmer W. R., DeGortari A. E., Bonney P.L., Knapp D. W. 2002. Effects of the cyclooxygenase inhibitor, piroxicam, on tumor response, apoptosis, and angiogenesis in a canine model of human invasive urinary bladder cancer. Cancer Res. 62, 356-358.

Namiecińska M., Marciniak K., Nowak J. Z. 2005. VEGF as an angiogenic, neurotropic, and neuroprotective factor. Post. Hig. Med. Dośw. 59, 573-583.

Nicosia R. F. 1998. What is the role of Vascular Endothelial Growth Factor-related molecules in tumor angiogenesis? Am. J. Pathol. 153, 11-16.

Olsson, A.K., A. Dimberg, J. Kreuger, and L. Claesson-Welsh. 2006. VEGF receptor signalling - in control of vascular function. Nat. Rev. Mol. Cell Biol. 7,359–371.

Olofsson B., Pajusola K., von Euler G., Chilov D., Alitalo K., Eriksson U. 1996.Genomic organization of the mouse and human genes for vascular endothelial growth factor B (VEGF-B) and characterization of a second splice isoform. J. Biol. Chem. 271, 19310-10317.

Olofsson B., Korpelainen E., Pepper M.S., Mandriota S.J., Aase K.,Kumar V., Gunji Y., Jeltsch M.M., Shibuya M., Alitalo K., Eriksson U. 1998. Vascular endothelial growth factor B (VEGF-B) binds to VEGF receptor-1and regulates plasminogen activator activity in endothelial cells. Proc. Natl. Acad. Sci. 95, 11709-11714.

Oshika Y., Nakamura M., Tokunaga T., Ozeki. Y, Fukushima Y., Hatanaka H., Abe Y., Yamazaki H., Kijima H., Tamaoki N., Ueyama Y. 1998. Expression of cell-associated isoform of vascular endothelial growth factor 189 and its prognostic relevance in non-small cell lung cancer. Int. J. Oncol. 12, 541-544.

Papetti M., Herman I. M. 2002. Mechanisms of normal and tumor-derived angiogenesis. Am. J. Physiol. Cell Physiol. 282, 947-970.

Plouët J., Schilling J., Gospodarowicz D. 1989. Isolation and characterization of a newly identified endothelial cell mitogen produced by AtT-20 cells. EMBO J. 8, 3801-3806

Poon R. T., Lau C. P., Cheung S. T., Yu W. C., Fan S.T. 2003. Quantitative correlation of serum levels and tumor expression of vascular endothelial growth factor in patients with hepatocellular carcinoma. Cancer Res. 63, 3121-3126.

Ranieri G., Coviello M., Chiriatti A., Stea B., Montemurro S., Quaranta M., Dittadi R., Paradiso A. 2004. Vascular endothelial growth factor assessment in different blood fractions of gastrointestinal cancer patients and healthy controls. Oncol. Rep. 11, 435-439.

Restucci B., Papparella S., Maiolino P., De Vico G. 2002. Expression of vascular endothelial growth factor in canine mammary tumors. Vet. Pathol. 39, 488-493.

Rofstad E. K, Halsor E. F. 2000. Vascular Endothelial Growth Factor, Interleukin 8, Platelet-derived Endothelial Cell Growth Factor, and Basic Fibroblast Growth Factor Promote Angiogenesis and Metastasis in Human Melanoma Xenografts. Cancer Res. 60, 4932-4938.

Rosen L. S. 2002. Clinical experience with angiogenesis signaling inhibitors: focus on vascular endothelial growth factor (VEGF) blockers. Cancer Control. 9, 36-44.

Roskoski R. Jr. 2007. Vascular endothelial growth factor (VEGF) signaling in tumor progression. Oncology/Hematology 62, 179–213.

Rydén L., Linderholm B., Nielsen N. H., Emdin S., Jönsson P. E., Landberg G. 2003. Tumor specific VEGF-A and VEGFR2/KDR protein are co-expressed in breast cancer. Breast Cancer Res Treat. 82, 147-54.

Scheidegger P., Weiglhofer W., Suarez S., Kaser-Hotz B., Steiner R., Ballmer-Hofer K., Jaussi R. 1999. Vascular endothelial growth factor (VEGF) and its receptors in tumor-bearing dogs. Biol. Chem. 380, 1449-1454.

Senger D. R., Galli S. J., Dvorak A. M., Perruzzi C. A., Harvey V. S., Dvorak H. F. 1983. Tumor cells secrete a vascular permeability factor that promotes accumulation of ascites fluid. Science 219, 983-985.

Senger D. R., Perruzzi C. A., Feder J., Dvorak H. F. 1986. A highly conserved vascular permeability factor secreted by a variety of human and rodent tumor cell lines. Cancer Res. 46, 5629-32.

Shibuya, M., Claesson-Welsh L. 2006. Signal transduction by VEGF receptorsin regulation of angiogenesis and lymphangiogenesis. Exp. Cell Res. 312, 549–560.

Sobczyńska-Rak A. 2009. Correlation between plasma VEGF and angiogenesis of skin and subcutaneous tissue cancer in dogs. Bull Vet Inst Pulawy 53, 503-506.

Stacker S.A., Stenvers K., Caesar C., Vitali A., Domagala T., Nice E., Roufail S., Simpson R.J., Moritz R., Karpanen T., Alitalo K., Achen M.G. 1999. Biosynthesis of vascular endothelial growth factor-D involves proteolytic processing which generates non-covalent homodimers. J. Biol. Chem. 274, 32127-32136.

Stępień-Wyrobiec O., Wyrobiec G., Rokicki W., Harabin-Słowińska M. 2007. Vascular endothelial growth factor (VEGF) - a regulator of angiogenesis. Ann. Acad. Med. Siles., 61, 152-160.

Sundar S. S., Ganesan T. S. 2007. Role of lymphangiogenesis in cancer. J Clin Oncol. 25, 4298-4307

Swidzińska E., Naumniuk E., Chyczewska E. 2006 Angiogenesis and neoangiogenesis - the role in lung cancer and other tumors. Pulmunol. Alergol. Pol. 74, 414-420.

Szala S. 2009. Angiogenesis and immune supression: yin and yang of tumor progression? Postepy Hig. Med. Dośw. 63, 598-612.

Szala S., Radzikowski Cz. 1997. Molecular basis of neoplastic angiogenesis. Nowotwory 47, 1-19.

Takahashi Y., Kitadi Y., Bucana C. D., Cleary K. R., Ellis L. M. 1995. Expresion of vascular endothelial growth facto rand its receptor, KDR, correlates with vascularity, metastasis, and proliferation of human colon cancer. Cancer Res. 55, 3964-3968.

Terman B. I., Stoletov K. V. 2001. VEGF and tumor angiogenesis. Jpn. J. Clin. Oncol. 18, 59-66.

Thielemann A., Kopczyński Z., Baszczuk A., Ćwiklińska K., Grodecka-Gazdecka S. 2010. Assessment of sVEGF-1 concentration In patients with breast cancer. Współczesna Onkologia 14, 189-195.

Troy G. C., Huckle W. R., Rossmeisl J. H., Panciera D., Lanz O., Robertson J. L., Ward D. L. 2006. Endostatin and vascular endothelial growth factor concentrations in healthy dogs, dogs with selected neoplasia, and dogs with nonneoplastic diseases. J. Vet. Intern. Med. 20, 144-150.

Volk L. D., Flister M. J., Bivens Ch. M., Stutzman A., Desai N., Trieu V., Ran S. 2008. Nab-paclitaxel efficacy in the orthotopic model of human breast cancer is significantly enhanced by concurrent anti-Vascular Endothelial Growth Factor A therapy. Neoplasia 10, 613-623.

Volk L. D., Flister M. J., Chihade D., Desai N., Trieu V., Ran S. 2001. Synergy of nab-paclitaxel and bevacizumab in eradicating large orthotopic breast tumors and preexisting metastases. Neoplasia 13, 327-338.

Waltenberger J., Claesson-Welsh L., Siegbahn A., Shibuya M., Heldin C. H. 1994. Different signal transduction properties of KDR and Flt1, two receptors for vascular endothelial growth factor. J. Biol. Chem. 269, 26988–26995.

Webb N. J. A., Myers C. R., Watson C. J., Bottomley M. J., Brenchley P. E. C. 1998. Activated human neurophilis express vascular endothelial growth factor (VEGF). Cytokine 10, 254-257.

Wergin M. C., Kaser - Hotz B. 2004. Plasma vascular endothelial growth factor (VEGF) measured in seventy dogs with spontaneously occurring tumours. In. Vivo. 18, 15-19.

Wergin M. C., Ballmer-Hofer K., Roos M., Achermann R. E., Inteeworn N., Akens M. K., Blattmann H., Kaser-Hotz B. 2004. Preliminary study of plasma vascular endothelial growth factor (VEGF) during low- and high-dose radiation therapy of dogs with spontaneous tumors. Vet. Radiol. Ultrasound. 45, 247-54.

Wojtukiewicz M. Z., Sierko E. 2009. The approach to antiangiogenic therapy in cancer patients. Onkol. Prak. Klin. 5, supl. 1–14.

Wójcik E., Sas-Korczyńska B., Stasik Z., Tarapacz J., Rychlik U., Kulpa J. K. 2010. MMP-9, TIMP-1 and VEGF in small cell lung cancer patients. J. Lab. Diagnost. 46, 299-305.

Xue Y., Chen F., Zhang D., Lim S., Cao Y. 2009. Tumor-derived VEGF modulates hematopoiesis. J. Angiogenes Res. 23, 1-9.

Yamada Y., Nezu J., Shimane M., Hirata Y. 1997. Molecular cloning of a novel vascular endothelial growth factor, VEGF-D. Genomics. 42, 483-8.

Yokoyama Y., Charnock-Jones D.S., Licence D., Yanaihara A., Hastings J.M., Holland C.M., Emoto M., Umemoto M., Sakamoto T., Sato S., Mizunuma H., Smith S.K. 2003. Vascular endothelial growth factor-D is an independent prognostic factor in epithelial ovarian carcinoma. Br. J. Cancer 88, 237-244

Yu J. L., Rak J. W., Klement G., Kebel R. S. 2002. Vascular endothelial growth factor isoform expression as a determinant of blood vessel patterning in human melanoma xenografts. Cancer Res. 62, 1838-1846.

Yuan B. A., Yu C. J., Kuo S. H., Chen W. J., Lin F. Y., Luh K. T., Yang P. C., Lee Y. C. 2001. Vascular endothelial growth factor 189 mRNA isoform expression specifically correlates with tumor angiogenesis, patient survival, and postpertive relapse in non-small-cell lung cancer. J. Clin. Oncol. 19, 432-441.

Zachary I. 2003. Biochem. Soc. Trans. 31, 1171–1177

Zheng S., Han M. Y., Xiao Z. X., Peng J. P., Dong Q. 2003. Clinical significance of vascular endothelial growth factor expression and neovascularization in collateral carcinoma. Gastroenterol. 9, 1227-1230.

Zhang F., Tang Z., Hou X., Lennartsson J., Li Y., Koch A. W., Scotney P., Lee C., Arjunan P., Dong L., Kumar A., Rissanen T. T., Wang B., Zhu C., Fariss R., Dong L., Tansey G., Raber J., Fong G., Ding H., Greenberg D., Becker K.G., Nash A., Cao Y., Watts R. J., Li X. 2009.VEGF-B is dispensable for blood vessel growth but critical for their survival, and VEGF-B targeting inhibits pathological angiogenesis. Proc. Natl. Acad. Sci. 106, 6152-6157.

9

Cancer Related Inflammation and Tumor Angiogenesis

Ping Wu
Department of Pathophysiology, Tongji Medical College,
Huazhong University of Science and Technology,
China

1. Introduction

Today, the relationship between inflammation and cancer has been widely accepted. Cancer-related inflammation (CRI) was even considered as 'the other half of the tumor'. Angiogenesis plays an important role in the evolution of both cancer and inflammatory diseases. It has been well established that inflammation is a defensive reaction of living tissue to injury which involves vascular response. The establishment of tumor also generates new blood vessel formation, mainly through hypoxia. In addition, the inflammatory cells infiltrating the tumor tissue, particularly tumor-associated macrophages (TAM), also contribute to tumor angiogenesis. Angiogenesis triggered by CRI has been considered as a potential target for cancer therapy.

As depicted in Fig. 1, the multistep development of cancer is thought to require six biological capabilities including: sustaining proliferative signaling, evading growth suppressors, resisting cell death, enabling replicative immortality, inducing angiogenesis, and activating invasion and metastasis [2]. Recently, cancer-related inflammation, a key component of tumor microenvironment, has been proposed to promote tumor progression and serve as the seventh hallmark of tumor (Fig. 1) [1].

Cancer inflammation has long been proposed as promoter of tumor growth. As early as in the 19th century, observations have been made that tumors often arose at sites of chronic inflammation, and that inflammatory cells were present in human tumors [3]. Although this idea has waned for a long time, a renaissance of the inflammation-cancer connection suggested by multiple lines of evidence has led to a currently accepted paradigm [3-5]. These lines of evidence categorized by Mantovani *et al.* [5] are listed below.

- Inflammatory diseases (e.g., inflammatory bowel disease) could increase the risk of developing different types of cancer including bladder, cervical, gastric, intestinal, esophageal, ovarian, prostate and thyroid tumors. Inflammatory cells, chemokines and cytokines are present in the microenvironment of all tumors in both experimental animal models and humans from the earliest stages of development. Signs of 'smoldering' inflammation are present even in tumors for which a firm causal relationship to infection has not been established (for example, breast tumors). Epidemiological studies have revealed that chronic inflammation predisposes to different types of cancer suggesting that underlying infections and inflammatory responses are linked [3].

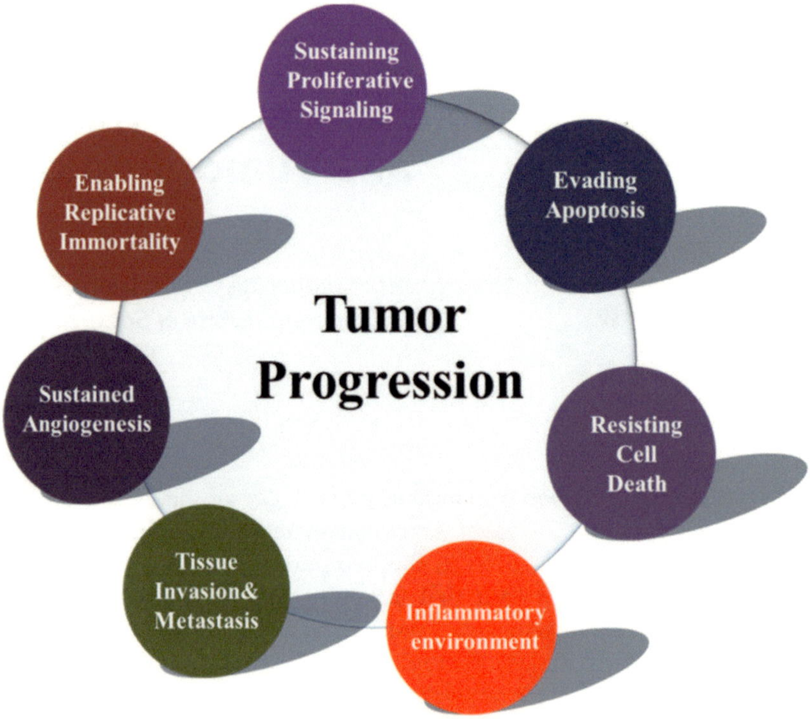

Fig. 1. Hallmarks of cancer [1].

- Signaling pathways involved in inflammation operate downstream of oncogenic mutations (such as mutations in the genes encoding RAS, MYC and RET).
- Adoptive transfer of inflammatory cells or overexpression of inflammatory cytokines promotes the development of tumors.
- Non-steroidal anti-inflammatory drugs (NSAIDs) reduce the risk of incidence of several tumors (e.g., colon and breast cancer) and mortality caused by these cancers. Protection offered by NSAIDs supports the idea that inflammation is a risk factor for certain cancers.
- The targeting of inflammatory mediators (e.g., TNF-α and IL-1β), key transcription factors involved in inflammation (e.g., NF-κB and STAT3) and tumor infiltration of inflammatory cells decreases the incidence and spread of various tumors.

2. Key factors and cells in cancer-related inflammation

In the tumor microenvironment, products of inflammatory cells influence almost every aspect of tumorigenesis and tumor progression [5]. Their effects on tumor angiogenesis will be discussed in more details in Part 3.

Two pathways have been schematically identified as the connection between initiation of cancer and inflammation, as intrinsic pathway and extrinsic pathway. In the intrinsic pathway, internal genetic events which cause neoplasia, at the same time, would trigger the expression of inflammation-related programs and then guide the construction of an

Factors	Biological activity
IL-1β	Elevated level in patient with leukoplakia and oral cancer [71]; Inducing chemical carcigenesis of fibrosarcomas, *in vivo* [72]; host derived or exogenous IL-1β enhancing tumor invasiveness and metastasis, *in vitro* and *in vivo* [73]
IL-6	Involved in tumor progression, such as in multiple myeloma, plasmacytomas, intestinal cancer, *in vitro* and *in vivo*, mainly through NF-κB and STAT3 [74]; Elevated IL-6 level be correlated with HCC, *in vivo* experiment and in clinical [75, 76]; Elevated level in patient with leukoplakia and oral cancer [71]
IL-23	Elevated in intestinal polyps and colorectal carcinoma [77]
IFN-γ	Enhancing the antitumor activity of alveolar macrophages, *in vitro* [78]
TNF-α	Elevated level in patient with leukoplakia and oral cancer [71]
LXs	Inhibiting the tumor growth of transplanted H22 in mice, *in vitro* and *in vivo* [79]; inhibiting hepatocyte growth factor-induced invasion of human hepatoma cells, in vitro [80]

Table 1. Effect of variety of inflammatory mediators on tumor progression.

inflammatory microenvironment inside tumor tissue. RET oncogene in papillary carcinoma of the thyroid is a typical example for this intrinsic pathway [6]. It should be noticed that although those oncogenes might be representative of different pro-inflammatory molecular classes and actions, they will share the capacity to orchestrate all CRI circuits [1].

As in the extrinsic pathway, inflammatory conditions would just help to facilitate tumor development. Chronic inflammation acts as a trigger to increase cancer risk or progression. Chronic inflammatory conditions associated with cancer development include chronic infections (e.g., Helicobacter pylori for gastric cancer and mucosal lymphoma; papilloma virus and hepatitis viruses for cervical and liver carcinoma, respectively), autoimmune diseases (e.g., inflammatory bowel disease for colon cancer) and inflammatory conditions of uncertain origin (e.g. prostatitis for prostate cancer) [2].

There is also close connection between inflammation and metastasis. A successful establishment of a metastatic lesion depends on both intrinsic properties of the tumor cells and factors derived from the tumor microenvironment that often contains secretory products of immune cells such as IL-1, IL-6, TNF and RANKL. All of these are known to augment tumor cells' ability to metastasize by affecting several steps in the cells' dissemination and implantation at secondary sites [7].

Notably, vascular endothelial growth factor-A (VEGF-A), one of the most important stimulators in tumor angiogenesis, is also an inflammatory factor inducing strong macrophages chemotaxis in tumor [8].

Besides the cytokines and chemokines mentioned above, in recent years, short noncoding RNAs termed microRNAs (miRNAs) have been described as a novel class of molecular promoters of neoplastic progression that control gene expression on the post-transcriptional level [9]. Some of the miRNAs play a crucial role both in inflammation and cancer. For example, miR-21 has been found to be deregulated in most types of cancers and therefore was classified as an onco-miR. Meanwhile, miR-21 also plays roles in chronic inflammatory diseases including cardiac and pulmonary fibrosis as well as myocardial infarction [10]. In contrast, miR-146a acts as a molecular brake on inflammation, myeloid cell proliferation, as well as oncogenic transformation [11].

3. Introduction about tumor angiogenesis

Although induction of new blood vessels by solid tumors had been first recognized by Virchow nearly 150 years ago [12], tumor angiogenesis is frequently linked to the name of Dr. Judah Folkman who founded this field nearly 40 years ago. Folkman proposed that the growth of all solid tumors is dependent on angiogenesis and suggested that suppression of tumor blood vessel growth would offer a new option for cancer therapy [13] .

Angiogenesis, the sprouting of new blood vessels from pre-existing endothelium, is an important component of various biological processes including embryonic vascular development, organ regeneration, wound healing, and recovery from myocardial ischemia or peptic ulcer. However, it is also a part of many pathologies that depend on neovascularization, such as diabetic retinopathy, rheumatoid arthritis and tumor growth [14]. The expansion of cancer requires the formation of new blood vessels due to oxygen and nutrients that can obtained by diffusion. Notably, the newly formed tumor vessels also provide a gateway for tumor cells to enter circulation and metastasize to distant organs [15]. Tumor vessels are characterized by lack of maturation, absence of smooth muscle cells, missing adrenergic innervation and lymphatic drainage, discontinuous endothelial lining, and sinusoidal vessel plexuses [16]. Tumor vasculature differs in many aspects from the vasculature of normal organs. The vessel diameter varies significantly in most tumors as compared with vessels in normal tissues. It is still unclear whether the vascular architecture of an individual tumor is tumor type-specific.

Our knowledge of the mechanisms underlying angiogenesis has increased dramatically in the past decades. Angiogenesis is a complex multistep process involving close orchestration of endothelial cells, soluble factors, and extracellular matrix. Usually, the vascular endothelium is a quiescent tissue with a very low turnover rate. However, in response to angiogenic factors, endothelial cells emerge from quiescence and become motile and proliferative. The initiation or termination of angiogenesis is tightly controlled by the net balance between positive and negative regulators. Positive factors include EC mitogenic factors such as fibroblast growth factor-1 and -2 (FGF-1, -2), transforming growth factor-α (TGF-α), VEGF-A and some non-mitogenic factors such as cytokines, CXC chemokines, and angiopoietins. Inhibitors of angiogenesis include the internal peptide fragments of extracellular matrix proteins (for instance, angiostatin and endostatin) [14, 17].

The complex steps in new vessel formation have been intensively investigated in recent years. The main steps are: (1) tipping the angiogenic balance, (2) destabilization of pre-existing blood vessels basement membrane by protease, (2) cell adhesion, (3) migration of EC toward the angiogenic stimulus, (4) proliferation, (5) formation of a capillary tubes, (6) loop formation by connection of individual sprouts, (7) vessel wall maturation (alignment of pericytes and smooth muscle), (7) formation of new basement membrane [14, 15, 18].

The ability of tumors to stimulate neovascularization is determined by their "angiogenic switch," of which the on/off is dictated by the inflammatory or hypoxic microenvironment inside tumor [15].

4. Inflammatory cells and cytokines in tumor angiogenesis

The above two processes, angiogenesis and inflammation, are closely linked in the following ways: (i) they are coupled in some chronic inflammatory diseases including Crohn disease, diabetes, psoriasis, rheumatoid arthritis, osteoarthritis, obesity, ocular diseases as well as cancer; (ii) inflammatory cells interact with endothelial cells, fibroblasts and ECM in the inflamed loci; and (iii) the same molecular events trigger both inflammation and angiogenesis (Table 2) [19].

Factors	Biological activity
VEGF	Inducing confluent microvascular ECs to invade collagen gels and form capillary like structures, *in vitro* [81] Angiogenic properties in the chick chorioallantoic membrane, the rabbit cornea and numerous mice xenograft models, *in vivo*[21] Elevated VEGF levels and its correlation with increased risk of metastasis and overall poor prognosis in different cancers, reviewed by Ferrara [82]
IL	IL-1β increasing EC outgrowth independently of VEGF, *in vivo* [83] IL-6 inducing vascular EC proliferation, tube formation and VEGF expression, *in vitro* [84]
Eicosanoids	12(S)-HETE and 15-HETEs as mediators of insulin and EGF-stimulated mammary epithelial cell proliferation and as synergistic effectors of bFGF- and PDGF-regulated growth of vascular endothelial cells, *in vitro* [15]
LXs	Synthetic analog of ATL inhibiting VEGF- and LTD4-stimulated angiogenesis, *in vitro* and *in vivo* [37, 85]; inhibiting actin cytoskeleton reorganization of EC stimulated with VEGF, *in vitro* [86] LXA_4 inhibiting proinflammatory cytokine responses; attenuating LTD4 and VEGF-stimulated proliferation and tube formation, *in vitro* [35]
Chemokines	CXCL8, induced by Ras to enhance VEGF-A and then acting on ECs to promote vessel formation, *in vitro* [39] CXCL12 promoting GSC-initiated angiogenesis by stimulating VEGF production, *in vitro* and *in vivo* [87]

Table 2. Effect of variety of inflammatory mediators on angiogenesis.

The role of inflammatory cells and cytokines in tumor angiogenesis is discussed in details in the following.

4.1 VEGF and tumor angiogenesis

VEGF-A, one of the most essential stimulators in tumor angiogenesis, was first reported by Senger, Dvorak and co-workers back in 1983 [20]. Collectively, the evidence from over 2 decades of experimental work together with the recent clinical results firmly put VEGF as the central mediator in promoting angiogenesis via a direct effect on ECs and mainly through its binding to VEGFR-2 [21]. Another major effect of VEGF-A in the angiogenesis, cancer and metastases process is the ability to increase vascular permeability. It has been postulated that VEGF increases permeability by increasing the vesico-vascular organelles, fenestrations and trans-cellular gaps [22, 23]. In cancer, under the influence of VEGF, metastases to the peritoneal cavity leads to vascularization and hyper-permeability leads to malignant ascites formation and death.

VEGF-A is up-regulated by transcription factor hypoxia inducible factor alpha (HIF1-α) in response to various stimuli including hypoxia, cytokines, growth factors and nitric oxide. As well documented, HIF1-α is central to oxygen homeostasis during embryonic development and postnatal life in both physiological and pathophysiological processes such as tumor growth, ischemia and tissue repair. It could respond to reduced oxygen tensions and control the expression of many genes involved in metabolism, angiogenesis, tumorigenesis, and metastasis [24]. The activity and amount of HIF-1α are regulated through proteasomal degradation by hydroxylation of its proline residues. Under hypoxia, a condition commonly occurring in growing solid tumors, the enzymatic activity of hydroxylases is limited. As a result, HIF1-α subunit is stabilized. This leads to formation of the dimer that enters the nucleus and binds to promoters of target genes, thereby inducing transcription of VEGF-A and other angiogenic factors [25].

4.2 Eicosanoids and tumor angiogenesis

Metabolism of archidonic acid (AA) through cyclooxygenase (COX), lipoxygenase (LOX), or P450 epoxygenase pathways leads to the formation of various eicosanoids that have potent biologic effects on a wide spectrum of physiological and pathological processes, including inflammation, fever, arthritis, and cancer. In the past decade, eicosanoids have emerged as key regulators of cancer progression. Studies using molecular and pharmacological approaches have found that enzymes involved in the eicosanoid production are overexpressed in cancer cells, enhance their angiogenic potential and simulate tumor growth *in vivo* [15].

Human prostate carcinoma (PCa) is a typical example to illustrate the influence of eicosanoids on tumor angiogenesis. It was indicated that the extent of angiogenesis is associated with PCa progression and the level of vascularization positively correlates with tumor stages [15]. There are several reports describing an increase in COX-2 expression in PCa tumors as compared with normal epithelial tissues [15]. Liu et al. examined the relationship between COX-2 expression and VEGF-A production under cobalt chloride ($CoCl_2$)-stimulated hypoxia in three human PCa cell lines. This study performed in a human metastatic prostate cancer cell line determined that VEGF-A induction by $CoCl_2$-induced hypoxia is maintained by a concomitant and persistent increase of COX-2 expression and sustained elevation of PGE_2 synthesis. This finding suggested that COX-2 activity, reflected by PGE_2 production, is involved in hypoxia-induced VEGF-A expression, which, in turn, modulates prostatic tumor angiogenesis [26]. They further tested the effect of COX-2 inhibitor, NS398, *in vivo*. NS398 efficiently inhibited growth of tumors from PC-3 cells in mice by decreasing angiogenesis and VEGF-A expression [27].

The pro-angiogenic effects of COX-2 are mediated primarily by three products of AA metabolism: thromboxane A_2 (TXA_2), prostaglandin E_2 (PGE_2), and prostaglandin I_2 (PGI_2). Downstream pro-angiogenic actions of these eicosanoid products include: (1) production of VEGF-A [28]; (2) promotion of vascular sprouting, migration, and tube formation [15]; (3) enhanced EC survival via Bcl-2 expression and Akt signaling [29]; (4) activation of epidermal growth factor receptor-mediated angiogenesis [30].

LOX is another lipid peroxidase dioxygenase family responsible for eicosanoids production. Overexpression of 12-LOX and 15-LOX in prostate cancer cells stimulates tumor angiogenesis and growth. For example, both EC migration and Matrigel implantation assays indicated that stable expression of 12-LOX in PC-3 cells increased their angiogenic potential compared with neomycin control [15]. These findings suggest that increased expression of 12-LOX in human PCa cells stimulates growth of prostate tumors by enhancing their angiogenicity. Similar observations regarding the role of 12-LOX in tumor angiogenesis were also made in breast cancer [31]. The product of 12-LOX, 12(S)-HETE, has been found to exert various effects on endothelial cells [15]. It was demonstrated that, when co-incubated with microvascular ECs, Lewis lung carcinoma cells or B16 melanoma (B16a) cells can synthesize 12(S)-HETE in sufficient amounts to induce EC retraction [32]. The fact that tumor cell–induced EC retraction could not be blocked by COX inhibitors, but by a specific LOX inhibitor, BHPP, provided further proof that LOX enzyme plays an important role in tumor angiogenesis [32]. Some studies indicated that 12(S)-HETE act as a mitogen for microvascular ECs. The expression of 15-LOX-1 in PC-3 tumors cells was also found to stimulate tumor angiogenesis and growth [33]. Besides 12-LOX and 15-LOX, 5-LOX was also shown to promote tumor development by potentiating the pro-angiogenic response [34].

More recent evidence has emerged the role of Lipoxins (LXs) and other lipid mediators, including the resolvins and neuroprotectins whose biosynthesis is linked in space and time to the resolution phase of an inflammatory response [35]. LXs have previously been shown to modulate responses of ECs including stimulation of prostacyclin production by human umbilical vein endothelial cell (HUVEC) [36]. Using HUVEC, Bake and his colleges demonstrated that LXA_4 inhibited VEGF-A-stimulated inflammatory responses including IL-6, TNF-α, IFN-β and IL-8 secretion, as well as endothelial ICAM-1 expression, and up-regulated an inflammatory inhibitor, IL-10. Consistent with these anti-inflammatory and pro-resolution responses to LXA_4, they found that LXA_4 inhibited leukotriene D4 and VEGF-A-stimulated proliferation and angiogenesis, as determined by tube formation of HUVEC. It was believed that the underlying molecular mechanisms is associated with the decrease of VEGF-A-stimulated VEGF receptor-2 (VEGFR-2) phosphorylation and downstream signaling events including activation of phospholipase C-γ, ERK1/2, and Akt [35]. Effects of LXA_4 on ECs may be of particular relevance given the biosynthesis of this agent within the inflamed vasculature. In human enterocytes and leukocytes, LXA_4 and its analogs inhibited the release of the cytokine IL-8 and IL-6, which has been recently reported to induce angiogenic activity in a carcinoma cell line. And, in an *in vivo* model, LXA_4 and its synthetic analogs stimulated the production of IL-4, a cytokine with anti-angiogenic properties. Furthermore, the proteolytic activity necessary to digest the basement membrane, a crucial step in the angiogenic process, can be regulated by LXs at nanomolar concentration through preventing the synthesis of metalloproteinases (MMP) and increasing the tissue inhibitor of metalloproteinase (TIMP-1) protein. Collectively, these data indicate that LXs regulate EC responses *in vitro* and *in vivo* which are relevant for tumor-angiogenesis [14].

Aspirin-triggered-15-epi-lipoxins (ATL) is one analogue of LXA_4. It is well known that aspirin's therapeutic mechanism of its anti-inflammatory action is through acetylation of COX-2 and inhibition of COX-2-derived eicosanoids. Furthermore, acetylated COX-2 could also induce the biosynthesis of ATL in different types of cell, including ECs [34]. ATL are generated *in vivo* during cell–cell interactions, that can involve, for example, EC–neutrophils, and display potent inhibitory actions in several key events in inflammation [14]. It is noteworthy that the modulation of EC proliferation and VEGF receptor signal transduction reported by Bake closely parallels the bioactions of the synthetic ATL which has been reported to inhibit VEGF-stimulated proliferation of HUVEC with a maximal effect of 50% at 10 nM , suggesting similar efficacy to LXA_4 [37].

4.3 Chemokines family and tumor angiogenesis

Chemokines govern directed chemotaxis in nearby responsive cells during immune responses and inflammatory reactions by signaling through corresponding G_i protein-coupled receptors of the CXC chemokine receptor (CXCR) and CC chemokine receptor

(CCR) family. In recently years, chemokine family, including ligands and receptors, has become the focus in anti-tumor research field.

CXCL8, one of glutamic acid-leucine-arginine (ELR$^+$) chemokine, is up-regulated in several types of cancers, including pancreatic, lung, melanoma, breast, prostate and ovarian cancers [38]. In human cervical epithelioid carcinoma HeLa cell, CXCL8 was also induced by Ras, which has been shown to enhance VEGF-A and then act on endothelial cells to promote vessel formation [39]. Conversely, inhibition of CXCL8 led to an increase in tumor necrosis consistent with a defect in tumor vasculature and paracrine mechanism of action.

Activation of CXCR by ELR$^+$ CXC chemokines would elicit a localized immune response, which could facilitate angiogenesis [4]. CXCR2 is proved to be a common receptor shared by most ELR$^+$ CXC chemokines. Activation of this receptor expressed in ECs had been shown to inhibit endothelial apoptosis, and induce migration and tube formation in ECs, processes linked to angiogenesis [40]. In a study on syngeneic murine Lewis lung cancer ectopic and orthotopic tumor model systems in CXCR2(+/+) and CXCR2(-/-) C57BL/6 mice, morphometric analysis of the primary tumors in CXCR2(-/-) mice demonstrated increased necrosis and reduced vascular density. These findings were further confirmed in CXCR2(+/+) mice using specific neutralizing antibody to CXCR2. The results of these studies support the notion that CXCR2 mediates the angiogenic activity of ELR(+) CXC chemokines in a preclinical model of lung cancer [41]. Similar effect of ELR(+) CXC chemokines and CXCR2 on tumor-associated angiogenesis was also shown in pancreatic cancer [42]. *In vitro*, ELR$^+$ CXC chemokines in supernatants from multiple pancreatic cancer cell lines had significantly higher level compared with an immortalized human pancreatic ductal epithelial cell line. Furthermore, both recombinant ELR$^+$ CXC chemokines and co-culturing with BxPC-3 significantly enhanced proliferation, invasion, and tube formation of HUVEC. These biological effects were significantly inhibited by treatment with a neutralizing antibody against CXCR2. *In vivo*, anti-CXCR2 antibody significantly reduced tumor volume as well as proliferation index and Factor VIII microvessel density.

CXCL12, ligand of CXCR4 receptor, also possesses angiogenic properties and is involved in the outgrowth and metastasis of CXCR4-expressing tumors and in certain inflammatory autoimmune disorders, such as rheumatoid arthritis [43].

4.4 Inflammation-related miRNA and tumor angiogenesis

In recent years, light has been shed on the connection between inflammation-related miRNA and tumor progression [9]. Two biologically active miRNAs, miR-126 and its complement miR-126*, have been reported to impair cancer progression through signaling pathways that control tumor cell proliferation, migration, invasion, and survival. Conversely, they may have a supportive role in the progression of cancer as well, which might be mediated by the promotion of blood vessel growth and inflammation. This effect of miR-126 and miR-126* on vascular functions could be explained by the fact that they are encoded by the intron 7 of the epidermal growth factor-like domain 7 (egfl7) gene. The endothelial cell-derived secreted protein EGFL7 has been suggested to control vascular tubulogenesis. Knock-out studies in zebrafish and mice suggested a major role of miR-126 in angiogenesis and vascular integrity, which was mediated by the repression of inhibitors of VEGF-A-induced proliferation in ECs.

4.5 Inflammatory cells and tumor angiogenesis

Tumor-associated macrophages (TAM) are prominent in the stromal compartment of virtually all types of malignancy. These highly versatile cells respond to the presence of stimuli in different parts of tumors with the release of a distinct repertoire of growth factors, cytokines, chemokines, and enzymes [44]. Plasticity and diversity have long been known as hallmarks of the monocyte-macrophage differentiation pathway under inflammatory conditions [45]. Inflammation-induced angiogenesis is accompanied by macrophage infiltration. M2-type macrophages support angiogenesis and lymphangiogenesis by releasing pro-angiogenic growth factors such as IL-8, VEGF-A, VEGF-C and EGF [46, 47]. In a pancreatic cancer model, IL-4 induced high expression of cathepsin in TAM that then mediated tumor growth, angiogenesis and invasion *in vivo* [48]. TAM have also been demonstrated as the main cells producing semaphorin 4D within the tumor stroma. The latter is critical for tumor angiogenesis and vessel maturation [49]. There is a significant correlation between the number of infiltrating macrophages and the microvascular density or tumor tumor progression levels in glioblastomas and melanoma [50, 51].

EC activation is manifested through chemokine production and up-regulation of surface adhesion molecules that facilitate adhesion of leukocytes that, in turn, cause more pronounced inflammation [52]., Leukocytes including TAM not only activate ECs but also promote and strengthen the entire process of tumor angiogenesis.

5. Oxidative stress in tumor angiogenesis

Dysregulation of redox status is a typical feature of many types of cancer [25]. It is widely accepted that the imbalance between the generation and clearance of reactive oxygen/nitrogen species (ROS/RNS) aids the development of the tumor mainly by inducing genomic instability. However, recent research has provided multiple evidences that ROS and other free radicals, such as nitric oxide, often produced at elevated levels within tumor tissue, may function as signaling molecules that initiate and/or modulate different regulatory pathways involved in tumorigenesis and metastasis [53]. High levels of ROS induce cell death, apoptosis and senescence; however, at the same time, low levels of ROS are important mediators in signaling pathways regulating growth and survival of endothelial and other cells [25, 54].

The role of ROS in angiogenesis is well established. ROS were demonstrated to trigger the secretion of the most potent angiogenic factor - VEGF-A, in many cell types and induce proliferation, migration, cytoskeletal reorganization and tubular morphogenesis in ECs in vitro [55-57]. Increased intracellular levels of ROS were demonstrated in different settings to stabilize HIF1-α, a key upstream regulatory of VEGF-A expression, not only under tumor hypoxia but also under normoxic conditions [58]. For example, up-regulation of HIF-1α in response to stimulation with angiotensin II (Ang II) and thrombin was shown to be dependent on the elevation of H_2O_2 levels and cells with compromised antioxidant capacity in normoxia [59].

6. Current treatments of inflammation-stimulated tumor angiogenesis

Folkman's original hypothesis has opened a new era in today's biomedical research and changed the face of cancer medicine [60]. Modulation of angiogenesis for disease therapy was proposed nearly 40 years ago. As a result, many protein-based and chemical anti-angiogenic drugs have been developed for treating human malignancies.

In fact, since the VEGF-A discovery and characterization and subsequent determination of its receptors/pathways involved, enormous effort has been put into developing enormous effort has been put into developing anti-VEGF agents.. In 2004, after 3-decades preclinical validation, bevacizumab, a humanized anti-VEGF-A neutralizing antibody, was approved by the US FDA for the clinical use to treat metastatic colorectal cancer in human patients [61]. This antibody was the first specific angiogenic inhibitor for use in clinical oncology. And following this initial success, bevacizumab has been expanded as one of the key component of the first-line therapeutic choices against various human cancers [60]. Clinical trials have reported positive response from patients treated with bevacizumab as a single agent or in combination with cytotoxic agents [62, 63].

Beside bevacizumab, various other types of molecules have been developed to target the VEGF pathway. These include proteins that bind VEGF such as VEGF trap, VEGF receptor antibody IMC-1121B or antagonists such as vatalinib, inhibitors of receptor tyrosine kinase such as sunitinib, sorafenib, and ZD6474 [64, 65]. There are also vaccines based on xenogeneic or non-xenogeneic homologous molecules targeting VEGF-A or VEGFR [66].

Unfortunately, patients with various types of tumors have different response to anti-angiogenic therapy. While a small fraction of most common solid tumors such as colorectal, lung and breast cancers respond, some cancer types show intrinsic refractoriness [60]. But, we should not forget that the effectiveness of almost all therapeutic modalities is influenced by the micro-architecture and the gradients of essential nutrients around vessels [16]. This has been the driving force in the fields of anti-angiogenic drug development in tumor therapy.

For prostate cancer, it has been shown that androgen regulates the expression of VEGF-A and that androgen withdrawal regresses prostate tumors, partly, by restraining their blood supply. Since prostate cancer eventually progresses to androgen independence, other mechanisms must take over at later stages of tumor [15]. *In vivo,* COX-2 inhibitor, NS398, efficiently inhibited growth of PC-3 tumors in mice and decreased angiogenesis. The same study showed that VEGF-A expression was also significantly down-regulated in the NS398-treated tumors [27]. Various well-documented clinical and experimental studies have also confirmed the effect of NSAIDs in the prevention of certain types [14]. The mechanism of aspirin acts to reduce the incidence and risk of these cancers is not clear but some articles indicated that it is result from the reduction of angiogenesis [67, 68]. Epidemiologic studies show that individuals taking nonselective COX inhibitor or NSAIDs, including aspirin, have a significant reduction in CRC mortality, compared with those who did not these drugs [69].

In vivo, anti-CXCR2 antibody significantly reduced tumor volume as well as proliferation index and Factor VIII microvessel density [42]. Thus, CXCR2 should be considered as a novel anti-angiogenic target in pancreatic cancer.

ROS scavenging by antioxidants was recently demonstrated to inhibit angiogenesis in a model of myocardial infarction in rats [11]. Current clinical anti-angiogenic approaches in oncology exploit VEGF-A-VEGFR-2 axis, with the application of VEGF-A neutralizing antibodies (bevacizumab) and small-molecule VEGFR-2 tyrosine kinase inhibitors (sorafenib, sunitinib) [21]. However, this treatment do not provide a cure but only moderately prolongs patients' lives [21, 70]. Recent progress in the understanding of redox modulation of regulation and signaling of VEGF-A may create possibilities to develop more universal anti-angiogenic drugs by targeting ROS.

Intensive research resulted in the development of several FDA-approved drugs on angiogenesis in tumor. However, most of the clinical trials of single anti-angiogenic agents in combination with traditional anticancer treatment yielded disappointing results. Thus, targeting multiple pathways regulating angiogenesis, such as inflammation, has been considered a promising target for therapeutic interventions. These clinically related issues need to be further addressed at molecular levels to understand the underlying mechanisms. Elucidation of molecular mechanisms linking cancer and inflammation may provide new targets for inhibition of angiogenesis and tumor progression.

7. Abbreviation

Arachidonic acid, AA;
Aspirin-triggered-15-epi-lipoxins, ATL;
Cancer-related inflammation, CRI;
Cyclooxygenase, COX;
CXC chemokine receptor, CXCR;
CC chemokine receptor, CCR;
Endothelial cell, EC;
Fibroblast growth factor, FGF;
Human umbilical vein endothelial cells, HUVEC;
Lipoxygenase, LOX;
Lipoxin, LX
Metalloproteinases, MMP;
Short noncoding RNAs termed microRNAs, miRNAs;
Non-steroidal anti-inflammatory drugs, NSAIDs;
Prostate carcinoma, PCa;
Prostaglandin E_2, PGE_2;
Prostaglandin I_2, PGI_2;
Tumor-associated macrophages, TAM;
Thromboxane A_2, TXA_2;
Tissue inhibititor of metalloproteinase , TIMP-1;
Transforming growth factor-*α*, TGF-*α*;
Vascular endothelial growth factor-A, VEGF-A;

8. References

[1] Colotta, F., et al., *Cancer-related inflammation, the seventh hallmark of cancer: links to genetic instability*. Carcinogenesis, 2009. 30(7): p. 1073-81.
[2] Hanahan, D. and R.A. Weinberg, *Hallmarks of cancer: the next generation*. Cell, 2011. 144(5): p. 646-74.
[3] Balkwill, F. and A. Mantovani, *Inflammation and cancer: back to Virchow?* Lancet, 2001. 357(9255): p. 539-45.
[4] Coussens, L.M. and Z. Werb, *Inflammation and cancer*. Nature, 2002. 420(6917): p. 860-7.
[5] Mantovani, A., et al., *Cancer-related inflammation*. Nature, 2008. 454(7203): p. 436-44.
[6] Borrello, M.G., et al., *Induction of a proinflammatory program in normal human thyrocytes by the RET/PTC1 oncogene*. Proc Natl Acad Sci U S A, 2005. 102(41): p. 14825-30.
[7] Mantovani, A., *Cancer: Inflaming metastasis*. Nature, 2009. 457(7225): p. 36-7.

[8] Cursiefen, C., et al., *VEGF-A stimulates lymphangiogenesis and hemangiogenesis in inflammatory neovascularization via macrophage recruitment.* J Clin Invest, 2004. 113(7): p. 1040-50.

[9] Porta, C., et al., *Tolerance and M2 (alternative) macrophage polarization are related processes orchestrated by p50 nuclear factor kappaB.* Proc Natl Acad Sci U S A, 2009. 106(35): p. 14978-83.

[10] Kumarswamy, R., I. Volkmann, and T. Thum, *Regulation and function of miRNA-21 in health and disease.* RNA Biol, 2011. 8(5).

[11] Boldin, M.P., et al., *miR-146a is a significant brake on autoimmunity, myeloproliferation, and cancer in mice.* J Exp Med, 2011. 208(6): p. 1189-201.

[12] Papoutsi, M., et al., *Development of an arterial tree in C6 gliomas but not in A375 melanomas.* Histochem Cell Biol, 2002. 118(3): p. 241-9.

[13] Folkman, J., *Tumor angiogenesis: therapeutic implications.* N Engl J Med, 1971. 285(21): p. 1182-6.

[14] Fierro, I.M., *Angiogenesis and lipoxins.* Prostaglandins Leukot Essent Fatty Acids, 2005. 73(3-4): p. 271-5.

[15] Kelm, J.M., et al., *Method for generation of homogeneous multicellular tumor spheroids applicable to a wide variety of cell types.* Biotechnol Bioeng, 2003. 83(2): p. 173-80.

[16] Konerding, M.A., et al., *Evidence for characteristic vascular patterns in solid tumours: quantitative studies using corrosion casts.* Br J Cancer, 1999. 80(5-6): p. 724-32.

[17] Folkman, J., *Role of angiogenesis in tumor growth and metastasis.* Semin Oncol, 2002. 29(6 Suppl 16): p. 15-8.

[18] Hall, K. and S. Ran, *Regulation of tumor angiogenesis by the local environment.* Front Biosci, 2010. 15: p. 195-212.

[19] Ono, M., *Molecular links between tumor angiogenesis and inflammation: inflammatory stimuli of macrophages and cancer cells as targets for therapeutic strategy.* Cancer Sci, 2008. 99(8): p. 1501-6.

[20] Senger, D.R., et al., *Tumor cells secrete a vascular permeability factor that promotes accumulation of ascites fluid.* Science, 1983. 219(4587): p. 983-5.

[21] Pourgholami, M.H. and D.L. Morris, *Inhibitors of vascular endothelial growth factor in cancer.* Cardiovasc Hematol Agents Med Chem, 2008. 6(4): p. 343-7.

[22] Dvorak, H.F., *Rous-Whipple Award Lecture. How tumors make bad blood vessels and stroma.* Am J Pathol, 2003. 162(6): p. 1747-57.

[23] Bates, D.O. and S.J. Harper, *Regulation of vascular permeability by vascular endothelial growth factors.* Vascul Pharmacol, 2002. 39(4-5): p. 225-37.

[24] Zhu, X.Y., et al., *Disparate effects of simvastatin on angiogenesis during hypoxia and inflammation.* Life Sci, 2008. 83(23-24): p. 801-9.

[25] Tertil, M., A. Jozkowicz, and J. Dulak, *Oxidative stress in tumor angiogenesis- therapeutic targets.* Curr Pharm Des, 2010. 16(35): p. 3877-94.

[26] Liu, X.H., et al., *Upregulation of vascular endothelial growth factor by cobalt chloride-simulated hypoxia is mediated by persistent induction of cyclooxygenase-2 in a metastatic human prostate cancer cell line.* Clin Exp Metastasis, 1999. 17(8): p. 687-94.

[27] Liu, X.H., et al., *Inhibition of cyclooxygenase-2 suppresses angiogenesis and the growth of prostate cancer in vivo.* J Urol, 2000. 164(3 Pt 1): p. 820-5.

[28] Inoue, H., et al., *Regulation by PGE2 of the production of interleukin-6, macrophage colony stimulating factor, and vascular endothelial growth factor in human synovial fibroblasts.* Br J Pharmacol, 2002. 136(2): p. 287-95.

[29] Nor, J.E., et al., *Up-Regulation of Bcl-2 in microvascular endothelial cells enhances intratumoral angiogenesis and accelerates tumor growth.* Cancer Res, 2001. 61(5): p. 2183-8.

[30] Pai, R., et al., *Prostaglandin E2 transactivates EGF receptor: a novel mechanism for promoting colon cancer growth and gastrointestinal hypertrophy.* Nat Med, 2002. 8(3): p. 289-93.

[31] Connolly, J.M. and D.P. Rose, *Enhanced angiogenesis and growth of 12-lipoxygenase gene-transfected MCF-7 human breast cancer cells in athymic nude mice.* Cancer Lett, 1998. 132(1-2): p. 107-12.

[32] Honn, K.V., et al., *Tumor cell-derived 12(S)-hydroxyeicosatetraenoic acid induces microvascular endothelial cell retraction.* Cancer Res, 1994. 54(2): p. 565-74.

[33] Kelavkar, U.P., et al., *Overexpression of 15-lipoxygenase-1 in PC-3 human prostate cancer cells increases tumorigenesis.* Carcinogenesis, 2001. 22(11): p. 1765-73.

[34] Romano, M., et al., *5-lipoxygenase regulates malignant mesothelial cell survival: involvement of vascular endothelial growth factor.* Faseb J, 2001. 15(13): p. 2326-36.

[35] Baker, N., et al., *Lipoxin a4: anti-inflammatory and anti-angiogenic impact on endothelial cells.* J Immunol, 2009. 182(6): p. 3819-26.

[36] Brezinski, M.E., et al., *Lipoxins stimulate prostacyclin generation by human endothelial cells.* FEBS Lett, 1989. 245(1-2): p. 167-72.

[37] Fierro, I.M., J.L. Kutok, and C.N. Serhan, *Novel lipid mediator regulators of endothelial cell proliferation and migration: aspirin-triggered-15R-lipoxin A(4) and lipoxin A(4).* J Pharmacol Exp Ther, 2002. 300(2): p. 385-92.

[38] O'Hayer, K.M., D.C. Brady, and C.M. Counter, *ELR+ CXC chemokines and oncogenic Ras-mediated tumorigenesis.* Carcinogenesis, 2009. 30(11): p. 1841-7.

[39] Rak, J., et al., *Oncogenes and tumor angiogenesis: differential modes of vascular endothelial growth factor up-regulation in ras-transformed epithelial cells and fibroblasts.* Cancer Res, 2000. 60(2): p. 490-8.

[40] Li, A., et al., *IL-8 directly enhanced endothelial cell survival, proliferation, and matrix metalloproteinases production and regulated angiogenesis.* J Immunol, 2003. 170(6): p. 3369-76.

[41] Keane, M.P., et al., *Depletion of CXCR2 inhibits tumor growth and angiogenesis in a murine model of lung cancer.* J Immunol, 2004. 172(5): p. 2853-60.

[42] Matsuo, Y., et al., *CXC-chemokine/CXCR2 biological axis promotes angiogenesis in vitro and in vivo in pancreatic cancer.* Int J Cancer, 2009. 125(5): p. 1027-37.

[43] Liekens, S., D. Schols, and S. Hatse, *CXCL12-CXCR4 axis in angiogenesis, metastasis and stem cell mobilization.* Curr Pharm Des, 2010. 16(35): p. 3903-20.

[44] Lewis, C.E. and J.W. Pollard, *Distinct role of macrophages in different tumor microenvironments.* Cancer Res, 2006. 66(2): p. 605-12.

[45] Biswas, S.K. and A. Mantovani, *Macrophage plasticity and interaction with lymphocyte subsets: cancer as a paradigm.* Nat Immunol, 2010. 11(10): p. 889-96.

[46] Mantovani, A., et al., *Macrophage polarization: tumor-associated macrophages as a paradigm for polarized M2 mononuclear phagocytes.* Trends Immunol, 2002. 23(11): p. 549-55.

[47] Schmidt, T. and P. Carmeliet, *Blood-vessel formation: Bridges that guide and unite.* Nature, 2010. 465(7299): p. 697-9.
[48] Gocheva, V., et al., *IL-4 induces cathepsin protease activity in tumor-associated macrophages to promote cancer growth and invasion.* Genes Dev, 2010. 24(3): p. 241-55.
[49] Sierra, J.R., et al., *Tumor angiogenesis and progression are enhanced by Sema4D produced by tumor-associated macrophages.* J Exp Med, 2008. 205(7): p. 1673-85.
[50] Nishie, A., et al., *Macrophage infiltration and heme oxygenase-1 expression correlate with angiogenesis in human gliomas.* Clin Cancer Res, 1999. 5(5): p. 1107-13.
[51] Torisu, H., et al., *Macrophage infiltration correlates with tumor stage and angiogenesis in human malignant melanoma: possible involvement of TNFalpha and IL-1alpha.* Int J Cancer, 2000. 85(2): p. 182-8.
[52] Pober, J.S. and W.C. Sessa, *Evolving functions of endothelial cells in inflammation.* Nat Rev Immunol, 2007. 7(10): p. 803-15.
[53] Trachootham, D., et al., *Redox regulation of cell survival.* Antioxid Redox Signal, 2008. 10(8): p. 1343-74.
[54] Storz, P., *Reactive oxygen species in tumor progression.* Front Biosci, 2005. 10: p. 1881-96.
[55] Birk, D.M., et al., *Current insights on the biology and clinical aspects of VEGF regulation.* Vasc Endovascular Surg, 2008. 42(6): p. 517-30.
[56] Luczak, K., et al., *Low concentration of oxidant and nitric oxide donors stimulate proliferation of human endothelial cells in vitro.* Cell Biol Int, 2004. 28(6): p. 483-6.
[57] Yasuda, M., et al., *Stimulation of in vitro angiogenesis by hydrogen peroxide and the relation with ETS-1 in endothelial cells.* Life Sci, 1999. 64(4): p. 249-58.
[58] Chandel, N.S., et al., *Mitochondrial reactive oxygen species trigger hypoxia-induced transcription.* Proc Natl Acad Sci U S A, 1998. 95(20): p. 11715-20.
[59] Gerald, D., et al., *JunD reduces tumor angiogenesis by protecting cells from oxidative stress.* Cell, 2004. 118(6): p. 781-94.
[60] Cao, Y., *Angiogenesis: What can it offer for future medicine?* Exp Cell Res, 2010. 316(8): p. 1304-8.
[61] Hurwitz, H., et al., *Bevacizumab plus irinotecan, fluorouracil, and leucovorin for metastatic colorectal cancer.* N Engl J Med, 2004. 350(23): p. 2335-42.
[62] Desjardins, A., et al., *Bevacizumab and daily temozolomide for recurrent glioblastoma.* Cancer, 2011.
[63] Cannistra, S.A., et al., *Phase II study of bevacizumab in patients with platinum-resistant ovarian cancer or peritoneal serous cancer.* J Clin Oncol, 2007. 25(33): p. 5180-6.
[64] Morabito, A., et al., *Tyrosine kinase inhibitors of vascular endothelial growth factor receptors in clinical trials: current status and future directions.* Oncologist, 2006. 11(7): p. 753-64.
[65] Hanrahan, E.O. and J.V. Heymach, *Vascular endothelial growth factor receptor tyrosine kinase inhibitors vandetanib (ZD6474) and AZD2171 in lung cancer.* Clin Cancer Res, 2007. 13(15 Pt 2): p. s4617-22.
[66] Pan, J., et al., *Anti-angiogenic active immunotherapy: a new approach to cancer treatment.* Cancer Immunol Immunother, 2008. 57(8): p. 1105-14.
[67] Wang, D. and R.N. Dubois, *Cyclooxygenase-2: a potential target in breast cancer.* Semin Oncol, 2004. 31(1 Suppl 3): p. 64-73.

[68] Shtivelband, M.I., et al., *Aspirin and salicylate inhibit colon cancer medium- and VEGF-induced endothelial tube formation: correlation with suppression of cyclooxygenase-2 expression.* J Thromb Haemost, 2003. 1(10): p. 2225-33.
[69] Koehne, C.H. and R.N. Dubois, *COX-2 inhibition and colorectal cancer.* Semin Oncol, 2004. 31(2 Suppl 7): p. 12-21.
[70] Backer, M.V., C.V. Hamby, and J.M. Backer, *Inhibition of vascular endothelial growth factor receptor signaling in angiogenic tumor vasculature.* Adv Genet, 2009. 67: p. 1-27.
[71] Brailo, V., et al., *Salivary and serum interleukin 1 beta, interleukin 6 and tumor necrosis factor alpha in patients with leukoplakia and oral cancer.* Med Oral Patol Oral Cir Bucal, 2011.
[72] Krelin, Y., et al., *Interleukin-1beta-driven inflammation promotes the development and invasiveness of chemical carcinogen-induced tumors.* Cancer Res, 2007. 67(3): p. 1062-71.
[73] Apte, R.N., et al., *The involvement of IL-1 in tumorigenesis, tumor invasiveness, metastasis and tumor-host interactions.* Cancer Metastasis Rev, 2006. 25(3): p. 387-408.
[74] Naugler, W.E. and M. Karin, *The wolf in sheep's clothing: the role of interleukin-6 in immunity, inflammation and cancer.* Trends Mol Med, 2008. 14(3): p. 109-19.
[75] Soresi, M., et al., *Interleukin-6 and its soluble receptor in patients with liver cirrhosis and hepatocellular carcinoma.* World J Gastroenterol, 2006. 12(16): p. 2563-8.
[76] Malaguarnera, M., et al., *[Role of interleukin 6 in hepatocellular carcinoma].* Bull Cancer, 1996. 83(5): p. 379-84.
[77] Lan, F., et al., *IL-23/IL-23R: potential mediator of intestinal tumor progression from adenomatous polyps to colorectal carcinoma.* Int J Colorectal Dis, 2011.
[78] Zhou, F., et al., *[Study of the antitumor activity of alveolar macrophages after transfected human INF-gamma gene].* Zhongguo Fei Ai Za Zhi, 2011. 14(5): p. 452-5.
[79] Chen, Y., et al., *Lipoxin A4 and its analogue suppress the tumor growth of transplanted H22 in mice: the role of antiangiogenesis.* Mol Cancer Ther, 2010. 9(8): p. 2164-74.
[80] Zhou, X.Y., et al., *Lipoxin A(4) inhibited hepatocyte growth factor-induced invasion of human hepatoma cells.* Hepatol Res, 2009. 39(9): p. 921-30.
[81] Pepper, M.S., et al., *Potent synergism between vascular endothelial growth factor and basic fibroblast growth factor in the induction of angiogenesis in vitro.* Biochem Biophys Res Commun, 1992. 189(2): p. 824-31.
[82] Ferrara, N., *Vascular endothelial growth factor: basic science and clinical progress.* Endocr Rev, 2004. 25(4): p. 581-611.
[83] Lavalette, S., et al., *Interleukin-1beta inhibition prevents choroidal neovascularization and does not exacerbate photoreceptor degeneration.* Am J Pathol, 2011. 178(5): p. 2416-23.
[84] Zhu, B.H., et al., *(-)-Epigallocatechin-3-gallate inhibits VEGF expression induced by IL-6 via Stat3 in gastric cancer.* World J Gastroenterol, 2011. 17(18): p. 2315-25.
[85] Cezar-de-Mello, P.F., et al., *ATL-1, an analogue of aspirin-triggered lipoxin A4, is a potent inhibitor of several steps in angiogenesis induced by vascular endothelial growth factor.* Br J Pharmacol, 2008. 153(5): p. 956-65.
[86] Cezar-de-Mello, P.F., et al., *Aspirin-triggered Lipoxin A4 inhibition of VEGF-induced endothelial cell migration involves actin polymerization and focal adhesion assembly.* Oncogene, 2006. 25(1): p. 122-9.

[87] Ping, Y.F., et al., *The chemokine CXCL12 and its receptor CXCR4 promote glioma stem cell-mediated VEGF production and tumour angiogenesis via PI3K/AKT signalling.* J Pathol, 2011. 224(3): p. 344-54.

10

Infantile Hemangiomas: A Disease Model in the Study of Vascular Development, Aberrant Vasculogenesis and Angiogenesis

Alvin Wong and June K. Wu
Department of Surgery, College of Physicians & Surgeons, New York, NY, USA

1. Introduction

Infantile hemangiomas (IHs) belong to a family of lesions called vascular anomalies. Vascular anomalies are classified into either vascular tumors or vascular malformations, with the IH being the most common vascular tumor, affecting approximately 5% of infants (Frieden, Haggstrom et al 2005). Despite their prevalence, the origin and pathogenesis of IHs remains poorly understood.

Clinically, IHs undergo a predictable course of rapid proliferation shortly after birth, followed by stabilization and involution throughout childhood. Occasionally, a fibrofatty residuum results after involution is complete. Despite its predictable clinical course, the regulatory mechanisms throughout different phases are only recently being elucidated (Frieden, Haggstrom et al. 2005).

During the proliferative phase, IH can cause serious morbidity and even mortality. Rapidly proliferating hemangiomas can be dangerous as they have potential to ulcerate and bleed. While disorganized, IHs are high-flow lesions; occasionally, life-threatening bleeding can occur. The location of the IH can also be detrimental. Hemangiomas in the peri-orbital area can cause obstructive amblyopia and astigmatism, and airway hemangiomas can cause stridor and respiratory distress. Visceral hemangiomas of the liver can cause congestive heart failure, hepatomegaly, and anemia; the mortality rate with treatment is significant, up to 30% (Arneja and Mulliken, 2010; Bitar et al., 2005; Boon et al., 1996; Ceisler & Blei, 2003; Chamlin et al., 2007; Haggstrom et al., 2006a; Schwartz et al., 2006).

In recent years, PHACE syndrome has been described and characterized. PHACE syndrome comprises a constellation of findings including **P**osterior fossa anomalies, large facial **H**emangioma, **A**rterial anomalies, **C**ardiac abnormalities/aortic **C**oarctation, and **E**ye anomalies (Frieden et al., 1996). Infants with PHACE syndrome are at increased risk for strokes, neurological and cardiac consequences (Burrows et al., 1998; Drolet et al., 2006).

Another syndrome featuring a large hemangioma over an area with aberrant underlying anatomical structures have also been described. PELVIS syndrome describes **P**erineal hemangioma, **E**xternal genitalia malformations, **L**ipomyelomeningocele, **V**esicorenal anomalies, **I**mperforate anus, and **S**kin tag (Girard et al., 2006). PHACE and PELVIS syndromes suggest that there may be an association between a cutaneous hemangioma and abnormal development of underlying anatomy. Given the existence of these syndromes, as well as the predisposition for hemangiomas to occur at the boundaries of developmental units near lines of fusion between mesenchymal growth plates (Waner et al., 2003), it seems likely that the formation of hemangiomas is closely related to the developmental events that take place during embryogenesis.

There are currently no FDA-approved treatments for IHs, (Acevedo and Cheresh 2008; Frieden et al., 2005) although corticosteroids and propanolol have been used with good control of problematic IHs. Laboratory studies have suggested that corticosteroids affect the vascular endothelial growth factor receptor (VEGFR) pathway (Greenberger et al., 2010), and *in vitro* studies have shown that propanolol can cause apoptosis in endothelial cells (Lamy et al., 2010). However, despite these laboratory studies, the exact mechanisms of action of these medications on IHs are still unknown. Occasionally, due to either failure of medical treatment or the urgency of the potential morbidity and mortality, an infant will require urgent surgical intervention (Arneja & Mulliken, 2010; Rabhar et al., 2004).

In summary, despite the prevalence and potential morbidities and mortalities, treatment of IHs relies on pharmacotherapy with poorly understood mechanisms of action, and surgical intervention when necessary. Part of the reason treatment for IHs is hampered is due to poor understanding of pathogenesis and regulatory signals governing its natural history. Therefore, understanding the pathogenesis and regulation of IH growth and involution will allow more directed therapy. Moreover, based on associations in PHACE and PELVIS syndromes the development of IH may be related to other abnormal anatomic developments during embryogenesis. Therefore, IH may be a useful disease model to study vascular development and vasculogenesis, as well as give insight to angiogenesis in pathologic settings.

2. Clinical course of IH

IHs typically affect the skin and occur in 4 to 10% of white infants (Holmdahl et al., 1955), with higher incidence in premature infants with low birth weight (Amir et al., 1986), high maternal age for the first baby, multiple gestation, complicated pregnancies with pre-eclampsia or placental abnormalities such as placenta previa. A lower rate is observed in dark-skinned children. There is a female predisposition of 3:1 to 5:1. IHs occur most often on the head and neck (60%), followed by the trunk (25%) and extremities (15%). Usually, cutaneous IHs arise as a single lesion; however, up to 20% of them occur as multiple lesions and are also more likely to involve the viscera. IH can develop in the GI tract, pancreas, kidney, lung, heart, mediastinum, meninges, and brain.

By definition, IHs occur after birth. Often, small telangiectasias or discoloration of the skin resembling a bruise herald the future development of the IH, but the frank lesion is not noticed until several weeks after birth. Congenital hemangiomas are vascular tumors that are fully developed at birth and do not have postnatal growth. They either involute rapidly (Rapidly Involuting Congenital Hemangiomas, RICH), or will not involute (Non-Involuting Congenital Hemangioma, NICH), RICHs and NICHs have a different clinical course from IHs and will not be discussed here.

After their initial appearance, IHs grow quickly over the first 6 to 8 weeks of the infant's life during the *proliferative phase*. Depending on their location within the dermis, IHs can vary in their appearance. Tumors within the dermis are characterized by a bright red coloration, are raised, and have a bosselated appearance [Figure 1].

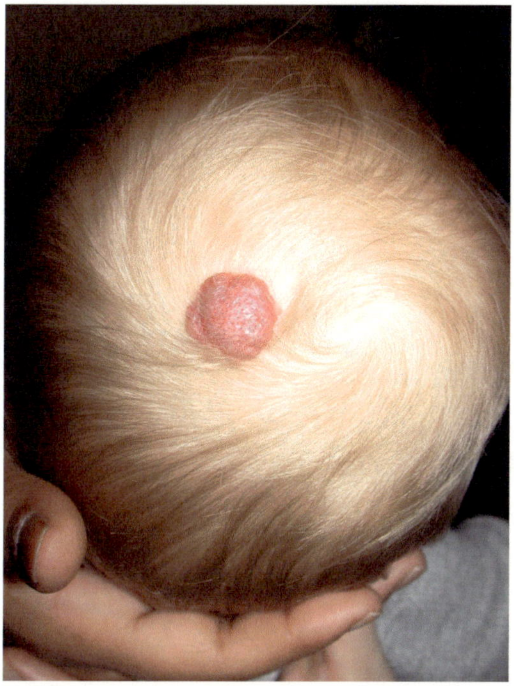

Fig. 1. Proliferating hemangioma of the scalp located in the dermis of an infant. Note the bright red color, elevation above the level of the normal surrounding skin, and raised, bosselated texture.

Those developing beneath the dermis in the subcuticular layer are usually only slightly raised and blue in color [Figure 2]. Growth usually plateaus before a year of age, but there are no reliable predictors for how large an IH can become in the first weeks of life.

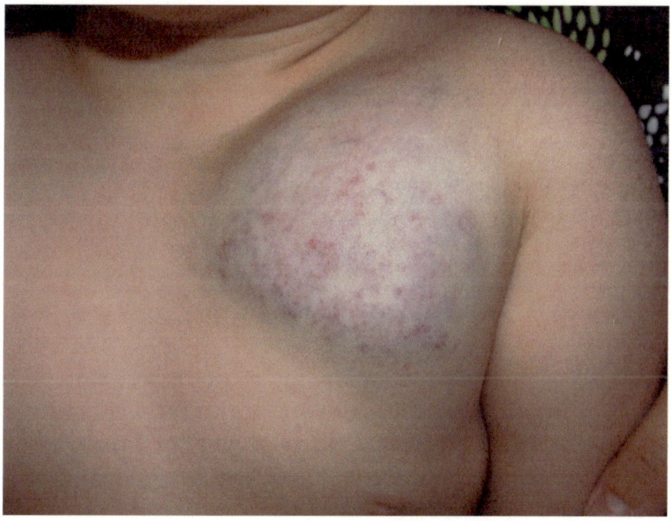

Fig. 2. Proliferating hemangioma located in the subcuticular layer of skin in an infant. Note the blue color, less prominent elevation, and smoother skin texture compared to Fig. 1.

During the *involuting phase*, generally from the age of 1 until 5 to 7 years, the IH continues to grow, although more slowly and in proportion with the child. Lesions located in the superficial dermis become less tense by palpation and a dull purple instead of crimson on visual inspection (Mulliken et al., 2000) [Figure 3].

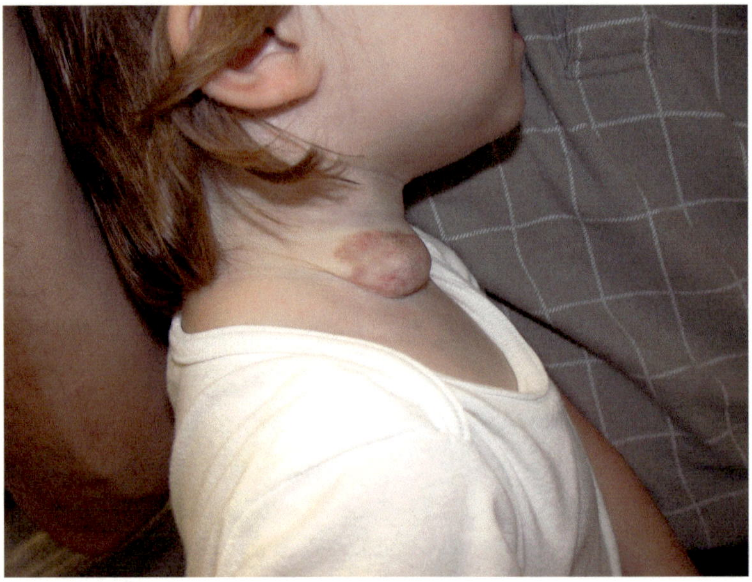

Fig. 3. Involuting hemangioma of the neck in a child. Note the mottled dull red and purple coloring compared to Fig. 1, as well as loose, extraneous skin and smoother texture.

The rate of this regression is difficult to predict, with no apparent links to appearance, location, gender, cutaneous depth, or size. However, involution is usually complete by 5 years of age in 50% of children, 7 years in 70%, and most by 10 to 12 years (Bowers et al., 1960).

3. Complications of IH

The potential morbidity and mortality that can occur as a result of IH is varied and ranges from life-threatening bleeding, airway obstruction, or threat to the visual axis during proliferation, to scarring and/or disfigurement during and after involution (Maguiness & Frieden, 2010).

Ulceration during proliferation occurs in 5% to 13% of all of IH and can cause significant morbidity for affected patients as a result of pain and scarring, as well as anxiety for parents [Figure 4].

Periorbital IHs can cause strabismus and amblyopia from the resultant obstruction of vision, and astigmatism can arise from a concomitant pressure or mass effect. If visual compromise is suspected, systemic therapy or surgical debulking is indicated. In patients in which amblyopia has already developed, the unaffected eye is patched (Ceisler & Blei, 2003; Ceisler et al., 2004; Schwartz et al., 2006).

Other potentially life-threatening complications include airway compromise in subglottic hemangiomas and symptomatic liver hemangiomas. Segmental hemangiomas, especially

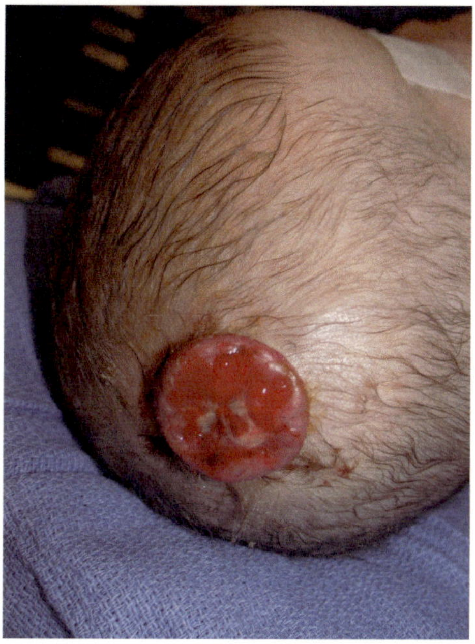

Fig. 4. Ulcerated proliferating hemangioma of the scalp in an infant.

those located in the mandibular region (classically referred to as having a "beard" distribution), have risk up to 63% of an associated airway hemangioma (Orlow et al., 1997). All patients with "beard distribution" hemangiomas should have an otolaryngologist evalutate him or her by laryngoscopy to rule out an airway hemangioma. Obstructive airway hemangiomas present with biphasic stridor. However, they may not be symptomatic until 6-8 weeks of life, when the airway hemangioma grows to a critical size that obstructs airflow. If the lesions are symptomatic, they may be treated with surgical or laser ablation, with or without systemic pharmacotherapy (Rahbar et al., 2004; Saetti et al., 2008).

Multifocal liver hemangiomas can cause high-output congestive right-sided heart failure, while diffuse liver hemangiomas, which fill the entire liver, can cause abdominal compartment syndrome and severe hypothyroidism with myxedema coma (Christison-Lagay et al., 2007). In these cases, aggressive management of the hypothyroidism is necessary, systemic or surgical therapy may be required, and rarely even a liver transplant is a therapeutic option (Maguiness & Frieden, 2010).

4. Associated syndromes

IH is also a prominent feature of two syndromes, PHACES and PELVIS. PHACES is a rare neurocutaneous syndrome that can include a constellation of problems such as **P**osterior fossa malformations, **H**emangiomas, **A**rterial anomalies, **C**oarctation of the aorta and cardiac defects, **E**ye abnormalities, and **S**ternal cleft or supraumbilical raphe defects. This syndrome involves a large facial hemangioma that is segmental in appearance, though the IH distribution does not follow dermatomes or Blaschko's lines (skin lines believed to trace the migration of embryonic cells). The pattern of appearance appears to follow developmental units, are reproducible, and have been categorized into segments. A segment 1 distribution involves the frontotemporal forehead and upper eye with extension to the scalp. Segment 2 distribution involves the maxilla, segment 3 is a mandibular or "beard" distribution, and the segment 4 distribution is frontonasal, involving a strip of skin from the superior forehead along the nose to the philtrum [Figure 5] (Haggstrom et al., 2006b).

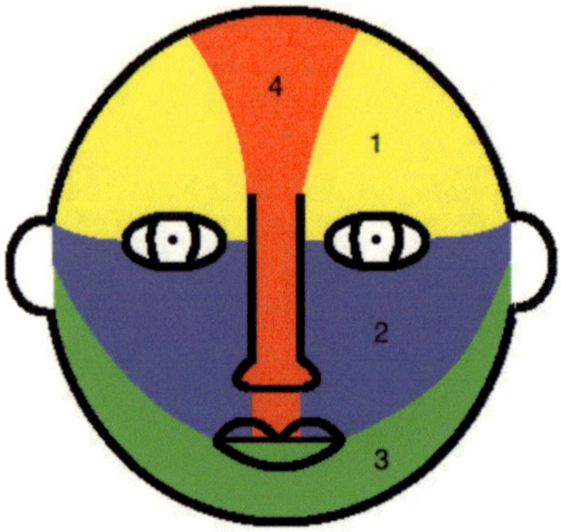

Fig. 5. Classification of facial segmental hemangioma localization into four areas based on observed distribution patterns, segments 1-4. Adapted from Haggstrom et al., 2006b.

Some of the most common and devastating of the congenital anomalies associated with PHACE syndrome are the structural brain and cerebrovascular anomalies (Drolet, et al., 2006; Metry et al., 2006; Metry et al., 2009). Structural anomalies of the brain parenchyma most commonly involve posterior fossa malformations such as Dandy-Walker syndrome, though other anomalies such as cerebral hypoplasia, microcephaly, heterotopia, and empty sella turcica have also been reported. The arterial anomalies associated with PHACE syndrome can manifest as the abnormal origin, abnormal course, hypoplasia, or absence of internal carotid or cerebral vasculature on the ipsilateral side of the facial hemangioma. Infants have also been reported to have an increased risk of vasculopathy and early stroke (Drolet et al., 2006).

Other conditions in which IH is associated with underlying structural defects include the well-described association of segmental lumbosacral hemangiomas with a tethered spinal cord, genitourinary anomalies, or both. Additionally, PELVIS syndrome (**P**erineal hemangioma-**E**xternal genitalia malformations-**L**ipomyelomeningocele-**V**esicorenal abnormalities-**I**mperforate anus-**S**kin tag) is similar to PHACES in that it too features a large hemangioma over an area with underlying structural and vascular aberrencies (Girard, Bigorre et al. 2006). In the case of PELVIS syndrome, patients present with a large segmental perineal hemangioma not localized to specific dermatomes. It is generally located from the sacral area to the thigh or pelvis, but also sometimes found to involve the vaginal wall, uterine horn, or fallopian tube. In addition, defects of the spine, genitourinary tract, and anus are found.

5. Treatment

First line medical treatment for problematic, proliferating IH is currently corticosteroids, though propranolol has become a favored mode of treatment recently. Intralesional corticosteroid injections are useful in small, well-localized tumors where the medication will be evenly distributed. Systemic treatment is indicated in cases where the IH may cause functional impairment or is life-threatening, or the large size of the hemangioma precludes local corticosteroid injection. Side effects of corticosteroids include gastrointestinal upset, weight gain, hypertension, adrenal suppression, immunosuppression, and growth delay (Maguiness & Frieden, 2010). However, most of these effects are reversed on cessation of treatment (Boon et al., 1999). Recently, propranolol has been shown to be an effective treatment in cases where steroids have been insufficient. Many authors have reported positive results in the treatment infants with rapidly proliferating IH, periorbital IH, subepiglottic IH, and visceral IH (Buckmiller et al., 2009; Holmes et al., 2010; Léauté-Labrèze et al., 2008; Leboulanger et al., 2010; Li et al., 2010; Mazereeuw-Hautier et al., 2010; Sans et al., 2009; Tan et al., 2010; Truong et al., 2010). Potential side effects include bradycardia, hypotension, and hypoglycemia. In infants with PHACE syndrome, the risk of stroke is theoretically increased if propranolol is administered. The efficacy and limitations of propanolol on IHs remains to be seen.

Vincristine is another alternative treatment modality that, while possessing many known side effects when used as a chemotherapy agent, has been demonstrated as an effective drug with a good safety profile (Maguiness & Frieden, 2010). In the past, interferon alpha (2a or 2b) has also been used in cases where corticosteroids were ineffective. However, due to the risk of spastic diplegia in children treated with interferon (Barlow et al., 1998), it is currently reserved to cases in which life-threatening IHs have not responded to other forms of treatment.

In summary, while most IHs are asymptomatic and require only monitoring and reassurance, there are subsets of IHs that will require aggressive intervention. Current medical treatments were discovered serendipitously and their mechanisms of action not well understood. Unless the pathogenesis and regulatory signaling mechanisms can be delineated, targeted therapy may not be possible. Despite our limited understanding, progress has been made in the basic science of IHs.

6. Pathophysiology of IHs

6.1 Past studies

Many descriptive studies have been published regarding hemangiomas. IHs have been described as a tumor of endothelial cells, but it is in fact made up of a heterogeneous group of cells including endothelial cells, myeloid cells, pericytes, and mast cells (Itinteang et al., 2011b; Tan et al., 2004; Ritter et al., 2006).

Histological studies have shown that endothelial cells in IHs are different from normal endothelial cells and vascular malformations (Mulliken & Glowacki, 1982). In addition to expressing CD31 and von Willebrand factor (vWF), hemangioma endothelial cells (HemECs) also express type IV collagenase, vascular endothelial growth factor, and insulin-like growth factor 2 at high levels during the proliferating phase, and high levels of tissue inhibitor of metalloproteinases 1 (TIMP1) during the involuting phase (Takahashi et al., 1994). E-selectin, urokinase and basic fibroblast growth factor are expressed at high levels in both phases. HemECs also express glucose transporter 1 (GLUT1) (North et al., 2000), merosin, Lewis Y antigen, and Fc gamma RII (Enjolras et al, 2007) at high levels. In particular, GLUT1 is of special interest as it is positive in 100% of IH endothelial cells, and not expressed in other infantile vascular tumors such as congenital hemangiomas, tufted angioma, kaposiform hemangioendothelioma, nor vascular malformations. GLUT1 is also expressed at high levels in the endothelial cells of barrier tissues such as placental endothelial cells and endothelial cells of the blood-brain barrier. The presence of GLUT1 is therefore useful as a diagnostic marker to confirm the histological diagnosis of IH (North et al., 2001). While these studies give valuable information to the unique appearance, history, and histological characteristics of IHs, they gave no insight into their developmental pathogenesis or regulatory mechanisms that govern the progression of IHs.

Due to the fact that endothelial cells in IHs express high levels of GLUT1, similar to placental endothelial cells, the "placental theory" of IH origin gained traction. In a study comparing the molecular gene expression profile of IHs to multiple different tissues, including brain, muscles, skin and placenta, it was found that the molecular profile of IH most closely resembled those of placental tissues (Barnés et al., 2005). Moreover, clinical observations of an association with IH incidence and exposure to chorionic villus sampling further lent credence to this theory (Bauland et al., 2010; Burton et al., 1995; Kaplan et al., 1990). Nonetheless, although these studies demonstrated an intriguing association between the placenta and IH, they have never definitively shown a causal role for the placenta in the formation of IH.

Studies in IHs have been further hampered by the lack of a viable animal model. Many studies have claimed to have a mouse model of hemangioma. A transgenic mouse with SV40 promoter-driven Polyomavirus Middle T gene demonstrated abnormal vascular proliferation with cavernous hemangioma-like structures in the skin, tongue, ear and gastric mucosa (Xu et al., 2009). The authors of this paper claimed that this was a model for IH; however, these tumors did not involute. Another xenograft model of infantile hemangioma onto nude mice did recapitulate the involuting phase, but is not an ideal laboratory model in that it has not been demonstrated that these cells can be passaged through mice and therefore requires fresh human sample tissue for each experiment (Peng et al., 2005; Tang et al., 2007). Furthermore, neither of these models recapitulate the proliferative phase of IH, and the authors of these reports did not report evidence of GLUT1 positivity.

Ritter et al (Ritter et al., 2002; 2003) was one of the first to employ microarrays in an attempt to quantify different genes that may be active in different phases of IHs. These studies showed that different genes had different expression levels in the proliferating phase versus the involuting phase. For instance, insulin-like growth factor 2 was suggested as a putative regulator of hemangioma proliferation, as its transcript levels were 10-fold higher than those in the involuting hemangiomas. However, these studies did not show causal relationships between the array data and IH behavior.

6.2 Intrinsic theory of hemangiomas

One important study of the basic science of IHs focused on the intrinsic vs. extrinsic origin theory, arguing that infantile hemangiomas arises from an intrinsic somatic mutation in an endothelial progenitor cell (Bischoff, 2002). By analyzing X-chromosome inactivation patterns using a polymorphism of the X-linked human androgen receptor gene (HUMARA), it was found that HemECs display a non-random pattern of X-chromosomal inactivation, demonstrating that each HemEC population was clonal and implicating a single progenitor cell as their origin. Additionally, non-endothelial cells isolated from hemangiomas did not display evidence of clonality, demonstrating that only endothelial cells within IHs are clonal.

Other studies have shown that the endothelial cells isolated from IHs behave abnormally when compared to isolated endothelial cells from foreskin/commercially available dermal microvascular endothelial cells. While HemECs display many of the same markers as normal endothelial cells such as CD31, vWF, and E-selectin (in response to LPS exposure), HemECs proliferate and migrate at a faster rate *in vitro* in response to treatment with exogenous VEGF-A when compared with human dermal microvascular endothelial cells (HDMECs) (Boye et al., 2001). A subsequent study showed that HemECs also possess properties similar to those of immature endothelial cells, cord blood endothelial progenitor cells (cbEPCs). When exposed to the angiogenesis inhibitor endostatin, cbEPCs paradoxically exhibited increased adhesion, proliferation and migration in response to a VEGF-A gradient, while HDMECs migrated more slowly in response to endostatin exposure. Eventually, the response of cbEPCs to the same experiments shifted to mirror that of mature endothelial cells as the cells were passaged in culture. HemECs exposed to endostatin also demonstrated behavior similar to that of cbEPCs, further demonstrating their abnormal behavior when compared with normal endothelial cells (Khan et al., 2006). Taken together, these data further support the theory that an anomaly intrinsic to the IH gives rise to the lesion.

Later investigations resulted in the isolation and characterization of a cell called the hemangioma stem cell (HemSC) (Khan et al., 2008). These HemSCs were demonstrated to be highly proliferative in culture, and capable of differentiating into endothelial, adipocyte, chondrocyte, osteocyte, and neuroglial lineages. Furthermore, when mixed with Matrigel and subsequently implanted as a subcutaneous Matrigel plug into the backs of nude mice, HemSCs formed $GLUT1^+$ endothelial cell-lined functional blood vessels during the first few weeks. Four weeks after implantation, however, the Matrigel plugs were instead found to contain adipocytes. This was the first valid published animal model of IH, and its recapitulation of the natural history of IH gave further credence to the intrinsic theory of IH as well as evidence for the new theory of a stem cell as the cellular origin of IHs.

Some evidence also points to a possible neural crest cell origin for IHs. Waner and colleagues were the first to notice that segmental hemangiomas tend to occur at regions of embryological fusion (Waner et al., 2003). Several years later, Haggstrom and colleagues conducted a larger study, finding that certain segmental facial hemangiomas tend to respect embryological boundaries such as the maxillary and mandibular promineces, while others did not (Haggstrom et al., 2006b). Using their observations, they grouped the distribution of facial hemangiomas into four segments. Given the pattern of distribution of segmental facial hemangiomas, these groups also postulated that facial hemangiomas may have a neural crest cell origin. Expression of a marker for neural crest stem cells, p75, has also been demonstrated in proliferating IH (Itinteang et al., 2010).

6.3 VEGF pathway

Different pathways have been suggested as possibly being involved in the pathogenesis and development of IHs. The VEGF pathway, as one of the most important signaling molecules in normal and pathophysiological angiogenesis, has been the subject of much study. VEGFR-1 and VEGFR-2 are both expressed in IH. However, Jinnin et al demonstrated that VEGFR-2 signaling is constitutively active in cultured HemECs in the presence of VEGF-A, and that this signaling is a result of downregulated VEGFR-1 expression. VEGFR-1 is expressed at much lower levels as a result of aberrant increased interaction of a mutated anthrax toxin receptor-1 (ANTXR-1) with b1-integrin and VEGFR-2. The increase in this complex formation in HemECs appears to suppress NFAT-promoted transcription of VEGFR-1. As both VEGFR-1 and VEGFR-2 proteins bind to VEGF-A, and VEGFR-1 is believed to act as a negative regulator of VEGFR-2 signaling through sequestration of VEGF-A, a decrease in VEGFR-1 expression would lead to constitutive VEGFR-2 signaling. This constitutive VEGFR-2 signaling in the presence of VEGF-A helps explain the aberrant overgrowth of endothelial cells in IH.

Studies involving treatment options for IH, such as corticosteroids and propranolol, serve to further highlight the importance of the VEGF pathway in IH pathogenesis. Corticosteroids have been one of the first-line medical treatments for problematic hemangiomas. Greenberger and colleagues demonstrated that dexamethasone treatment of mice implanted with HemSCs in a Matrigel plug with led to a dose-dependent inhibition of microvessel density in those plugs. Pre-treating HemSCs with dexamethasone, or silencing VEGF-A expression in HemSCs using shRNA lentiviral particles, before implantation into mice also gave similar results. Furthermore, *in vitro* administration of dexamethasone to HemSCs resulted in a significant decrease in both mRNA transcript and protein expression levels of VEGF-A. The authors also showed that VEGF-A expression is present in IHs in the proliferating phase, but not in those in the involuting phase, strongly suggesting that early expression of VEGF-A by HemSCs has a crucial role in the pathogenesis of IH. (Greenberger et al., 2010b). In a subsequent study, the same authors demonstrated that treatment of HemSCs with dexamethasone suppresses the activity of nuclear factor kappa-light-chain-enhancer of activated B cells (NF-κB). They also showed that direct suppression of NF-κB activity leads to decreased VEGF-A mRNA and protein expression, suggesting that NF-κB regulates VEGF-A expression in HemSCs and providing a plausible mechanism explaining the clinical effect of corticosteroids on IH (Greenberger et al., 2010a).

Recently, propranolol has been demonstrated to be an effective drug for the treatment of IH. In 2008, Léauté-Labrèze and colleagues reported a dramatic response to propranolol treatment in a small cohort of eleven patients with IH (Léauté-Labrèze et al., 2008). However, the molecular mechanisms behind this effect are of considerable interest. Recent work by Lamy and colleagues in HUVECs has demonstrated that treatment with propranolol inhibited proliferation, chemotactic migration, and tube formation *in vitro*, as well as inhibition of VEGF-A-induced tyrosine phosphorylation of VEGFR-2 (Lamy et al., 2010). While this study demonstrates that propranolol can interfere with some of the important steps involved in angiogenesis, shortcomings of this study include lack of *in vivo* data and the fact that none of the experiments were conducted in HemECs and limits the application of the group's conclusions to IHs. More work is needed to elucidate the mechanism of action of propranolol on the accelerated involution of IH.

6.4 TIE/Angiopoietin signaling

The tyrosine kinase with immunoglobulin-like and EGF-like domains 2 (TIE2)/angiopoietin signaling pathway is also another putative regulator of IH pathogenesis. Tie1, Tie2, and angiopoietin-2 (Ang2) are strongly expressed in cultured HemECs, with low expression of Ang1. Relative to human dermal microvascular endothelial cells (HDMECs), Tie2 mRNA and protein expression are increased in HemECs, and HemECs also demonstrate a concomitant increase in cellular responsiveness to Ang1 as measured by cellular proliferation and migration. Altered regulation of Ang2 has also been observed, with Ang2 mRNA expression in HemECs down-regulated in response to serum relative to HDMECs. Thus Tie2 and its ligands Ang1 and Ang2 likely have an important role in the pathogenesis of hemangioma (Acevedo & Cheresh, 2008; Jinnin et al., 2008; Yu, et al., 2001).

6.5 Notch signaling

Recent studies have also focused on the Notch signaling pathway, a highly conserved juxtacrine signaling pathway that is involved in cell fate determination during embryogenesis. Four Notch receptor genes (Notch1-4) were found to be expressed in IHs, as well as 2 Notch ligands, Jagged-1 and Delta-like-4 (Dll-4) (Wu & Kitajewski, 2009). Moreover, the Notch expression profile of proliferating hemangiomas is different than that of hemangiomas undergoing involution, with involuting hemangiomas demonstrating increased expression of Notch4 and Jagged-1 when compared with proliferating hemangiomas. HemSCs and HemECs also demonstrate completely different Notch expression profiles, with HemSCs expressing higher levels of Notch2 and Notch3, but lower levels of Notch1, Notch4, Jagged-1, and Dll-4 compared to HemECs (Wu et al., 2010). These data suggest a possible role for Notch signaling in the maintanence of HemSC pluripotency and differentiation into HemEC phenotype.

6.6 Renin-angiotensin system

Another area of focus on pathogenesis of IH is the renin-angiotensin system (Itinteang et al., 2011a). Proliferating hemangioma has been demonstrated to express both angiotensin-converting enzyme (ACE) and angiotensin receptor 2. Blast-like structures isolated from IH using an *in vitro* explant model expressed CD133, CD34, and VEGFR-2, as well as ACE. These blast-like structures increased in number following angiotenisin II treatment in a dose-response manner. The authors postulate that treatment of IH with propranolol exerts its effects at least partially through downregulation of renin activity of the kidney, leading to decreased conversion of angiotensinogen to angiotensin I and ultimately to decreased angiotensin II levels, thereby decreasing proliferation of IH. While interesting, whether or how the renin-angiotensin system contributes to the pathogenesis or development of IHs remain to be seen.

6.7 Tumor endothelial cells

It has long been known that as tumors develop and increase in size, they recruit blood vessels from their host in order to attempt to meet their increased metabolized demands by a process termed angiogenesis. The resultant vasculature is abnormal, and characterized by tortuous vessels, a disorganized sprouting, vessel leakiness, and loose associations between the vessels' endothelial cells and the basement membrane and pericytes that cover them. While an abnormal vasculature is a hallmark of solid tumors, it is only recently that there has been evidence suggesting that these blood vessels are composed of endothelial cells that are in and of themselves intrinsically abnormal as well. Endothelial cells isolated from human renal cell carcinoma have been reported to be more resistant to serum starvation and vincristine-induced apoptosis when compared to normal endothelial cells, exhibit enhanced Akt activation and decreased expression of the tumor suppressor gene PTEN, and do not undergo senescence (Bussolati et al., 2003). Murine Lewis lung carcinoma endothelial cells were characterized by a comparatively elongated cellular morphology, fewer cell-cell contacts, and increased levels of a host of endothelial cell-surface markers (Allport & Weissleder, 2003).

Hida and colleagues purified murine endothelial cells from human xenograft models of melanoma and liposarcoma and compared them with murine endothelial cells isolated from normal murine skin and adipose tissue. They found that endothelial cells isolated from tumors were cytogenetically different when compared to normal endothelial cells, displaying larger, heterogenous nuclei and aneuploidy that was exacerbated by passage in culture. Abnormal multiple centrosomes were also seen, and FISH analysis showed that the structural chromosomal aberrations were heterogenous, indicating that the mutations were not clonal (Hida et al., 2004). Possible mechanisms for this cytogenetic instability include the unique growth factor milieu in the tumor environment causing genetic instability; loss of tumor suppressor and checkpoint activity; uptake of human tumor oncogenes by fusion or phagocytosis of apoptotic bodies; and transdifferentiation of tumor cells into endothelial cells.

Xiong and colleages isolated endothelial cells from human hepatocellular carcinoma (HCC) and adjacent normal tissue, and reported that HCC endothelial cells demonstrate enhanced angiogenic activity including enhanced proliferation, resistance to apoptosis in the absence of serum, enhanced migration, and enhanced ability to form tubes when implanted into Matrigel in the absence of serum. These cells were also relatively resistant to chemotherapeutic drugs including adriamycin and 5-fluorouracil, and the antiangiogenic drug sorafenib. Tumor endothelial cells share many of the same characteristics of HemECs, and further research comparing the similarities and differences between the two cell types may give insight both into the origin of IHs and the unique properties of tumor endothelial cells (Xiong et al., 2009).

Interestingly, Dudley and colleagues have recently reported that tumor endothelial cells isolated from a transgenic mouse model in which the mice develop prostate adenocarcinoma at puberty demonstrate some of the features of mesenchymal stem cells. When cultured *in vitro* and stimulated with osteogenic medium, clonal populations of these prostate tumor endothelial cells demonstrated alkaline phosphatase activity, expressed bone-specific markers such as osteopontin and osteocalcin, and underwent mineralization. These same cells formed cartilage-like tissues when cultured in chondrogenic medium, with concomitant upregulation of cartilage-specific genes. However, these tumor endothelial cells could not be differentiated to form adipocytes, distinguishing them from normal mesenchymal stem cells and HemSCs (Dudley et al., 2008).

7. Conclusion

IHs remain poorly understood but may have serious clinical consequences. While many details of their pathogenesis and regulatory mechanisms are still not known, they most likely originate from a hemangioma stem cell (HemSC) that abnormally differentiate into hemangioma endothelial cells (HemEC). These HemECs are different from mature endothelial cells in that they retain features of immature endothelial progenitor cells, suggesting an abnormality in stem cell differentiation. In addition, many different signaling mechanisms have been studied as potential candidates for regulating the transition of IH from the proliferating to involuting phase, and from HemSC to HemEC.

Understanding the mechanisms that regulate IHs will allow directed therapy for affected infants. Moreover, IHs also serve as a model of aberrant vasculogenesis and allow for greater understanding of vascular development, including the role of the VEGF, Notch, and renin-angiotensin signaling pathways. These mechanisms may give insight into hematopoietic differentiation and should be investigated for their potential role in normal vasculogenesis. IHs also share many similarities with tumor endothelial cells, and further study and comparison with the unique characteristics of tumor endothelial cells could lead to new insights into tumor angiogenesis.

8. References

Acevedo, L. M. & Cheresh, D. A. (2008). Suppressing NFAT increases VEGF signaling in hemangiomas. *Cancer Cell*, Vol. 14, No. 6, December 2009, pp. 429-430.

Allport, J.R. & Wiessleder, R. (2003). Murine Lewis lung carcinoma-derived endothelium expresses markers of endothelial activation and requires tumor-specific extracellular matrix in vitro. *Neoplasia*, Vol. 5, No. 3, May-June 2003, pp. 205-217.

Amir, J., Metzker, A.; Krikler, R. & Reisner, S.H. (1986). Strawberry hemangioma in preterm infants. *Pediatric Dermatology*, Vol. 3, No. 4, September 1986, 331-332.

Arneja, J. S. & Mulliken, J. B. (2010). Resection of amblyogenic periocular hemangiomas: indications and outcomes. *Plastics and Reconstructive Surgery*, Vol. 125, No. 1, January 2010, pp. 274-281.

Barnés C.M.; Huang, S.; Kaipainen, A.; Sanoudou, D.; Chen, E.J.; Eichler, G.S.; Guo, Y.; Yu, Y.; Ingber, D.E.; Mulliken, J.B.; Beggs, A.H.; Folkman, J. & Fishman, S.J. Evidence by molecular profiling for a placental origin of infantile hemangioma. *Proceedings of the National Academy of Sciences of the United States of America*, Vol. 102, No. 52, December 2005, pp. 19097-19102.

Barlow, C.F.; Priebe, C.J.; Mulliken, J.B.; Barnes, P.D.; MacDonald, D.; Folkman, J. & Ezekowitz, R.A. Spastic diplegia as a complication of interferon alfa-2a treatment of hemangiomas of infancy. *The Journal of Pediatrics*, Vol. 132, No. 3 Pt 1, March 1998, pp. 527-530.

Bauland, C.G.; Smit, J.M.; Bartelink, L.R.; Zondervan, H.A. & Spauwen, P.H. (2010). Hemangioma in the newborn: increased incidence after chorionic villus sampling. *Prenatal Diagnosis*, Vol. 30, No. 10, October 2010, pp. 913-917.

Bischoff, J. Monoclonal expansion of endothelial cells in hemangioma: an intrinsic defect with extrinsic consequences? *Trends in Cardiovascular Medicine*, Vol. 12, No. 5, July 2002, pp. 220-204.

Bitar, M. A.; Moukarbel, R.V. & Zalzal, G.H. (2005). Management of congenital subglottic hemangioma: trends and success over the past 17 years. *Otolaryngology – Head and Neck Surgery*, Vol. 132, No. 2, February 2005, pp. 226-231.

Boon, L. M.; Burrows, P. E.; Paltiel, H.J.; Lund, D.P.; Ezekowitz, R.A.B.; Folkman, J. & Mulliken, J.B. (1996). Hepatic vascular anomalies in infancy: a twenty-seven-year experience. *The Journal of Pediatrics*, Vol. 129, No. 3, September 1996, pp. 346-354.

Boon, L.M.; MacDonald, D.M. & Mulliken, J.B. (1999). Complications of systemic corticosteroid therapy for problematic hemangioma. *Plastic and Reconstructive Surgery*, Vol. 104, No. 6, November 1999, pp. 1616-1623.

Bowers, R.E.; Graham, E.A. & Tomlinson, K.M. The natural history of the strawberry nevus. *Archives of Dermatology*, Vol. 82, No. 5, 1960, pp. 667-680.

Boye, E.; Yu, Y.; Paranya, G.; Mulliken, J.B.; Olsen, B.R.; Bischoff, J. (2001). Clonality and altered behavior of endothelial cells from hemangiomas. *The Journal of Clinical Investigation*, Vol. 107, No. 6, March 2001, pp. 745-752.

Buckmiller, L.; Dyamenahalli, U. & Richter, G.T. Propranolol for airway hemangiomas: Case report of novel treatment. (2009). *Laryngoscope*, Vol. 119, No. 10, October 2009, pp. 2051-2054.

Bussolati, B.; Deambrosis, I.; Russo, S.; Deregibus, M.C. & Camussi, G. Altered angiogenesis and survival in human tumor-derived endothelial cells. The *FASEB Journal*, Vol. 17, No. 9, June 2003, pp. 1159-1161.

Burrows, P.E.; Robertson, R.L.; Mulliken, J.B.; Beardsley, D.S.; Chaloupka J.C.; Ezekowitz, R.A. & Scott, R.M. (1998). Cerebral vasculopathy and neurologic sequelae in infants with cervicofacial hemangioma: report of eight patients. *Radiology*, Vol. 207, No. 3, June 1998, pp. 601–607.

Burton, B.K.; Schulz, C.J.; Angle, B. & Burd, L.I. (1995). An increased incidence of haemangiomas in infants born following chorionic villus sampling (CVS). *Prenatal Diagnosis*, Vol. 15, No. 3, March 1995, pp. 209-214.

Ceisler, E. & Blei, F. (2003). Ophthalmic issues in hemangiomas of infancy. *Lymphatic Research and Biology*, Vol. 1, No. 4, 2003, pp. 321-330.

Ceisler, E.; Santos, L. & Blei, F. Periocular hemangioma: what every physician should know. (2004). *Pediatric Dermatology*, Vol. 21, No. 1, January-February 2004, pp. 1-9.

Chamlin, S. L.; Haggstrom, A. N.; Drolet, B.A.; Baselga, E.; Frieden, I.J.; Garzon, M.C.; Horii, K.A.; Lucky, A.W.; Metry, D.W.; Newell, B.; Nopper, A.J. & Mancini, A.J. (2007). Multicenter prospective study of ulcerated hemangiomas. *The Journal of Pediatrics*, Vol. 151, No. 6, December 2007, pp. 684-689.

Christison-Lagay, E.R.; Burrows, P.E.; Alomari, A; Dubois, J.; Kozakewich, H.P.; Lane, T.S.; Paltiel, H.J.; Klement, G.; Mulliken, J.B.& Fishman, S.J. (2007). Hepatic hemangiomas: Subtype classification and development of a clinical practice algorithm and registry. *Journal of Pediatric Surgery*, Vol. 42, No. 1, January 2007, pp. 62-67.

Drolet, B.A.; Dohil, M.; Golomb, M.R.; Wells, R.; Murowski, L.; Tamburro, J.; Sty, J. & Friedlander, S.F. (2006). Early stroke and cerebral vasculopathy in children with facial hemangiomas and PHACE association. *Pediatrics*, Vol. 117, No. 3, March 2006, pp. 959–964.

Dudley, A.C.; Khan, Z.A.; Shih, S.C.; Kang, S.Y.; Zwaans, B.M.M.; Bischoff, J. & Klagsbrun, M. (2008). Calcification of multipotent prostate tumor endothelium. *Cancer Cell*, Vol. 14, No. 3, September 2008, pp. 201-211.

Enjolras, O.; Wassef, M. & Chapot, R. (May 2007). *Color Atlast of Vascular Tumors and Vascular Malformations*, Cambridge University Press, ISBN 978-0-521-84851-0, New York, NY.

Frieden, I. J.; Haggstrom, A. N.; Drolet, B.A.; Mancini, A.J.; Friedlander, S.F.; Boon, L.; Chamlin, S.L.; Baselga E.; Garzon, M.C.; Nopper A.J.; Siegel, D.H.; Mathes, E.W.; Goddard, D.S.; Bischoff, J.; North, P.E. & Esterly, N.B. (2005). Infantile hemangiomas: current knowledge, future directions. Proceedings of a research workshop on infantile hemangiomas, April 7-9, 2005, Bethesda, Maryland, USA. *Pediatric Dermatology*, Vol. 22, No. 5, September-October 2005, pp. 383-406.

Frieden, I.J.; Reese, V. & Cohen, D. (1996). PHACE syndrome. The association of posterior fossa brain malformations, hemangiomas, arterial anomalies, coarctation of the aorta and cardiac defects, and eye abnormalities. *Archives of Dermatology*, Vol. 132, No. 3, March 1996, pp. 307-311.

Greenberger, S.; Adini, I.; Boscolo, E.; Mulliken, J.B.; Bischoff, J. (2010). Targeting NF-κB in infantile hemangioma-derived stem cells reduces VEGF-A expression. *Angiogenesis*, Vol. 13, No. 4, December 2010, pp. 327-335.

Greenberger, S.; Boscolo, E.; Adini, I.; Mulliken, J.B. & Bischoff, J. (2010). Corticosteroid suppression of VEGF-A in infantile hemangioma-derived stem cells. *The New England Journal of Medicine*, Vol. 362, No. 11, March 2010, pp. 1005-13.

Girard, C.; Bigorre, M.; Guillot, B. & Bessis, D. (2006). PELVIS Syndrome. *Archives of Dermatology*, Vol. 142, No. 7, July 2006, pp. 884-888.

Haggstrom, A. N.; Drolet, B. A.; Baselga, E.; Chamlin, S.L.; Garzon, M.C.; Horii, K.A.; Lucky, A.W.; Mancini, A.J.; Metry, D.W.; Newell, B.; Nopper, A.J. & Frieden, I.J. (2006). Prospective study of infantile hemangiomas: clinical characteristics predicting complications and treatment. *Pediatrics*, Vol. 118, No. 3, September 2006, pp. 882-887.

Haggstrom, A. N.; Lammer, E.J.; Schneider, R.A.; Marcucio, R. & Frieden, I.J. (2006). Patterns of infantile hemangiomas: new clues to hemangioma pathogenesis and embryonic facial development. *Pediatrics*, Vol. 117, No. 3, March 2006, pp. 698-703.

Hida, K.; Hida, Y.; Amin, D.N.; Flint, A.F.; Panigrahy, D.; Morton, C.C. & Klagsbrun, M. (2004). Tumor-associated endothelial cells with cytogenetic abnormalities. *Cancer Research*, Vol. 64, No. 22, November 2004, pp. 8249-8255.

Holmdahl, K. (1955). Cutaneous hemangiomas in premature and mature infants. *Acta Paediatrica*, Vol. 44, No. 4, July 1955, pp. 370-379.

Holmes, W.J.M.; Mishra, A.; Gorst, C. & Liew, S.H. (2010). Propranolol as first-line treatment for rapidly proliferating infantile hemangiomas. *Journal of Plastic, Reconstructive, & Aesthetic Surgery*, Vol. 64, No. 4, April 2011, pp. 445-451.

Itinteang, T.; Brasch, H.D.; Tan, S.T. & Day, D.J. (2011). Expression of components of the renin-angiotensin system in proliferating infantile hemangioma may account for the propranolol-induced accelerated involution. *Journal of Plastic, Reconstructive, & Aesthetic Surgery*, Vol. 64, No. 6, June 2011, pp. 759-765.

Itinteang, T.; Tan, S.T.; Brasch, H. & Day, D.J. (2010). Primitive mesodermal cells with a neural crest stem cell phenotype predominate proliferating infantile haemangioma. *Journal of Clinical Pathology*, Vol. 63, No. 9, September 2010, pp. 771-776.

Itinteang, T.; Vishvanath, A.; Day, D.J. & Tan, S.T. (2011). Mesenchymal stem cells in infantile haemangioma. *Journal of Clinical Pathology*, Vol. 64, No. 3, March 2011, pp. 232-236.

Jinnin, M.; Medici, D.; Park, L.; Limaye, N.; Liu, Y.; Boscolo, E.; Bischoff, J.; Vikkula, M.; Boye, E. & Olsen, B.R. (2008). Suppressed NFAT-dependent VEGFR1 expression and constitutive VEGFR2 signaling in infantile hemangioma. *Nature Medicine*, Vol. 14, No. 11, November 2008, pp. 1236-1246.

Kaplan, P.; Normandin, J. Jr.; Wilson, G.N.; Plauchu, H.; Lippman, A. & Vekemans, M. (1990). Malformations and minor anomalies in children whose mothers had prenatal diagnosis: comparison between CVS and amniocentesis. *American Journal of Medical Genetics*, Vol. 37, No. 3, pp. 366-370.

Khan, Z.A.; Boscolo, E.; Picard, A.; Psutka, S.; Melero-Martin, J.M.; Bartch, T.C.; Mulliken, J.B.; Bischoff, J. (2008). Multipotential stem cells recapitulate human infantile hemangioma in immunodeficient mice. *The Journal of Clinical Investigation*, Vol. 118, No. 7, July 2008, pp. 2592-2599.

Khan, Z.A.; Melero-Martin, J.M.; Wu, X.; Paruchuri, S.; Boscolo, E.; Mulliken, J.M. & Bischoff, J. (2006). Endothelial progenitor cells from infantile hemangioma and umbilical cord blood display unique cellular responses to endostatin. *Blood*, Vol. 108, No. 3, August 2006, pp. 915-921.

Lamy, S.; Lachambre, M.P.; Lord-Dufour, S. & Béliveau, R. (2010). Propranolol suppresses angiogenesis in vitro: inhibition of proliferation, migration, and differentiation of endothelial cells. *Vascular Pharmacology*, Vol. 53, No. 5-6, November-December 2010, pp. 200-8.

Léauté-Labrèze, C.; Dumas de la Roque, E.; Hubiche, T.; Boralevi, F.; Thambo, J.B.; Taïeb, A. (2008). Propranolol for sever hemangiomas of infancy. *The New England Journal of Medicine*, Vol. 358, No. 24, June 2008, pp. 2649-2651.

Leboulanger, N.; Fayoux, P.; Teissier, N.; Cox, A.; Van Den Abbeele, T.; Carrabin, L.; Couloigner, V.; Nicollas, R.; Triglia, J.M.; Ayari, S.; Froehlich, P.; Lescanne, E.; Marianowski, R.; Mom, T.; Mondain, M.; Marie, J.P.; Roger, G.; Garabédian, E.N. & Denoyelle, F. Propranolol in the therapeutic strategy of infantile laryngotracheal hemangioma: a preliminary retrospective study of French experience. (2010). *The International Journal of Pediatric Otorhinolaryngology*, Vol. 74, No. 11, November 2010, pp. 1254-1257.

Li, Y.C.; McCahon, E.; Rowe, N.A.; Martin, P.A.; Wilcsek, G.A. & Martin, F.J. (2010). Successful treatment of infantile hemangiomas of the orbit with propranolol. *Clinical & Experimental Ophthalmology*, Vol. 38, No. 6, August 2010, pp. 554-559.

Maguiness, S.M., & Frieden, I.J. (2010). Current management of infantile hemangiomas. *Seminars in Cutaneous Medicine and Surgery*, Vol. 29, No. 2, June 2010, pp. 106-114.

Mazereeuw-Hautier, J.; Hoeger, P.H.; Benlahrech, S.; Ammour, A.; Broue, P.; Vial, J.; Ohanessian, G.; Léauté-Labrèze, C.; Labenne, M.; Vabres, P.; Rössler, J. & and Bodemer, C. (2010). Efficacy of Propranolol in Hepatic Infantile Hemangiomas with Diffuse Neonatal Hemangiomatosis. *The Journal of Pediatrics*, Vol. 157, No. 2, pp. 340-342.

Metry, D.W.; Haggstrom, A.N.; Drolet, B.A.; Baselga, E.; Chamlin, S.; Garzon, M.; Horil, K.; Lucky, A.; Mancini, A.J.; Newell, B.; Nopper, A.; Heyer, G. & Frieden, I.J. (2006). A prospective study of PHACE syndrome in infantile hemangiomas: demographic features, clinical findings, and complications. *American Journal of Medical Genetics*, Vol. 140, No. 9, May 2006, pp. 975-986.

Metry, D.; Heyer, G.; Hess, C.; Garzon, M.; Haggstrom, A.; Frommelt, P.; Adams, D.; Siegel, D.; Hall, K.; Powell, J.; Frieden, I. & Drolet, B. (2009). Consensus Statement on Diagnostic Criteria for PHACE Syndrome. *Pediatrics*, Vol. 124, No. 5, November 2009, pp. 1447-1456.

Mulliken, J.M.; Fishman, S.J. & Burrows, P.E. (2000). Vascular anomalies. *Current Problems in Surgery*, Vol. 37, No. 8, August 2000, pp. 517-584.

Mulliken, J.M. & Glowacki, J. (1982). Hemangiomas and vascular malformations in infants and children: a classifcation based on endothelial characteristics. *Plastic and Reconstructive Surgery*, Vol. 69, No. 3, March 1982, pp. 412-422.

North, P.E.; Waner, M.; Mizeracki, A.; Mrak, R.E.; Nicholas, R.; Kincannon, J.; Suen, J.Y. & Mihm, M.C. Jr. (2001). A unique microvascular phenotype shared by juvenile hemangiomas and human placenta. *Archives of Dermatology*, Vol. 137, No. 5, May 2001, pp. 559-70.

North, P.E.; Waner, M.; Mizeracki, A. & Mihm, M.C. Jr. GLUT1: a newly discovered immunohistochemical marker for juvenile hemangiomas. *Human Pathology*, Vol. 31, No. 1, January 2000, pp. 11-22.

Orlow, S.J.; Isdoff, M.S. & Blei, F. (1997). Increased risk of symptomatic hemangiomas of the airway in association with cutaneous hemangiomas in a "beard" distribution. *The Journal of Pediatrics*, Vol. 131, No. 4, October 1997, pp. 643–646.

Peng, Q.; Liu, W.; Tang, Y. & Yu, S. (2005). The establishment of the hemangioma model in a nude mouse. *Journal of Pediatric Surgery*, Vol. 40, No. 7, July 2005, pp. 1167-1172.

Rahbar, R.; Nicollas, R.; Roger, G.; Triglia, J.M.; Garabedian, E.N.; McGill, T.J. & Healy, G.B. (2004). The biology and management of subglottic hemangioma: past, present, future. *The Laryngoscope*, Vol. 114, No. 11, November 2004, pp. 1180-1891.

Ritter, M.R.; Dorrell, M.I.; Edmonds, J.; Friedlander, S.F. & Friedlander, M. (2002). Insulin-like growth factor 2 and potential regulators of hemangioma growth and involution identified by large-scale expression analysis. *Proceedings of the National Academy of Sciences of the United States of America*, Vol. 99, No. 11, May 2002, pp. 7455-7460.

Ritter, M.R.; Moreno, S.K.; Dorrell, M.I.; Rubens, J.; Ney, J.; Friedlander, D.F.; Bergman, J.; Cunningham, B.B.; Eichenfield, L.; Reinisch, J.; Cohen, S.; Veccione, T.; Holmes, R.; Friedlander, S.F. & Friedlander, M. (2003). Identifying potential regulators of infantile hemangioma progression through large-scale expression analysis: a possible role for the immune system and indoleamine 2,3 dioxygenase (IDO) during involution. *Lymphatic Research and Biology*, Vol. 1, No. 4, 2003, pp. 291-299.

Ritter, M.R.; Reinisch, J.; Friedlander, S.F. & Friedlander, M. (2006). Myeloid cells in infantile hemangioma. *The American Journal of Pathology*, Vol. 168, No. 2, February 2006, pp. 621-8.

Saetti, R.; Silvestrini, M.; Cutrone, C. & Name, S. (2008). Treatment of congenital subglottic hemangiomas: Our experience compared with reports in the literature. *Archives of Otolaryngology – Head and Neck Surgery*, Vol. 134, No. 8, August 2008, pp.848-851.

Sans, V.; de la Roque, E.D.; Berge, J.; Grenier, N.; Boralevi, F.; Mazereeuw-Hautier, J.; Lipsker, D.; Dupuis, E.; Ezzedine, K.; Vergnes, P.; Taïeb, A. & Léauté-Labrèze, C. (2009). Propranolol for severe infantile hemangiomas: follow-up report. *Pediatrics*, Vol. 124, No. 3, September 2009, pp. e423-431.

Schwartz, S. R.; Blei, F.; Ceisler, E.; Steel, M.; Furlan, L. & Kodsi, S. (2006). Risk factors for amblyopia in children with capillary hemangiomas of the eyelids and orbit. *Journal of AAPOS*, Vol. 10, No. 3, June 2006, pp. 262-268.

Takahashi, K.; Mulliken, J.B., Kozakewich, H.P.; Rogers, R.A.; Folkman, J. & Ezekowitz, R.A. (1994). Cellular markers that distinguish the phases of hemangioma during infancy and childhood. *The Journal of Clinical Investigation*, Vol. 93, No. 6, June 1994, pp. 2357-2364.

Tan, S.T.; Itinteang, T. & Leadbitter, P. (2010). Low-dose propranolol for infantile haemangioma. *Journal of Plastic, Reconstructive, & Aesthetic Surgery*, Vol. 64, No. 3, March 2011, pp. 292-299.

Tan, S.T.; Wallis, R.A.; He, Y. & Davis, P.F. (2004). Mast cells and hemangioma. *Plastic and Reconstructive Surgery*, Vol. 113, No. 3, March 2004, pp. 999-1011.

Tang, Y.; Liu, W.; Yu, S.; Wang, Y.; Peng, Q.; Xiong, Z.; Wang, Y. & Wei, T. (2007) A novel in vivo model of human hemangioma: xenograft of human hemangioma tissue on nude mice. *Plastic and Reconstructive Surgery*, Vol. 120, No. 4, September 2007, pp. 869-878.

Truong, M.T.; Perkins, J.A.; Messner, A.H. & Chang, K.W. (2010). Propranolol for the treatment of airway hemangiomas: a case series and treatment algorithm. *International Journal of Pediatric Otorhinolaryngology*, Vol. 74, No. 9, September 2010, pp. 1043-1048.

Waner, M.; North, P.E.; Scherer, K.A.; Frieden, I.J.; Waner, A. & Mihm, M.C. Jr. (2003). The nonrandom distribution of facial hemangiomas. *Archives of Dermatology*, Vol. 139, No. 7, July 2003, pp. 869-875.

Wu, J.K.; Adepoju, O.; De Silva, D.; Baribault, K.; Boscolo, E.; Bischoff, J. & Kitajewski, J. (2010). A switch in notch gene expression parallels stem cell to endothelial cell transition in infantile hemangioma. *Angiogenesis*, Vol. 13, No. 1, March 2010, pp. 15-23.

Wu, J.K. & Kitajewski, J.K. (2009). A potential role for notch signaling in the pathogenesis and regulation of hemangiomas. *The Journal of Craniofacial Surgery*, Vol. 20, Suppl 1, March 2009, pp. 698-702.

Xiong, Y.Q.; Sun, H.C.; Zhang, W.; Zhu, X.D.; Zhuang, P.Y.; Zhang, J.B.; Wang, L.; Wu, W.Z.; Qin, L.X. &Tang, Z.Y. (2009). Human hepatocellular carcinoma tumor-derived endothelial cells manifest increased angiogenesis capability and drug resistance compared with normal endothelial cells. *Clinical Cancer Research*, Vol. 15, No. 15, August 2009, pp. 4838-4846.

Xu, Q.; Chen, W.; Wang, Z.; Zheng, J. & Zhang, Z. (2009). Mice transgenic with SV40-late-promoter-driven polyomavirus middle T oncogene exclusively develop hemangiomas. *Transgenic Research*, Vol. 18, No. 3, June 2009, pp. 399-406.

Yu Y.; Varughese, J.; Brown, L.F.; Mulliken, J.B. & Bischoff, J. Increased Tie2 expression, enhanced response to angiopoietin-1, and dysregulated angiopoietin-2 expression in hemangioma-derived endothelial cells. *The American Journal of Pathology*, Vol. 159, No. 6, December 2001, pp. 2271-2280.

11

MicroRNAs Regulation of Tumor Angiogenesis

Munekazu Yamakuchi
Aab Cardiovascular Research Institute,
University of Rochester School of Medicine and Dentistry,
USA

1. Introduction

In the 1970s, Dr. Judah Folkman proposed that many solid tumors require angiogenesis to grow beyond 2 mm in size (Folkman, 1971). His theory held that solid tumors could grow without additional blood vessels up to 1-2 mm, obtaining oxygen and nutrients by diffusion. However, these tumors could undergo an angiogenic switch, releasing substances that would induce new capillary sproutings from existing blood vessels, which would increase oxygen and nutrient delivery to the tumor, permitting tumor expansion. Since Dr. Folkman's hypothesis, assays for angiogenesis have been developed, new angiogenic molecules such as VEGF and VEGF receptors have been discovered, endogenous inhibitors of angiogenesis such as angiostatin have been defined, and anti-angiogenic drugs have been developed to treat cancers (Ferrara, 2002; Ferrara and Kerbel, 2005; Kerbel, 2008). However, the biology of human tumor angiogenesis is poorly understood, and the molecular mechanisms that modulate the angiogenic switch are not well characterized.

MicroRNAs (miRNAs) are small non-coding RNAs that regulate gene expression in a post-transcriptional manner (Bartel, 2004). miRNAs regulate physiological processes such as cell proliferation, apoptosis, and differentiation (Ambros, 2004; Bartel, 2004; He and Hannon, 2004). However, miRNAs are also involved in pathophysiological processes such as oncogenesis (Croce, 2008, 2009). Recent studies unveiled new functions of miRNAs that control angiogenesis and those miRNAs are thought to be new tools for manipulating tumor angiogenic balance. In this chapter, I summarize how a set of miRNAs can regulate tumor angiogenesis, reviewing the current findings and our data.

I first describe the biogenesis and function of miRNAs and briefly review general roles of miRNAs in cancer. Next I classify a set of miRNAs that positively or negatively regulate tumor angiogenesis and add current progress in this area. Lastly I focus on hypoxia inducible factors as key molecule of hypoxia signaling and tumor angiogenesis in a view of regulation by miRNAs.

2. microRNAs (miRNAs)

Non-coding RNA (ncRNA), lin-4 and lin-14, were first identified to regulate larval developmental timing in *C. elegance* in 1993 (Lee et al., 1993; Wightman et al., 1993). By now, thousands of miRNAs have been discovered in many organisms and mammalian miRNAs are predicted to alter the activity of about 50% of all protein coding genes (Filipowicz et al., 2008). miRNAs control gene expression by destabilizing or inhibiting transcription, involving in a variety of biological processes. According to mapping of 186 miRNAs and comparison of locations of previous reported nonrandom genetic alterations, Calin et al. discovered that miRNA genes are frequently (more than 50%) located at fragile sites, in minimal regions of loss of heterozygosity, in minimal regions of amplification or in common breakpoint regions (Calin et al., 2004b). As the diverse functions of miRNAs are further studied, our understanding of the molecular pathways of cancers becomes more complicated (Nana-Sinkam and Croce).

2.1 miRNA biogenesis

Figure 1 illustrates intergenic miRNA biogenesis. First mRNAs are transcribed into primary miRNAs (pri-miRNAs) by RNA polymerase II. These long pri-miRNAs contain stem-loop hairpin structures, which are cleaved into smaller pieces (pre-miRNA) by RNase III Drosha and DiGeorge syndrome critical region 8 (DGCR8) complex. Pre-miRNA is transported from nucleus into cytoplasm by exportin 5 and then diced into double stranded mature miRNAs by Dicer and TAR RNA-binding protein 2 (TRBP2) complex. Both or one strand of single mature miRNAs is incorporated into Argonaute containing RNA-induced silencing complex (RISC), which bind to target mRNAs and dampen their expression.

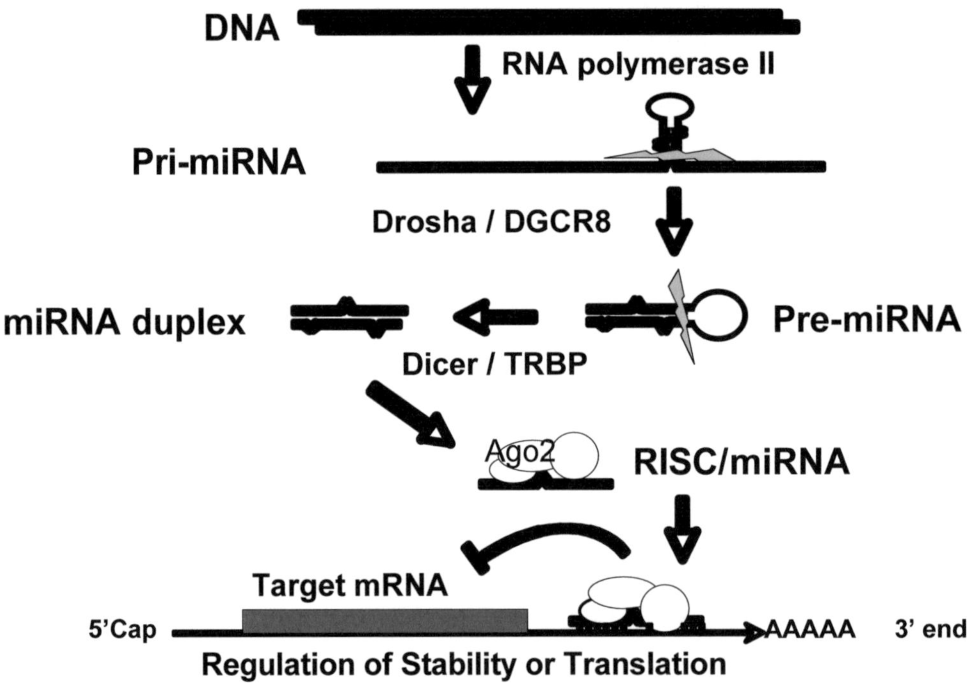

Fig. 1. miRNA biogenesis. DNA is transcribed into a primary micro-RNA (pri-miR). The pri-miR is processed into a 70 nt precursor micro-RNA (pre-miR). The pre-miR is processed into a 22 nt long micro-RNA (miRNA). A single strand of the mature miRNA is loaded onto a nucleoprotein RISC complex that silences target messenger RNAs.

MiRNAs suppress target mRNA expression in two ways, Argonaute-catalyzed cleavage of mRNA or mRNA destabilization (Filipowicz et al., 2008). If the seed sequence of a particular miRNA perfectly matches the sequence of a target mRNA, then the target mRNA is degraded. Sequence identity between micro-RNA and mRNA often occur in plants. In mammalian cells, there are very few reports about miRNA cleavage of target mRNA (Davis et al., 2005; Jones-Rhoades et al., 2006). Instead, the seed sequence of miRNA usually has homology but not identity to target mRNA in mammalian cells. This imperfect match represses translation by decreasing mRNA stability. The match sequences of 2nd to 6th nucleotide position in 5′ end of miRNAs (seed sequence) are sufficient to suppress gene expressions. Some miRNAs suppress target mRNAs expression unless the seed sequence does not completely match to target mRNA target (Bartel, 2009; Shin et al.). Moreover miRNAs can reduce not only the expressions of protein from the target mRNAs, but also the levels of their target transcripts (Lim et al., 2005).

To accomplish miRNA searches, accurate methods for target prediction are required. There are many miRNA target prediction programs available on-line (Hofacker, 2007; Sethupathy et al., 2006). These prediction systems depend on algorithms of miRNA and mRNA (especially region of seed sequence) and evolutionarily conservation. Targetscan, miRanda, and PicTar are commonly used tools for target prediction. Those programs provided a lot of information for potential target genes, but the false positive rate were calculated about 24-70% (Thomson et al.). To avoid false positive target genes, overlapped targets from those three prediction programs are generally chosen as more convincing potential target genes.

2.2 miRNAs function in cancer

Genomic alterations of miRNAs are associated with human cancers (Calin et al., 2004a; Iorio et al., 2005). MiR-15a and miR-16a are frequently downregulated in patients with B cell chronic lymphocytic leukemia (Calin et al., 2004b). Lu et al. performed miRNA expression profiling of 334 human cancer samples and showed the feasibility of classification tumor types and stages on miRNA profiles (Lu et al., 2005). This suggested that monitoring the expression of miRNAs in human cancer is very informative for cancer diagnosis. There have been many studies focusing on this diagnostic role of miRNAs and on the association between cancer specific miRNAs and their function. Let-7 family members regulate the human RAS oncogene; and human lung tumor tissues displayed reduced levels of let-7 and increased levels of RAS protein compared to normal lung tissues, suggesting that let-7 might control oncogenesis in humans (Johnson et al., 2005). Furthermore, p53 upregulated the expression of miR-34 family members, which functions as a tumor suppressor (Chang et al., 2007; He et al., 2007; Raver-Shapira et al., 2007).

3. miRNAs and tumor angiogenesis

Distinct miRNAs regulate tumor angiogenesis in diverse pathways. These miRNAs that regulate angiogenesis are classified into three groups; (1) miRNAs that are not altered under hypoxic condition, (2) hypoxia regulated miRNAs, and (3) miRNAs that regulate HIF-1 signaling molecules. I address functions of each miRNA and discuss two types of angiogenesis miRNAs; pro-angiogenic miRNAs and anti-angiogenic miRNAs (Figure 2).

3.1 Hypoxia independent miRNAs

3.1.1 miR-126

Several studies of miRNA profiling revealed that miR-126 is expressed specifically in endothelial cells (Harris et al., 2008; Kuehbacher et al., 2007). MiR-126 is encoded on an

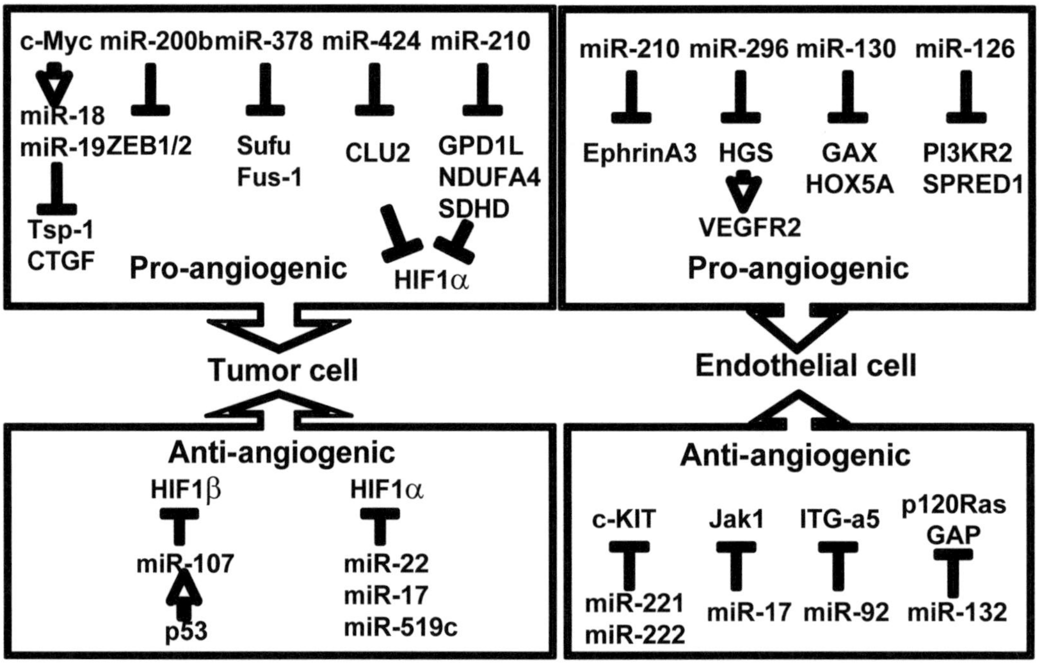

Fig. 2. Role of miRNAs in tumor angiogenesis. Different miRNAs contribute to angiogenic response in tumor cells and endothelial cells.

intron of Egfl7 gene and Egfl7 knockout mice displays vascular abnormalities (Schmidt et al., 2007). Endothelial outgrowth was impaired in aortic rings from *miR-126*$^{-/-}$ mice and endothelial cells from *miR-126*$^{-/-}$ mice diminished angiogenic response to FGF-2, suggesting that miR-126 knockout endothelial cells are defective in angiogenesis (Fish et al., 2008; Wang et al., 2008). Moreover Sprouty-related EVH domain-containing protein (Spred-1) and PI3K regulatory subunit 2 (PIK3R2) were defined as target gene of miR-126. Therefore, pro-angiogenic activity of miR-126 is mediated via the increase of MAP kinase and PI3K signaling in response to angiogenic growth factors. In cancer cells, miR-126 behaves as an anti-tumor miRNA. MiR-126 inhibited metastasis in human breast cancer and tumorigenesis in colon cancer and lung cancer (Crawford et al., 2008; Guo et al., 2008; Tavazoie et al., 2008), but the non-cell-autonomous effects of miR-126 in tumor on angiogenesis are still unclear.

3.1.2 miR-132

MiR-132 has been recognized as an angiogenic growth factor inducible miRNA in endothelial cells. In normal endothelial cells, the level of miR-132 is very low, but miR-132 is highly expressed in human tumors and hemangiomas. VEGF and bFGF or conditioned media from tumors activated cAMP-response element binding protein (CREB) and increased miR-132 levels in various types of endothelial cells (Anand et al.; Lagos et al.). Interestingly neurotropic growth factors also induced miR-132, promoting dendritic growth and spine formation in neuronal culture (Magill et al.). MiR-132 facilitated pathological angiogenesis by suppressing p120RasGAP, a molecular brake for RAS. Knockdown of miR-132 decreased angiogenesis in tumor models (Anand et al.). Moreover, endothelial cells from several pathological human and mouse tissues including tumors had a dramatic decrease in p120RasGAP expression and a corresponding increase in miR-132 level (Anand and Cheresh). These findings suggest that miR-132 controls an angiogenic switch in tumor cells.

3.1.3 miR-296

The upregulation of growth factor receptors on endothelial cells is an important step in angiogenesis. Angiogenic growth factors increased the expression of miR-296 in human brain microvascular endothelial cells and knockdown of miR-296 inhibited endothelial cell migration and tube formation by modulating hepatocyte growth factor-regulated tyrosine kinase substrate (HGS) (Wurdinger et al., 2008). HGS mediated the sorting of growth factor receptors (PDGFR-ß and VEGFR2) to lysosomes to degrade them (Ewan et al., 2006; Takata et al., 2000). Inhibition of miR-296 showed significant decrease glioma angiogenesis in vivo, suggesting that miR-296 acts as a pro-angiogenic miRNA in endothelial cells.

Loss of miR-296 expression was observed during tumor progression in human cancers (Hong et al.). One of potential target proteins was Scribble (Scrib) and overexpression of Scrib in human mammary epithelial cells (HMEC) inhibited cell migration and invasion (Vaira et al.). The levels of Scrib were upregulated in primary lesions and distant metastases of liver, colon, lung, breast and stomach cancer, but the exact function in tumors has been not determined. Another target, high-motility group AT-hook gene 1 (HMGA1) was identified in prostate cancer (Wei et al.). HMGA1 expression was associated with high-grade prostate cancer and proliferative and metastatic potential in vitro (Diana et al., 2005). These findings indicate that inhibition of miR-296 cell-autonomously downregulates tumor angiogenesis.

3.1.4 miR-378

MiR-378 enhanced cell survival and promotes tumor growth and angiogenesis. Knockdown of miR-378 decreased cell survival in U87 glioma cells. Injection of miR-378 overexpressed U87 cells into nude mice increased tumor volume and elevated the size of blood vessels (Lee et al., 2007). At least two potential targets of miR-378 were identified; suppressor of fused (Sufu) and tumor suppressor candidate 2 (Fus-1). Sufu is a negative regulator of sonic hedgehog signaling pathway (Yue et al., 2009). Sonic hedgehog pathway is a crucial regulator of angiogenesis and metastasis and increases angiogenic factors such as angiopoietin-1 and angiopoietin-2 (Pola et al., 2001). Sonic hedgehog promotes capillary morphogenesis, induced endothelial cell migration, and increased the expression of MMP-9 and osteopontin in endothelial cells via Rho kinase (Renault et al.). These data suggested that miR-378 might control not only angiogenic potential in tumor cells but also angiogenic activity in endothelial cells.

3.1.5 miR-17-92 in tumors

The miR-17-92 cluster is a polycistronic miRNA gene, containing six mature miRNAs (miR-17, miR-18a, miR-19a, miR-19b-1, miR-20a, and miR-92) on *c13orf25* transcript (He et al., 2005; Tanzer and Stadler, 2004). These six miRNAs and two miR-17-92 cluster paralogs (miR-106a-363 and miR-106b-25) are categorized into four families by their seed sequences; (1) miR-17 family (miR-17, -20a, -20b, -106a, -106b, and -93), (2) miR-18 family (miR-18a and miR-18b), (3) miR-19 family (miR-19a, -19b-1, and -19b-2), and (4) miR-92 family (miR-92a-1, -92a-2, -383, and -25) (Figure 3A).

The transcripts of region containing miR-17-92 precursor were elevated n various cancers, such as B-cell lymphoma, multiple myeloma, thyroid cancer, and lung cancer (Hayashita et al., 2005; Inomata et al., 2009; Pichiorri et al., 2008; Takakura et al., 2008). This elevation of miR-17-92 contributes to tumor growth partially by enhancing tumor angiogenesis (Dews et al., 2006).

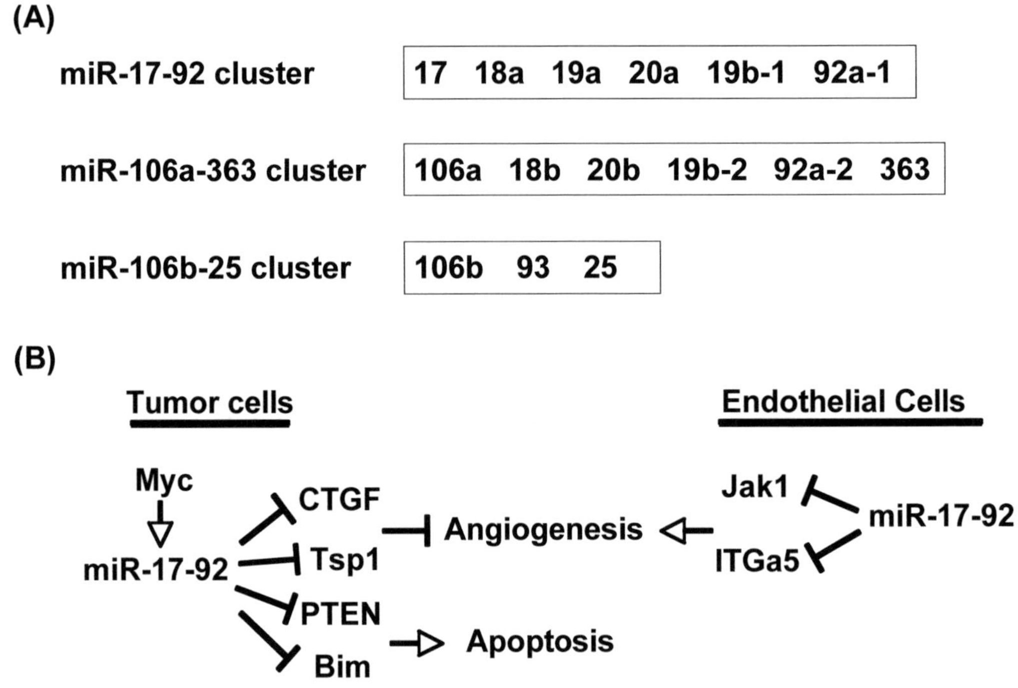

Fig. 3. The pleiotropic functions of miR-17-92 cluster. (A) Primary transcripts of miR-17-92 cluster and its paralogs. (B) Mir-17-92 can promote proliferation and increase angiogenesis in cancer cells. In endothelial cells, miR-17-92 inhibits angiogenesis.

miR-17-92 cluster has been identified as a direct transcriptional target of c-Myc by using a spotted oligonucleotide array (O'Donnell et al., 2005). c-Myc is a helix-loop-helix oncogenic transcription factor that regulates cell proliferation and transformation and activated in many human cancers (Dang, 1999). Myc binds to E-box element with Max, driving cell cycle progression. Myc also negatively regulates some gene transcriptions with Miz-1. Dews et al. have shown that Myc-overexpressing tumors possessed more robust neovascularization and miR-17-92 mediated tumor angiogenesis by Myc (Dews et al., 2006). They also found that miR-17-92 targeted two anti-angiogenic factors, thrombospondin-1 (TSP-1) and connective tissue growth factor (CTGF) expression in RasGfpMyc colonocytes.

Another transcription factor that regulates miR-17-92 cluster has been reported. E2F1 and E2F3 also directly activated miR-17-92 transcription as well as turns on the progression of the cell cycle (Sylvestre et al., 2007; Woods et al., 2007). MiR-17 and miR-20 inhibited the expression of E2F1, E2F2, and E2F3 (O'Donnell et al., 2005). These data suggested a negative feedback loop between miR-17-92 cluster, E2F, and Myc.

The regulation and function of miR-17-92 have become more complicated. Each miRNAs in this cluster works cooperatively and independently. Each individual miRNA has different target genes because of their own seed sequences. For example, miR-19, which is thought to be a major oncogenic component of miR-17-92 cluster, suppressed PTEN expression (Olive et al., 2009). In the Eμ-myc model of Burkitt's lymphoma, miR-19 was necessary and sufficient for mir-17-92 to promote c-Myc-induced B lymphomagenesis. MiR-17, miR-20, and miR106b regulate cell cycle progression through the inhibition of cyclin dependent kinase inhibitor, p21 (Ivanovska et al., 2008).

3.1.6 miR-17-92 in endothelial cells

The miR-17-92 cluster is highly expressed in endothelial cells (Kuehbacher et al., 2007). Overexpression of miR-92a inhibited angiogenesis in endothelial cells in part by repressing integrin α5 (ITGa5). Inhibition of miR-92a in a mouse model of hind limb ischemia augmented neovascularization and functional recovery of damaged tissue (Bonauer et al., 2009). The same research group has explored the role of the other miRNAs of miR-17-92 cluster in endothelial cells as well (Doebele et al.). Overexpression of all individual members of miR-17-92 cluster (miR-17, miR-18a, miR-19a, and miR-20a) inhibited endothelial proliferation and migration in vitro, in contrast, and individual knockdown enhanced migration and proliferation. MiR-17 and miR-20 were particularly potent inhibitors of endothelial migration, and their effects were mediated in part through the tyrosine kinase Jak1 (Doebele et al.).

These data indicate that individual miRNAs in miR-17-92 cluster suppress angiogenesis of normal endothelial cells in vivo. What about their effect upon angiogenesis of endothelial cells in tumors in vivo? Although inhibitors of miR-17 and miR-20 increased vascularization of Matrigel plugs in mice, but these same inhibitors did not affect tumor angiogenesis (Doebele et al.). These results show that specific miRNAs can regulate angiogenesis in one context (Matrigel plugs) but have no effect upon angiogenesis in another context (tumor angiogenesis). One possible explanation is that different sets of genes modulate angiogenesis in different physiological situations (Figure 3B). Suarez et al. showed that reduction of miRNAs by knockdown of Dicer in endothelial cells impaired angiogenic response and reconstitution of individual miRNAs in miR-17-92 cluster rescued angiogenic inhibition (Suarez et al., 2008). These results show that endothelial miRNAs are important for angiogenesis.

In summary, contradictory data show that miR-17 inhibits angiogenesis following hind limb ischemia, but all miRNAs together promote angiogenesis in hind limb ischemia. The individual contribution to angiogenesis of distinct miRNA inside endothelial cells is not fully known.

3.1.7 miR-221/222

miR-221 and miR-222 are abundant in endothelial cells, and they affect angiogenic activity of stem cell factor (SCF) by modulating the level of its receptor c-Kit (Poliseno et al., 2006). miR-221 strongly upregulated GAX expression by inhibiting ZEB2, a modulator of the epithelial-mesenchymal transition (Chen et al.). GAX is a regulatory gene controlling the angiogenic phenotype in endothelial cells. In several solid tumors, miR-221/222 is highly expressed (le Sage et al., 2007; Medina et al., 2008) and regulated by proto-oncogene ETS-1, involving in the pathogenesis of cancers (Mattia et al.). In melanoma progression, ETS-1 is directly targeted by miR-222, but not by miR-221, which makes a complex ETS-1/miR-222 co-regulatory loop. miR-222 might inhibit angiogenesis by repressing Ets signaling in endothelial cells.

3.2 Hypoxia-regulated miRNAs

3.2.1 miR-210

Hypoxia promotes tumor angiogenesis. Hypoxia induced miRNAs are identified both in cancer and endothelial cells. Hypoxia dramatically increased miR-210 expression (Huang et al., 2009). The expression of miR-210 is higher in many solid tumors and correlates with poor survival in cancer patients (Greither et al.; Huang et al., 2009; Puissegur et al.). Overexpression of miR-210 in endothelial cells stimulated angiogenesis and migration and inhibition of miR-210 decreased hypoxia induced tube formation of endothelial cells (Fasanaro et al., 2008). MiR-210 targeted the receptor tyrosine kinase Ephrin-A3 that involves in vascular remodeling. Glycerol-3-phosphate dehydrogenase (GPD1L) was identified as another direct target of miR-210 in cancer cells (Kelly et al.). GPD1L is linked to the stability of HIF-1α protein through the activity of prolyl hydroxylases (PHDs). Hypoxia triggered accumulation of miR-210 and increased miR-210 inactivates PHDs by decreasing GPD1L protein, which blocked HIF-1α degradation. MiR-210 also targeted specific mitochondrial components with consequences on the regulation of cell death and survival and the modulation of HIF-1 activity (Puissegur et al.). Overexpression of miR-210 directly repressed two members of electron transport chain (ETC) complexes: NADH dehydrogenase (ubiquinone) 1 alpha subcomplex 4 (NDUFA4), a subunit of ETC complex I, and succinate dehydrogenase complex, subunit D (SDHD), a subunit of the ETC complex II and induced mitochondrial dysfunctions, which accumulated succinate, inhibiting PHDs activity, then increasing HIF-1α. These two models represent a positive feedback loop. These data suggest that miR-210 has pro-angiogenic activity. This hypoxia-induced miRNA could be one of promising tumor markers.

3.2.2 miR-424

Hypoxia increased miR-424 level in endothelial cells and in ischemic tissues undergoing vascular remodeling and angiogenesis. Increased level of miR-424 led to degradation of an ubiquitin ligase scaffold protein cullin-2 (CLU2), which prevented HIF-1α downregulation by destabilizing the E3-ligase assembly (Ghosh et al., 2010). The expression of miR-424 was regulated by C/EBP-α/RUNX-1–mediated transactivation of PU.1. This finding indicates that miR-424 acts as a pro-angiogenic factor.

3.2.3 miR-200b

MiR-200b, one of five members of miR-200 family inhibited cell migration and epithelial-mesenchymal transition (EMT) in epithelial cancer cells by modulating the expression of zinc finger E-box-binding homeobox 1 and 2 (ZEB1 and ZEB2) (Burk et al., 2008; Park et al., 2008). The miR-200 family is regulated by transforming growth factor β 1 (TGF-β1) and platelet-derived growth factor (PDGF) (Gregory et al., 2008). MiR-200b is inducible by hypoxia and down-regulates v-ets erythroblastosis virus E26 oncogene homolog 1 (ETS-1), promoting angiogenesis activity in endothelial cells (Chan et al., 2011).

3.3 HIF-1 and miRNAs

Continued tumor growth depends upon obtaining oxygen and nutrients. As tumor grows, the center of tumor becomes hypoxic, causing an angiogenic switch (Kaelin, 2005). In the presence of oxygen, prolyl hydroxylase domain protein 2 (PHD2 or EGLN1) hydroxylates prolyl residues on hypoxia-inducible factor-1 alpha (HIF-1α) (Semenza, 2007). After prolyl hydroxylation, HIF-1α binds to a complex containing von Hippel-Lindau (VHL) which leads to HIF-1α degradation. However, under hypoxic conditions, HIF-1α is not prolyl hydroxylated. Instead, HIF-1α interacts with its partner HIF-1 beta (HIF-1β), and the HIF-1 complex translocates to the nucleus, binds to hypoxia responsive element (HRE), and regulates transcription of hundreds of genes. Genes transactivated by HIF-1 help to adapt the cells to low oxygen levels, controlling erythropoiesis, glycolysis, and angiogenesis (Harris, 2002; Semenza, 2003). Interest in the role of HIF-1 in cancer has been growing and HIF-1 is thought to be a therapeutic target of cancer progression (Semenza, 2003). Therefore we demonstrate a set of miRNAs that affect HIF-1 complex (Figure 4).

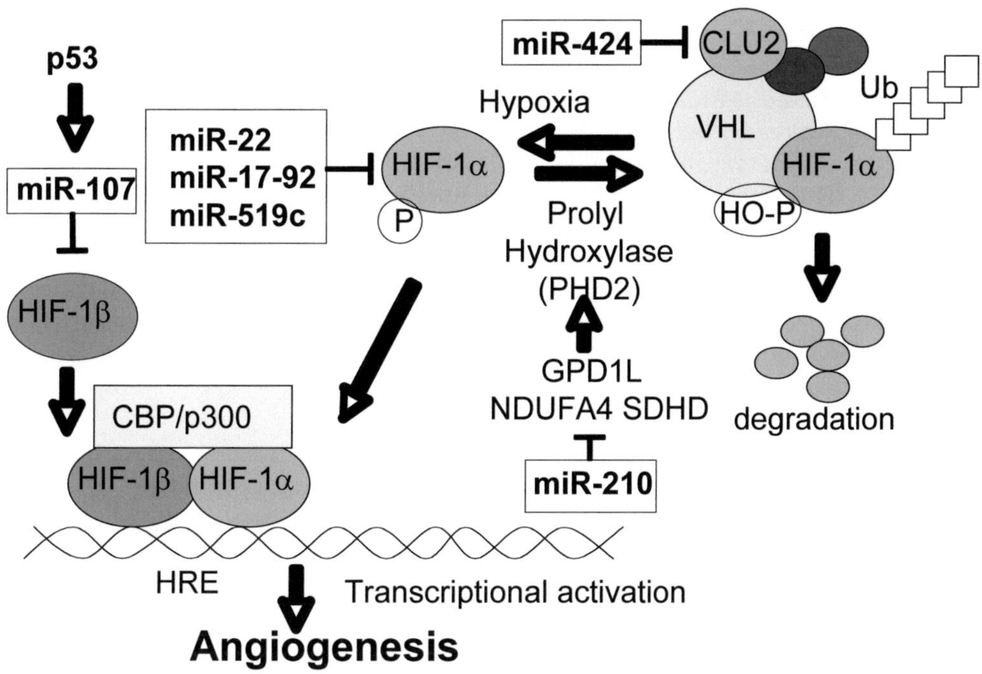

Fig. 4. Regulation of hypoxia signaling via miRNAs. Normally prolyl hydroxylase (PHD) hydroxylates HIF-1α on prolyl residues, marking HIF-1α for destruction through pVHL. However, during hypoxia, HIF-1α is not hydroxylated, and instead HIF-1α binds to HIF-1β, translocates to the nucleus, and activates gene transcription. A set of miRNAs regulates hypoxia signaling.

3.3.1 HIF-1α

HIF-1α expression is associated with poor prognosis in a variety of cancer such as breast, ovary, and brain cancer (Semenza, 2003). There are several miRNAs that regulate HIF-1α. First HIF-1α was reported as the target of miR-17-92 miRNA cluster in lung cancer cells (Taguchi et al., 2008). Taguchi et al. performed proteomic comparison between a miR-17-92–transfected clone and an empty vector–transfected clone from normal human bronchial epithelial cell line and then found that miR-17-92 targets HIF-1α. MiR-20b, located on 106a-

363 cluster, a member of miR-17-92 family, was also shown to regulate HIF-1α expression (Lei et al., 2009). The inhibition of miR-20b increased HIF-1α protein and VEGF in normoxic tumor cells. In contrast, the increase of miR-20b in hypoxic tumor cells decreased the expression of HIF-1α and VEGF. HIF-1α, VEGF, and STAT3 are identified to be direct targets of miR-20b (Cascio et al.; Lei et al., 2009). As describing above, the miR-17-92 family has a complicated network to control tumor angiogenesis.

MiR-519c reduced tumor angiogenesis through direct binding to the HIF-1α 3′ UTR (Cha et al.). Mice injected with lung adenocarcinoma cells overexpressing miR-519c suppressed tumor angiogenesis, growth, and metastasis. Interestingly hepatocyte growth factor (HGF) suppressed miR-519c expression. The expression of miR-519c was closely correlated with tumor progression in human lung cancer tissues.

We found that miR-22 regulated HIF-1α in HCT116, human colon cancer cells (Yamakuchi et al.). Overexpression of miR-22 decreased transactivation of the 3′UTR of HIF-1α. In contrast, miR-22 did not alter transactivation of HIF-1a when the miR-22 binding site within the 3′ UTR of HIF-1α is mutated. Thus miR-22 directly regulates expression of HIF-1α. The function of miR-22 varies between different cancer types. The human miR-22 gene is located within a loss of heterozygosity region (LOH) in several cancer cells (Calin et al., 2004b; Xiong et al.). Ectopic expression of miR-22 suppressed proliferation in breast cancer cells (Xiong et al.). In contrast, knockdown of miR-22 increases apoptosis in human bronchial epithelial cells (Liu et al.). We found that miR-22 downregulated VEGF secretion and inhibited endothelial cell migration, suggesting that miR-22 acts as an anti-angiogenesis factor in colon cancer cell lines. Moreover the expression of miR-22 is inversely correlated to the level of VEGF in human colon cancer (Yamakuchi et al.), supporting the idea that miR-22 has an anti-angiogenic effect.

3.3.2 HIF-1β

We recently reported that miR-107 regulated tumor angiogenesis in colon cancer (Yamakuchi et al.). First we performed miRNAs profiling to identify miRNAs expressed in human colon cancer samples and found several miRNAs that are highly expressed in human colon cancer specimen such as miR-923, miR-1826, and miR-1915. The tumor suppressor gene p53 is mutated in more than half of all human cancer (Vogelstein and Kinzler, 2004). Since anti-angiogenic therapy is more effective in tumors with wild-type p53 than in tumors with mutant p53, p53 plays an important role in the regulation of tumor angiogenesis. Therefore we selected miRNAs regulated by p53. In the colon cancer cell line HCT116, we've identified several miRNAs induced by p53 (Chang et al., 2007). Furthermore we searched for miRNAs that can target HIF-1 signaling genes using prediction programs described above. Finally we've chosen miR-23a, miR-26, miR-103, and miR-107 as candidate regulators of tumor angiogenesis. Among these miRNAs, only miR-107 could regulate hypoxia signaling and was regulated by p53 in vitro. HIF-1β was shown to be a target gene of miR-107 by Western blotting and reporter gene assay. HIF-1β (also called ARNT, dioxin receptor) is a basic helix-loop-helix transcription factor and a counterpart of HIF-1α (Fukunaga et al., 1995; Reisz-Porszasz et al., 1994). Homozygous knockout of HIF-1β in mice was lethal because of poor placentation and decreased branching of the placental vasculature (Kozak et al., 1997; Maltepe et al., 1997). One of the interesting points in our findings is the regulation of HIF-1β. HIF-1β has been thought to be constitutively expressed in many cells (Wang et al., 1995). Our data indicated that miR-107 modulated the expression of HIF-1β, following tumor angiogenesis.

miR-107 controlled tumor angiogenesis through suppressing HIF-1β in vivo. HCT116 tumor cells overexpressing miR-107 subcutaneously implanted in nude mice grew slower than control cells. To exclude the effect of p53, p53 genetically knockout HCT116 cells were used. Injection of p53 knockout HCT116 cells obtained bigger tumor compared to p53 wild type HCT116 cells. When p53 knockout HCT116 cells with overexpressing miR-107 were injected, the size of tumor and the number of vessels in tumor were significantly decreased compared to p53 knockout HCT116 cells transduced with scramble miRNA.
In human colon cancer, there was a negative correlation between the expression of miR-107 and VEGF level. Data from both clinical studies and experimental models suggested that miR-107 is an anti-angiogenic miRNA.

3.3.3 HIF-2α and HIF-3α

HIF-2α and HIF-3α has been identified as partners with HiF-1β. HIF-2α is closely related to HIF-1α, and both activate HRE-dependent gene transcription (Wenger, 2002). HIF-3α lacks structures for transactivation existed in the C-termini of HIF-1α and HIF-2α. HIF-2α might contribute to tumor angiogenesis in some cells (Burkitt et al., 2009; Favier et al., 2007; Giatromanolaki et al., 2006). However regulation of HIF-2α or HIF-3α by miRNAs has not reported yet.

4. Conclusion

Tumor angiogenesis is a complex process, consisting of a balance between pro-angiogenic factors and anti-angiogenic factors. Since Dr. Folkman generated the hypothesis that tumors will die without an adequate blood supply, anti-angiogenic therapies for cancer patients have been rapidly developed. Research into miRNA has produced new insights into tumorigenesis. New data on regulation of tumor angiogenesis by miRNAs suggest that miRNAs are promising therapeutic molecules to prevent and treat cancer.

5. Acknowledgment

I thank Dr. Charles J. Lowenstein for discussing the details of this work. This work was supported by Scientist Development Grant 835446N from American Heart Association.

6. References

Ambros, V. (2004). The functions of animal microRNAs. Nature *431*, 350-355.

Anand, S., and Cheresh, D.A. MicroRNA-mediated regulation of the angiogenic switch. Curr Opin Hematol *18*, 171-176.

Anand, S., Majeti, B.K., Acevedo, L.M., Murphy, E.A., Mukthavaram, R., Scheppke, L., Huang, M., Shields, D.J., Lindquist, J.N., Lapinski, P.E., *et al.* MicroRNA-132-mediated loss of p120RasGAP activates the endothelium to facilitate pathological angiogenesis. Nat Med *16*, 909-914.

Bartel, D.P. (2004). MicroRNAs: genomics, biogenesis, mechanism, and function. Cell *116*, 281-297.

Bartel, D.P. (2009). MicroRNAs: target recognition and regulatory functions. Cell *136*, 215-233.

Bonauer, A., Carmona, G., Iwasaki, M., Mione, M., Koyanagi, M., Fischer, A., Burchfield, J., Fox, H., Doebele, C., Ohtani, K., *et al.* (2009). MicroRNA-92a controls angiogenesis and functional recovery of ischemic tissues in mice. Science *324*, 1710-1713.

Burk, U., Schubert, J., Wellner, U., Schmalhofer, O., Vincan, E., Spaderna, S., and Brabletz, T. (2008). A reciprocal repression between ZEB1 and members of the miR-200 family promotes EMT and invasion in cancer cells. EMBO Rep *9*, 582-589.

Burkitt, K., Chun, S.Y., Dang, D.T., and Dang, L.H. (2009). Targeting both HIF-1 and HIF-2 in human colon cancer cells improves tumor response to sunitinib treatment. Mol Cancer Ther *8*, 1148-1156.

Calin, G.A., Liu, C.G., Sevignani, C., Ferracin, M., Felli, N., Dumitru, C.D., Shimizu, M., Cimmino, A., Zupo, S., Dono, M., *et al.* (2004a). MicroRNA profiling reveals distinct signatures in B cell chronic lymphocytic leukemias. Proc Natl Acad Sci U S A *101*, 11755-11760.

Calin, G.A., Sevignani, C., Dumitru, C.D., Hyslop, T., Noch, E., Yendamuri, S., Shimizu, M., Rattan, S., Bullrich, F., Negrini, M., *et al.* (2004b). Human microRNA genes are frequently located at fragile sites and genomic regions involved in cancers. Proc Natl Acad Sci U S A *101*, 2999-3004.

Cascio, S., D'Andrea, A., Ferla, R., Surmacz, E., Gulotta, E., Amodeo, V., Bazan, V., Gebbia, N., and Russo, A. miR-20b modulates VEGF expression by targeting HIF-1 alpha and STAT3 in MCF-7 breast cancer cells. J Cell Physiol *224*, 242-249.

Cha, S.T., Chen, P.S., Johansson, G., Chu, C.Y., Wang, M.Y., Jeng, Y.M., Yu, S.L., Chen, J.S., Chang, K.J., Jee, S.H., *et al.* MicroRNA-519c suppresses hypoxia-inducible factor-1alpha expression and tumor angiogenesis. Cancer Res *70*, 2675-2685.

Chan, Y.C., Khanna, S., Roy, S., and Sen, C.K. (2011). miR-200b targets Ets-1 and is down-regulated by hypoxia to induce angiogenic response of endothelial cells. J Biol Chem *286*, 2047-2056.

Chang, T.C., Wentzel, E.A., Kent, O.A., Ramachandran, K., Mullendore, M., Lee, K.H., Feldmann, G., Yamakuchi, M., Ferlito, M., Lowenstein, C.J., *et al.* (2007). Transactivation of miR-34a by p53 broadly influences gene expression and promotes apoptosis. Mol Cell *26*, 745-752.

Chen, Y., Banda, M., Speyer, C.L., Smith, J.S., Rabson, A.B., and Gorski, D.H. Regulation of the expression and activity of the antiangiogenic homeobox gene GAX/MEOX2 by ZEB2 and microRNA-221. Mol Cell Biol *30*, 3902-3913.

Crawford, M., Brawner, E., Batte, K., Yu, L., Hunter, M.G., Otterson, G.A., Nuovo, G., Marsh, C.B., and Nana-Sinkam, S.P. (2008). MicroRNA-126 inhibits invasion in non-small cell lung carcinoma cell lines. Biochem Biophys Res Commun *373*, 607-612.

Croce, C.M. (2008). Oncogenes and cancer. N Engl J Med *358*, 502-511.

Croce, C.M. (2009). Causes and consequences of microRNA dysregulation in cancer. Nat Rev Genet *10*, 704-714.

Dang, C.V. (1999). c-Myc target genes involved in cell growth, apoptosis, and metabolism. Mol Cell Biol *19*, 1-11.

Davis, E., Caiment, F., Tordoir, X., Cavaille, J., Ferguson-Smith, A., Cockett, N., Georges, M., and Charlier, C. (2005). RNAi-mediated allelic trans-interaction at the imprinted Rtl1/Peg11 locus. Curr Biol *15*, 743-749.

Dews, M., Homayouni, A., Yu, D., Murphy, D., Sevignani, C., Wentzel, E., Furth, E.E., Lee, W.M., Enders, G.H., Mendell, J.T., *et al.* (2006). Augmentation of tumor angiogenesis by a Myc-activated microRNA cluster. Nat Genet *38*, 1060-1065.
Diana, F., Di Bernardo, J., Sgarra, R., Tessari, M.A., Rustighi, A., Fusco, A., Giancotti, V., and Manfioletti, G. (2005). Differential HMGA expression and post-translational modifications in prostatic tumor cells. Int J Oncol *26*, 515-520.
Doebele, C., Bonauer, A., Fischer, A., Scholz, A., Reiss, Y., Urbich, C., Hofmann, W.K., Zeiher, A.M., and Dimmeler, S. Members of the microRNA-17-92 cluster exhibit a cell-intrinsic antiangiogenic function in endothelial cells. Blood *115*, 4944-4950.
Ewan, L.C., Jopling, H.M., Jia, H., Mittar, S., Bagherzadeh, A., Howell, G.J., Walker, J.H., Zachary, I.C., and Ponnambalam, S. (2006). Intrinsic tyrosine kinase activity is required for vascular endothelial growth factor receptor 2 ubiquitination, sorting and degradation in endothelial cells. Traffic *7*, 1270-1282.
Fasanaro, P., D'Alessandra, Y., Di Stefano, V., Melchionna, R., Romani, S., Pompilio, G., Capogrossi, M.C., and Martelli, F. (2008). MicroRNA-210 modulates endothelial cell response to hypoxia and inhibits the receptor tyrosine kinase ligand Ephrin-A3. J Biol Chem *283*, 15878-15883.
Favier, J., Lapointe, S., Maliba, R., and Sirois, M.G. (2007). HIF2 alpha reduces growth rate but promotes angiogenesis in a mouse model of neuroblastoma. BMC Cancer *7*, 139.
Ferrara, N. (2002). VEGF and the quest for tumour angiogenesis factors. Nat Rev Cancer *2*, 795-803.
Ferrara, N., and Kerbel, R.S. (2005). Angiogenesis as a therapeutic target. Nature *438*, 967-974.
Filipowicz, W., Bhattacharyya, S.N., and Sonenberg, N. (2008). Mechanisms of post-transcriptional regulation by microRNAs: are the answers in sight? Nat Rev Genet *9*, 102-114.
Fish, J.E., Santoro, M.M., Morton, S.U., Yu, S., Yeh, R.F., Wythe, J.D., Ivey, K.N., Bruneau, B.G., Stainier, D.Y., and Srivastava, D. (2008). miR-126 regulates angiogenic signaling and vascular integrity. Dev Cell *15*, 272-284.
Folkman, J. (1971). Tumor angiogenesis: therapeutic implications. N Engl J Med *285*, 1182-1186.
Fukunaga, B.N., Probst, M.R., Reisz-Porszasz, S., and Hankinson, O. (1995). Identification of functional domains of the aryl hydrocarbon receptor. J Biol Chem *270*, 29270-29278.
Ghosh, G., Subramanian, I.V., Adhikari, N., Zhang, X., Joshi, H.P., Basi, D., Chandrashekhar, Y.S., Hall, J.L., Roy, S., Zeng, Y., *et al.* (2010). Hypoxia-induced microRNA-424 expression in human endothelial cells regulates HIF-alpha isoforms and promotes angiogenesis. J Clin Invest *120*, 4141-4154.
Giatromanolaki, A., Sivridis, E., Fiska, A., and Koukourakis, M.I. (2006). Hypoxia-inducible factor-2 alpha (HIF-2 alpha) induces angiogenesis in breast carcinomas. Appl Immunohistochem Mol Morphol *14*, 78-82.
Gregory, P.A., Bert, A.G., Paterson, E.L., Barry, S.C., Tsykin, A., Farshid, G., Vadas, M.A., Khew-Goodall, Y., and Goodall, G.J. (2008). The miR-200 family and miR-205 regulate epithelial to mesenchymal transition by targeting ZEB1 and SIP1. Nat Cell Biol *10*, 593-601.

Greither, T., Wurl, P., Grochola, L., Bond, G., Bache, M., Kappler, M., Lautenschlager, C., Holzhausen, H.J., Wach, S., Eckert, A.W., *et al.* Expression of microRNA 210 associates with poor survival and age of tumor onset of soft-tissue sarcoma patients. Int J Cancer.

Guo, C., Sah, J.F., Beard, L., Willson, J.K., Markowitz, S.D., and Guda, K. (2008). The noncoding RNA, miR-126, suppresses the growth of neoplastic cells by targeting phosphatidylinositol 3-kinase signaling and is frequently lost in colon cancers. Genes Chromosomes Cancer *47*, 939-946.

Harris, A.L. (2002). Hypoxia--a key regulatory factor in tumour growth. Nat Rev Cancer *2*, 38-47.

Harris, T.A., Yamakuchi, M., Ferlito, M., Mendell, J.T., and Lowenstein, C.J. (2008). MicroRNA-126 regulates endothelial expression of vascular cell adhesion molecule 1. Proc Natl Acad Sci U S A *105*, 1516-1521.

Hayashita, Y., Osada, H., Tatematsu, Y., Yamada, H., Yanagisawa, K., Tomida, S., Yatabe, Y., Kawahara, K., Sekido, Y., and Takahashi, T. (2005). A polycistronic microRNA cluster, miR-17-92, is overexpressed in human lung cancers and enhances cell proliferation. Cancer Res *65*, 9628-9632.

He, L., and Hannon, G.J. (2004). MicroRNAs: small RNAs with a big role in gene regulation. Nat Rev Genet *5*, 522-531.

He, L., He, X., Lim, L.P., de Stanchina, E., Xuan, Z., Liang, Y., Xue, W., Zender, L., Magnus, J., Ridzon, D., *et al.* (2007). A microRNA component of the p53 tumour suppressor network. Nature *447*, 1130-1134.

He, L., Thomson, J.M., Hemann, M.T., Hernando-Monge, E., Mu, D., Goodson, S., Powers, S., Cordon-Cardo, C., Lowe, S.W., Hannon, G.J., *et al.* (2005). A microRNA polycistron as a potential human oncogene. Nature *435*, 828-833.

Hofacker, I.L. (2007). How microRNAs choose their targets. Nat Genet *39*, 1191-1192.

Hong, L., Han, Y., Zhang, H., Li, M., Gong, T., Sun, L., Wu, K., Zhao, Q., and Fan, D. The prognostic and chemotherapeutic value of miR-296 in esophageal squamous cell carcinoma. Ann Surg *251*, 1056-1063.

Huang, X., Ding, L., Bennewith, K.L., Tong, R.T., Welford, S.M., Ang, K.K., Story, M., Le, Q.T., and Giaccia, A.J. (2009). Hypoxia-inducible mir-210 regulates normoxic gene expression involved in tumor initiation. Mol Cell *35*, 856-867.

Inomata, M., Tagawa, H., Guo, Y.M., Kameoka, Y., Takahashi, N., and Sawada, K. (2009). MicroRNA-17-92 down-regulates expression of distinct targets in different B-cell lymphoma subtypes. Blood *113*, 396-402.

Iorio, M.V., Ferracin, M., Liu, C.G., Veronese, A., Spizzo, R., Sabbioni, S., Magri, E., Pedriali, M., Fabbri, M., Campiglio, M., *et al.* (2005). MicroRNA gene expression deregulation in human breast cancer. Cancer Res *65*, 7065-7070.

Ivanovska, I., Ball, A.S., Diaz, R.L., Magnus, J.F., Kibukawa, M., Schelter, J.M., Kobayashi, S.V., Lim, L., Burchard, J., Jackson, A.L., *et al.* (2008). MicroRNAs in the miR-106b family regulate p21/CDKN1A and promote cell cycle progression. Mol Cell Biol *28*, 2167-2174.

Johnson, S.M., Grosshans, H., Shingara, J., Byrom, M., Jarvis, R., Cheng, A., Labourier, E., Reinert, K.L., Brown, D., and Slack, F.J. (2005). RAS is regulated by the let-7 microRNA family. Cell *120*, 635-647.

Jones-Rhoades, M.W., Bartel, D.P., and Bartel, B. (2006). MicroRNAS and their regulatory roles in plants. Annu Rev Plant Biol *57*, 19-53.

Kaelin, W.G. (2005). The von Hippel-Lindau tumor suppressor protein: roles in cancer and oxygen sensing. Cold Spring Harb Symp Quant Biol *70*, 159-166.

Kelly, T.J., Souza, A.L., Clish, C.B., and Puigserver, P. A Hypoxia-Induced Positive Feedback Loop Promotes Hypoxia-Inducible Factor 1{alpha} Stability through miR-210 Suppression of Glycerol-3-Phosphate Dehydrogenase 1-Like. Mol Cell Biol *31*, 2696-2706.

Kerbel, R.S. (2008). Tumor angiogenesis. N Engl J Med *358*, 2039-2049.

Kozak, K.R., Abbott, B., and Hankinson, O. (1997). ARNT-deficient mice and placental differentiation. Dev Biol *191*, 297-305.

Kuehbacher, A., Urbich, C., Zeiher, A.M., and Dimmeler, S. (2007). Role of Dicer and Drosha for endothelial microRNA expression and angiogenesis. Circ Res *101*, 59-68.

Lagos, D., Pollara, G., Henderson, S., Gratrix, F., Fabani, M., Milne, R.S., Gotch, F., and Boshoff, C. miR-132 regulates antiviral innate immunity through suppression of the p300 transcriptional co-activator. Nat Cell Biol *12*, 513-519.

le Sage, C., Nagel, R., Egan, D.A., Schrier, M., Mesman, E., Mangiola, A., Anile, C., Maira, G., Mercatelli, N., Ciafre, S.A., *et al.* (2007). Regulation of the p27 (Kip1) tumor suppressor by miR-221 and miR-222 promotes cancer cell proliferation. Embo J *26*, 3699-3708.

Lee, D.Y., Deng, Z., Wang, C.H., and Yang, B.B. (2007). MicroRNA-378 promotes cell survival, tumor growth, and angiogenesis by targeting SuFu and Fus-1 expression. Proc Natl Acad Sci U S A *104*, 20350-20355.

Lee, R.C., Feinbaum, R.L., and Ambros, V. (1993). The C. elegans heterochronic gene lin-4 encodes small RNAs with antisense complementarity to lin-14. Cell *75*, 843-854.

Lei, Z., Li, B., Yang, Z., Fang, H., Zhang, G.M., Feng, Z.H., and Huang, B. (2009). Regulation of HIF-1alpha and VEGF by miR-20b tunes tumor cells to adapt to the alteration of oxygen concentration. PLoS One *4*, e7629.

Lim, L.P., Lau, N.C., Garrett-Engele, P., Grimson, A., Schelter, J.M., Castle, J., Bartel, D.P., Linsley, P.S., and Johnson, J.M. (2005). Microarray analysis shows that some microRNAs downregulate large numbers of target mRNAs. Nature *433*, 769-773.

Liu, L., Jiang, Y., Zhang, H., Greenlee, A.R., Yu, R., and Yang, Q. miR-22 functions as a micro-oncogene in transformed human bronchial epithelial cells induced by anti-benzo[a]pyrene-7,8-diol-9,10-epoxide. Toxicol In Vitro *24*, 1168-1175.

Lu, J., Getz, G., Miska, E.A., Alvarez-Saavedra, E., Lamb, J., Peck, D., Sweet-Cordero, A., Ebert, B.L., Mak, R.H., Ferrando, A.A., *et al.* (2005). MicroRNA expression profiles classify human cancers. Nature *435*, 834-838.

Magill, S.T., Cambronne, X.A., Luikart, B.W., Lioy, D.T., Leighton, B.H., Westbrook, G.L., Mandel, G., and Goodman, R.H. microRNA-132 regulates dendritic growth and arborization of newborn neurons in the adult hippocampus. Proc Natl Acad Sci U S A *107*, 20382-20387.

Maltepe, E., Schmidt, J.V., Baunoch, D., Bradfield, C.A., and Simon, M.C. (1997). Abnormal angiogenesis and responses to glucose and oxygen deprivation in mice lacking the protein ARNT. Nature *386*, 403-407.

Mattia, G., Errico, M.C., Felicetti, F., Petrini, M., Bottero, L., Tomasello, L., Romania, P., Boe, A., Segnalini, P., Di Virgilio, A., *et al.* Constitutive activation of the ETS-1-miR-222 circuitry in metastatic melanoma. Pigment Cell Melanoma Res.

Medina, R., Zaidi, S.K., Liu, C.G., Stein, J.L., van Wijnen, A.J., Croce, C.M., and Stein, G.S. (2008). MicroRNAs 221 and 222 bypass quiescence and compromise cell survival. Cancer Res *68*, 2773-2780.

Nana-Sinkam, S.P., and Croce, C.M. MicroRNA dysregulation in cancer: opportunities for the development of microRNA-based drugs. IDrugs *13*, 843-846.

O'Donnell, K.A., Wentzel, E.A., Zeller, K.I., Dang, C.V., and Mendell, J.T. (2005). c-Myc-regulated microRNAs modulate E2F1 expression. Nature *435*, 839-843.

Olive, V., Bennett, M.J., Walker, J.C., Ma, C., Jiang, I., Cordon-Cardo, C., Li, Q.J., Lowe, S.W., Hannon, G.J., and He, L. (2009). miR-19 is a key oncogenic component of mir-17-92. Genes Dev *23*, 2839-2849.

Park, S.M., Gaur, A.B., Lengyel, E., and Peter, M.E. (2008). The miR-200 family determines the epithelial phenotype of cancer cells by targeting the E-cadherin repressors ZEB1 and ZEB2. Genes Dev *22*, 894-907.

Pichiorri, F., Suh, S.S., Ladetto, M., Kuehl, M., Palumbo, T., Drandi, D., Taccioli, C., Zanesi, N., Alder, H., Hagan, J.P., *et al.* (2008). MicroRNAs regulate critical genes associated with multiple myeloma pathogenesis. Proc Natl Acad Sci U S A *105*, 12885-12890.

Pola, R., Ling, L.E., Silver, M., Corbley, M.J., Kearney, M., Blake Pepinsky, R., Shapiro, R., Taylor, F.R., Baker, D.P., Asahara, T., *et al.* (2001). The morphogen Sonic hedgehog is an indirect angiogenic agent upregulating two families of angiogenic growth factors. Nat Med *7*, 706-711.

Poliseno, L., Tuccoli, A., Mariani, L., Evangelista, M., Citti, L., Woods, K., Mercatanti, A., Hammond, S., and Rainaldi, G. (2006). MicroRNAs modulate the angiogenic properties of HUVECs. Blood *108*, 3068-3071.

Puissegur, M.P., Mazure, N.M., Bertero, T., Pradelli, L., Grosso, S., Robbe-Sermesant, K., Maurin, T., Lebrigand, K., Cardinaud, B., Hofman, V., *et al.* miR-210 is overexpressed in late stages of lung cancer and mediates mitochondrial alterations associated with modulation of HIF-1 activity. Cell Death Differ *18*, 465-478.

Raver-Shapira, N., Marciano, E., Meiri, E., Spector, Y., Rosenfeld, N., Moskovits, N., Bentwich, Z., and Oren, M. (2007). Transcriptional activation of miR-34a contributes to p53-mediated apoptosis. Mol Cell *26*, 731-743.

Reisz-Porszasz, S., Probst, M.R., Fukunaga, B.N., and Hankinson, O. (1994). Identification of functional domains of the aryl hydrocarbon receptor nuclear translocator protein (ARNT). Mol Cell Biol *14*, 6075-6086.

Renault, M.A., Roncalli, J., Tongers, J., Thorne, T., Klyachko, E., Misener, S., Volpert, O.V., Mehta, S., Burg, A., Luedemann, C., *et al.* Sonic hedgehog induces angiogenesis via Rho kinase-dependent signaling in endothelial cells. J Mol Cell Cardiol *49*, 490-498.

Schmidt, M., De Maziere, A., Smyczek, T., Gray, A., Parker, L., Filvaroff, E., French, D., van Dijk, S., Klumperman, J., and Ye, W. (2007). The role of Egfl7 in vascular morphogenesis. Novartis Found Symp *283*, 18-28; discussion 28-36, 238-241.

Semenza, G.L. (2003). Targeting HIF-1 for cancer therapy. Nat Rev Cancer *3*, 721-732.

Semenza, G.L. (2007). Hypoxia-inducible factor 1 (HIF-1) pathway. Sci STKE *2007*, cm8.

Sethupathy, P., Megraw, M., and Hatzigeorgiou, A.G. (2006). A guide through present computational approaches for the identification of mammalian microRNA targets. Nat Methods *3*, 881-886.

Shin, C., Nam, J.W., Farh, K.K., Chiang, H.R., Shkumatava, A., and Bartel, D.P. Expanding the microRNA targeting code: functional sites with centered pairing. Mol Cell *38*, 789-802.

Suarez, Y., Fernandez-Hernando, C., Yu, J., Gerber, S.A., Harrison, K.D., Pober, J.S., Iruela-Arispe, M.L., Merkenschlager, M., and Sessa, W.C. (2008). Dicer-dependent endothelial microRNAs are necessary for postnatal angiogenesis. Proc Natl Acad Sci U S A *105*, 14082-14087.

Sylvestre, Y., De Guire, V., Querido, E., Mukhopadhyay, U.K., Bourdeau, V., Major, F., Ferbeyre, G., and Chartrand, P. (2007). An E2F/miR-20a autoregulatory feedback loop. J Biol Chem *282*, 2135-2143.

Taguchi, A., Yanagisawa, K., Tanaka, M., Cao, K., Matsuyama, Y., Goto, H., and Takahashi, T. (2008). Identification of hypoxia-inducible factor-1 alpha as a novel target for miR-17-92 microRNA cluster. Cancer Res *68*, 5540-5545.

Takakura, S., Mitsutake, N., Nakashima, M., Namba, H., Saenko, V.A., Rogounovitch, T.I., Nakazawa, Y., Hayashi, T., Ohtsuru, A., and Yamashita, S. (2008). Oncogenic role of miR-17-92 cluster in anaplastic thyroid cancer cells. Cancer Sci *99*, 1147-1154.

Takata, H., Kato, M., Denda, K., and Kitamura, N. (2000). A hrs binding protein having a Src homology 3 domain is involved in intracellular degradation of growth factors and their receptors. Genes Cells *5*, 57-69.

Tanzer, A., and Stadler, P.F. (2004). Molecular evolution of a microRNA cluster. J Mol Biol *339*, 327-335.

Tavazoie, S.F., Alarcon, C., Oskarsson, T., Padua, D., Wang, Q., Bos, P.D., Gerald, W.L., and Massague, J. (2008). Endogenous human microRNAs that suppress breast cancer metastasis. Nature *451*, 147-152.

Thomson, D.W., Bracken, C.P., and Goodall, G.J. Experimental strategies for microRNA target identification. Nucleic Acids Res.

Vaira, V., Faversani, A., Dohi, T., Montorsi, M., Augello, C., Gatti, S., Coggi, G., Altieri, D.C., and Bosari, S. miR-296 regulation of a cell polarity-cell plasticity module controls tumor progression. Oncogene.

Vogelstein, B., and Kinzler, K.W. (2004). Cancer genes and the pathways they control. Nat Med *10*, 789-799.

Wang, G.L., Jiang, B.H., Rue, E.A., and Semenza, G.L. (1995). Hypoxia-inducible factor 1 is a basic-helix-loop-helix-PAS heterodimer regulated by cellular O2 tension. Proc Natl Acad Sci U S A *92*, 5510-5514.

Wang, S., Aurora, A.B., Johnson, B.A., Qi, X., McAnally, J., Hill, J.A., Richardson, J.A., Bassel-Duby, R., and Olson, E.N. (2008). The endothelial-specific microRNA miR-126 governs vascular integrity and angiogenesis. Dev Cell *15*, 261-271.

Wei, J.J., Wu, X., Peng, Y., Shi, G., Olca, B., Yang, X., Daniels, G., Osman, I., Ouyang, J., Hernando, E., *et al.* Regulation of HMGA1 expression by microRNA-296 affects prostate cancer growth and invasion. Clin Cancer Res *17*, 1297-1305.

Wenger, R.H. (2002). Cellular adaptation to hypoxia: O2-sensing protein hydroxylases, hypoxia-inducible transcription factors, and O2-regulated gene expression. Faseb J *16*, 1151-1162.

Wightman, B., Ha, I., and Ruvkun, G. (1993). Posttranscriptional regulation of the heterochronic gene lin-14 by lin-4 mediates temporal pattern formation in C. elegans. Cell *75*, 855-862.

Woods, K., Thomson, J.M., and Hammond, S.M. (2007). Direct regulation of an oncogenic micro-RNA cluster by E2F transcription factors. J Biol Chem *282*, 2130-2134.

Wurdinger, T., Tannous, B.A., Saydam, O., Skog, J., Grau, S., Soutschek, J., Weissleder, R., Breakefield, X.O., and Krichevsky, A.M. (2008). miR-296 regulates growth factor receptor overexpression in angiogenic endothelial cells. Cancer Cell *14*, 382-393.

Xiong, J., Yu, D., Wei, N., Fu, H., Cai, T., Huang, Y., Wu, C., Zheng, X., Du, Q., Lin, D., *et al.* An estrogen receptor alpha suppressor, microRNA-22, is downregulated in estrogen receptor alpha-positive human breast cancer cell lines and clinical samples. Febs J *277*, 1684-1694.

Yamakuchi, M., Lotterman, C.D., Bao, C., Hruban, R.H., Karim, B., Mendell, J.T., Huso, D., and Lowenstein, C.J. P53-induced microRNA-107 inhibits HIF-1 and tumor angiogenesis. Proc Natl Acad Sci U S A *107*, 6334-6339.

Yamakuchi, M., Yagi, S., Ito, T., and Lowenstein, C.J. MicroRNA-22 Regulates Hypoxia Signaling in Colon Cancer Cells. PLoS One *6*, e20291.

Yue, S., Chen, Y., and Cheng, S.Y. (2009). Hedgehog signaling promotes the degradation of tumor suppressor Sufu through the ubiquitin-proteasome pathway. Oncogene *28*, 492-499.

12

New Molecular Targets for Anti-Angiogenic Therapeutic Strategies

Amanda G. Linkous[1] and Eugenia M. Yazlovitskaya[2]
[1]*Neuro-Oncology Branch, National Cancer Institute, National Institutes of Health*
[2]*Department of Medicine, Vanderbilt-Ingram Cancer Center, Vanderbilt University*
USA

1. Introduction

The concept of targeting tumor blood vessel formation, i.e. tumor angiogenesis, has long been accepted as a potential strategy for controlling tumor growth. Characterized by the ability to supply oxygen, growth factors, hormones and nutrients, tumor vasculature has been identified as a key factor for the maintenance and progression of many solid tumors. The development of tumor vasculature is regulated by a highly complex network of signal transduction pathways involving pro- and anti-angiogenic factors. This delicate, yet dynamic balance between the promotion and inhibition of vascularization provides an abundance of molecular targets for therapeutic intervention.

Since more than 85% of cancer mortality results from solid tumors, the continual development of anti-vascular agents remains an important goal in the quest for novel anti-cancer therapies (Jain, 2005). Despite its supporting role in the nutrition and viability of human cancers, however, tumor angiogenesis was not always considered a hallmark of tumor progression (Hanahan & Folkman, 1996). Initial skepticism centered on the hypothesis that angiogenesis was only critical in the early phase of tumor development. Thus, many opponents believed that angiogenic inhibition would be largely ineffective in most late-stage cancers. Other skeptics argued that the concept of anti-angiogenic therapy was counterintuitive because destruction of the tumor vasculature would significantly compromise the delivery of cytotoxic agents to the tumor (Jain, 2005). Though these concerns are not without merit, an overwhelming body of evidence in early-stage and established tumors demonstrates a synergistic effect when inhibitors of angiogenesis are combined with chemotherapy and/or radiotherapy.

Despite the advantages of anti-angiogenic therapy, some have proposed that vascular destruction promotes the increased adaptation of tumor cells to areas of insufficient vascularization. The basis for this concern can be found through closer examination of the vascular abnormalities often identified in the tumor microenvironment. Characterized by aberrant morphology and increased compression of blood and lymphatic vessels, the tumor vascular network is an environment of interstitial hypertension and hypoxia (low oxygen availability) (Hanahan & Folkman, 1996; Jain, 2005). While some cancer cells are able to survive these harsh conditions of nutrient deprivation and impaired oxygenation, many of these tumor cells undergo programmed cell death. Nevertheless, anti-vascular therapy is feared to select for tumor cells with enhanced invasive and metastatic potential. Equipped with a more malignant phenotype characterized by high degrees of resilience, such tumor cells could plausibly disseminate into surrounding tissue and co-opt preexisting vessels that are resistant to angiogenesis inhibitors. Appropriately, an extensive number of studies have been conducted to address this issue. Fortunately, data collected from a variety of research groups indicate that the expansion of metastatic tumor cells to distant organ sites is predominantly dependent on angiogenesis (Hanahan & Folkman, 1996). Thus, pharmacological intervention with tumor angiogenic processes may still prove to be an effective method for controlling metastatic growth.

Tumor blood vessel formation is a highly dynamic process that is regulated by a balance of pro- and anti-angiogenic factors. The search for angiogenic inducers first began after the initial observation that capillary growth was stimulated even when tumors were implanted into avascular regions such as the cornea. This evidence of capillary sprouting in areas of absent or quiescent vasculature bolstered the hypothesis that tumor cells release diffusible triggers of vascularization.

The first discovered inducer of angiogenesis was basic fibroblast growth factor, known as bFGF or FGF-2 (Hanahan & Folkman, 1996). FGF-2 was soon accompanied by the isolation of the closely related FGF-1 or acidic FGF (aFGF). Although both proteins lack traditional signal sequences for secretion, each growth factor can be released upon exposure to cell stress. One angiogenic protein that is readily secreted from tumor cells is vascular endothelial growth factor (VEGF). Originally identified as vascular permeability factor (VPF), VEGF is a potent promoter of tumor vascularization and is a primary target of anti-angiogenic therapy. Other promoters of angiogenesis include angiopoietins and members of the Ephrin family of ligands.

Over the years, a number of pro-angiogenic factors have been discovered. Since physiological blood vessel formation is well-coordinated and tightly controlled, experts within the field hypothesized that tumor angiogenesis may also be a balance of pro- and anti-angiogenic factors. Experiments designed to address the existence of endogenous inhibitors of angiogenesis revealed that the mutational inactivation of a tumor suppressor gene initiated tumorigenesis in a previously nontumorigenic hamster cell line (Rastinejad et al., 1989). A secreted glycoprotein that mediates cell-cell interaction, thrombospondin-1 (TSP-1) was shown to strongly inhibit endothelial cell chemotaxis as well as vascularization of the cornea. Interestingly, the regulation of TSP-1 levels is dependent on the tumor suppressor protein p53; TSP-1 production is dramatically lower in cells with impaired p53 function (Rastinejad et al., 1989). This intricate relationship between tumor suppressors and regulators of angiogenesis further emphasizes the pivotal role of vascularization in tumor progression.

Although both truncated and full-length TSP-1 can strongly attenuate vascular formation, many other negative regulators of angiogenesis remain sequestered as inactive components of larger molecules (Hanahan & Folkman, 1996). Upon receipt of the signal to limit or terminate vascular growth, potent inhibitory fragments of intact molecules are then released. An example of this quiescent storage can be found in fibronectin. Despite its abundance in the circulatory system, full-length fibronectin is not an inhibitor of angiogenesis. However, a 29 kDa fragment of the intact molecule substantially inhibited endothelial cell proliferation. Similarly, a 16 kDa fragment of prolactin and a fragment of plasminogen known as angiostatin are highly effective inhibitors of the angiogenic process.

This pattern of storing inhibitory fragments within physiologically abundant proteins represents a key mechanism by which angiogenic processes can be turned on or off. In addition, overwhelming evidence suggests that the balance of inducers and inhibitors is critical for promoting vascular quiescence over new capillary formation (**Figure 1**) (Hanahan & Folkman, 1996). Not surprisingly, a primary focus within the field of tumor angiogenesis is to prevent the angiogenic switch through the modulation of endogenous factors.

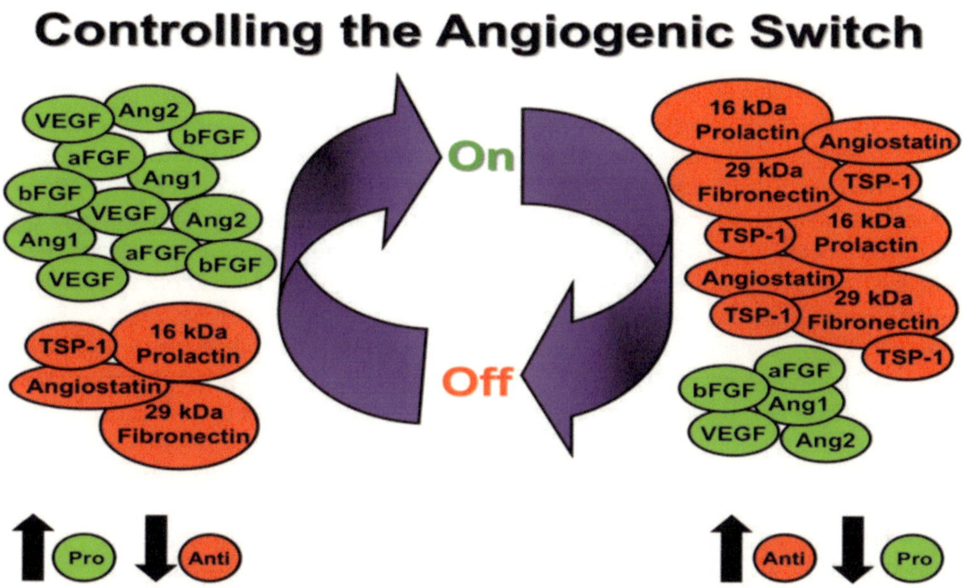

Fig. 1. Controlling the Angiogenic Switch (Hanahan & Folkman, 1996).

Both positive and negative regulators control the balance between normal quiescent vasculature and active blood vessel formation. Enhanced levels of pro-angiogenic molecules ("Pro", green) in combination with reduced levels of anti-angiogenic molecules ("Anti", red) activate the angiogenic switch. Alternatively, a reduction in the pro-angiogenic factors with an accompanying increase in angiogenesis inhibitors blocks neovascularization.

In addition to their active involvement in the response to cytotoxic therapies, tumor vascular endothelial cells are also preferred targets due to their genetic stability. In contrast to tumor cells, which harbor a wide variety of genetic alterations, cytogenetic abnormalities within tumor endothelium are fairly limited. This substantial lack of mutations renders the tumor vasculature network less susceptible to acquired drug resistance (Kerbel, 1991).

2. Response of tumor vasculature to radiation therapy

Since its inception, anti-angiogenic therapy has evolved from a relatively unclear concept to a widely-accepted strategy for restricting tumor progression. The inhibition of tumor neovascularization has uncovered a new role for vascular endothelial cells as active participants in the response to conventional treatments such as chemotherapy and ionizing radiation. Today, anti-angiogenesis therapy is recognized as a standard modality of cancer treatment in addition to surgery and cytotoxic therapies.

A potential role for vascular endothelial cells in the response to radiation therapy is particularly relevant for radioresistant cancers. Administered to two thirds of all cancer patients, ionizing radiation induces DNA damage in rapidly dividing tumor cells, causing them to undergo mitotic catastrophe or apoptotic cell death. Although modifications in therapeutic protocols have improved tumor response, local recurrence presents an ongoing challenge for treatment-resistant tumors like lung cancer and glioblastoma (GBM) (Clamon et al., 1999; DeAngelis, 2001; Lee et al., 1999; Wagner, 2000). Both tumors are quite recalcitrant to radiation, and treatment of these malignancies is, therefore, highly problematic. Attempts to improve the treatment efficacy in GBM patients have yielded intensified forms of radiotherapy including brachytherapy and radioactive seeds implanted in the tumor bed that deliver an additional dose of radiation (up to 60 Gy). Unfortunately, none have significantly improved survival (DeAngelis, 2001; Suh & Barnett, 1999; Videtic et al., 1999). Brachytherapy has been replaced by noninvasive stereotactic radiosurgery, which alleviates many of the complications involved in the administration of radiation. However, stereotactic radiosurgery is only amenable to tumors 3 cm or less in diameter, and only if they are not located immediately adjacent to critical structures such as the optic nerve or brain stem (Tokuuye et al., 1998). Despite aggressive treatment, most glioblastoma patients die of the disease, with median survival of about one year.

Poor overall survival also remains a concern for lung cancer. Despite surgery and radiation treatment, approximately 30 to 40% of patients with non–small-cell lung cancer (NSCLC) who have discrete lesions and histologically negative lymph nodes die of recurrent disease (Brock et al., 2008; Hoffman et al., 2000). It has become obvious, therefore, that additional treatments are necessary to achieve improved survival benefit for these patients. Currently, the most common approach to enhance the efficiency of radiotherapy is to combine radiation with chemotherapeutic agents (Dietz et al., 2008; Forastiere et al., 2006; Iranzo et al., 2009; McGinn et al., 1996; Stratford, 1992). Regrettably, many of the platinum-based chemotherapeutic agents used as standard treatment for cancer also exhibit toxicity within normal tissues. Therefore, the development of non-toxic, yet effective molecular-targeted radiosensitizers may have a positive impact on the therapeutic ratio.

Understanding the response of the tumor microenvironment to ionizing radiation is fundamental for the design of novel and efficient radiosensitizing agents. The effectiveness of radiotherapy is often limited by the response of tumor vasculature, specifically vascular endothelium. Several studies have demonstrated that clinically relevant doses of ionizing radiation (2-5 Gy) elicit the activation of both PI3K/Akt and MAPK pro-survival signaling pathways in vascular endothelium (Dent et al., 2003; Linkous et al., 2009; Yazlovitskaya et al., 2008; Zhan & Han, 2004; Zingg et al., 2004). The result of such activation is increased radioresistance within the tumor blood vessels. Since destruction of the tumor vascular network enhances the treatment of cancer (Folkman, 1971; Strijbos et al., 2008), radiosensitizers that target these survival pathways could improve the outcome of cancer patients.

Upon irradiation, signal transduction is generated during the interaction of ionizing radiation with cellular membranes (Haimovitz-Friedman et al., 1994; Valerie et al., 2007). In our laboratory, we demonstrated that ionizing radiation interacts with vascular endothelial cell membranes to activate an enzyme known as cytosolic phospholipase A2 ($cPLA_2$) (**Figure 2**) (Linkous et al., 2009; Yazlovitskaya et al., 2008). As an 85-kDa Ca^{2+}-sensitive protein, $cPLA_2$ belongs to a superfamily of PLA_2 enzymes that are responsible for the hydrolysis of the sn-2 acyl bond of glycerophospholipids on the cell membrane. As a result of this hydrolysis, both free fatty acid and lysophospholipids are generated. Calcium binding to the amino-terminal CalB domain of $cPLA_2$ promotes the translocation of the ubiquitously distributed $cPLA_2$ from the cytosol to the cell membrane. Once there, $cPLA_2$ then specifically cleaves the acyl ester bond of phosphatidylcholine (PC) to produce lysophospholipids and release arachidonic acid (AA) (Hirabayashi et al., 1999; Hirabayashi et al., 2004; Hirabayashi & Shimizu, 2000).

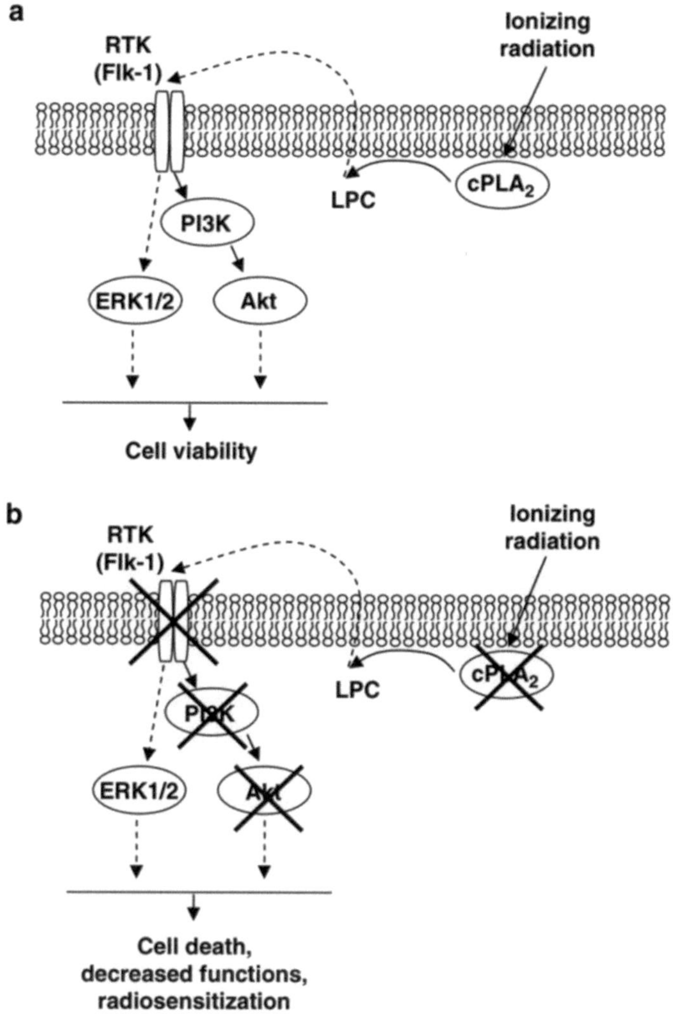

Fig. 2. Proposed sequence of molecular events in irradiated vascular endothelium (Yazlovitskaya et al., 2008). (a) Ionizing radiation triggers the activation of cytosolic phospholipase A2 ($cPLA_2$) followed by increased production of lysophosphatidylcholine (LPC), activation of Flk-1 (VEGFR-2) and phosphorylation of Akt and extracellular signal-regulated kinase (ERK) 1/2 leading to cell viability. (b) Inhibition of this survival pathway at the level of various components (indicated by crosses) leads to cell death, decreased endothelial function, and increased radiosensitization.

This cytosolic form of PLA_2 has been implicated in diverse cellular responses such as mitogenesis, differentiation, and inflammation. Radiation-induced activation of $cPLA_2$ in vascular endothelial cells resulted in the increased production of LPC, a lipid-derived second messenger which triggered Akt and ERK1/2 phosphorylation (Linkous et al., 2009;

Yazlovitskaya et al., 2008). Influencing a wide range of cell types within the vascular system, LPC can modulate a variety of biological functions including cytokine synthesis, chemotaxis, and endothelial growth factor expression (Fujita et al., 2006). Not surprisingly, radiation-induced activation of the $cPLA_2$-LPC signaling cascade contributes to the survival and overall radioresistance of vascular endothelial cells (**Figure 2**).

Additional evidentiary support for a direct role of tumor endothelial cells in the response to radiation therapy was demonstrated in irradiated MCA/729 fibrosarcomas and B16F1 melanomas (Garcia-Barros et al., 2003). Using mice deficient in acid sphingomyelinase and Bax, two major participants of programmed cell death, Garcia-Barros et al. demonstrated that, due to lack of endothelial apoptosis in the host component, tumors grew 200-400% more rapidly than tumors containing wild-type vasculature. In addition, tumors implanted in apoptosis-resistant mice were refractory to single-dose radiation up to 20 Gy (Garcia-Barros et al., 2003).

3. Targeting the VEGF-VEGFR pathway

Without question, the most widely studied and well-known target of anti-angiogenesis therapy is VEGF. The mammalian VEGF-related family of angiogenic and lymphangiogenic growth factors consists of five glycoproteins referred to as VEGF-A, VEGF-B, VEGF-C, VEGF-D, and placental growth factor 1 and 2 (PGF-1 and PGF-2) (Ellis & Hicklin, 2008; Hicklin & Ellis, 2005). Existing in both soluble and extracellular matrix-bound forms, VEGF promotes endothelial cell growth, migration, and survival in a variety of human cancers including breast, colorectal, and glioblastoma multiforme (GBM).

Predominantly produced by tumor cells, VEGF ligands exert their pro-angiogenic effects on endothelial cells through the binding and activation of receptor tyrosine kinases known as VEGFR-1, VEGFR-2, and VEGFR-3. Each of the VEGF family ligands has a specific binding affinity for the different receptor tyrosine kinases. VEGF-A binds to both VEGFR-1 and VEGFR-2, while VEGF-B binds exclusively to VEGFR-1. VEGF-C and VEGF-D preferentially bind to VEGFR-3, however, proteolytic processing allows both family members to bind to VEGFR-2 as well (Ellis & Hicklin, 2008). Thus, members of the same glycoprotein family are responsible for a diverse range of functions. Since the interaction of VEGF ligands with their respective receptors can trigger the activation of multiple signaling pathways, the VEGF-VEGFR axis has become the most heavily targeted pathway in anti-angiogenesis therapy (Ellis & Hicklin, 2008; Hicklin & Ellis, 2005).

Initial approaches to impair VEGF-VEGFR signaling focused on the development of neutralizing antibodies to VEGF ligands. Attempts at pharmacological intervention have led to the discovery of a humanized monoclonal antibody known as bevacizumab **(Table 1)**. Recognized for its ability to bind and sequester circulating VEGF-A, bevacizumab was recently approved by the US Food and Drug Administration (FDA) for the clinical treatment of patients with glioma and cancers of the colon, lung, and breast. Additional treatments including sorafenib and sunitinib (inhibitors of VEGF receptor tyrosine kinases) are also currently approved for cancer therapy (Ellis & Hicklin, 2008; Hicklin & Ellis, 2005).

Data collected from human glioma specimens has shown a direct correlation between VEGF-A production and degree of malignancy; VEGF-A levels are 10 times higher in high-grade tumors in comparison to low-grade glioma (Linkous & Yazlovitskaya, 2011; Norden et al., 2009; Plate et al., 1994; Plate et al., 1992; Schmidt et al., 1999). In addition, other principal contributors like neuropilins and angiopoietin-2 (ANG-2) promote angiogenesis through the potentiation of VEGF signaling.

Angiogenic Target	Inhibitors	Treated Cells or Tumors	References
VEGF-A	Bevacizumab	Glioma, colon cancer, lung cancer, and breast cancer	(Ellis & Hicklin, 2008; Hicklin and Ellis, 2005)
VEGF receptor tyrosine kinases	Sorafenib	Renal cell carcinoma, glioma, colon cancer, lung cancer, and breast cancer	(Bhargava & Robinson, 2011; Ellis & Hicklin, 2008; Hicklin & Ellis, 2005)
VEGF receptor tyrosine kinases	Sunitinib	Renal cell carcinoma, glioma, colon cancer, lung cancer, and breast cancer	(Bhargava & Robinson, 2011; Ellis & Hicklin, 2008; Hicklin & Ellis, 2005)
VEGF receptor tyrosine kinases	Tivozanib	Renal cell carcinoma, metastatic breast cancer, and advanced colorectal cancer	(Bhargava & Robinson, 2011)
VEGF receptor tyrosine kinases	Axitinib	Lung cancer, metastatic breast cancer, pancreatic cancer, and advanced gastric cancers	(Bhargava & Robinson, 2011)
Protein kinase D1-3 (PKD1, PKD2, and PKD3)	CRT0066101	Pancreatic cancer	(LaValle *et al.*, 2010)
Rho-associated coiled-coil-forming kinase (ROCK)	HA1077 (Fasudil)	Vascular endothelial cells, breast cancer, and metastatic lung cancer	(van der Meel *et al.*, 2011)
Rac1	NSC23766	T-cell lymphoma and prostate cancer	(van der Meel *et al.*, 2011)
Cytosolic phospholipase A2 ($cPLA_2$)	Arachidonyltrifluorometh yl Ketone ($AACOCF_3$)	Vascular endothelial cells, mouse models of lung and ovarian cancers	(Yazlovitskaya *et al.*, 2008; Linkous *et al.*, 2009; Schulte *et al.*, 2011; Farooqui *et al.*, 2006)
Cytosolic phospholipase A2 ($cPLA_2$)	Methyl Arachidonyl Fluorophosphonate (MAFP)	Vascular endothelial cells	(Yazlovitskaya *et al.*, 2008; Farooqui *et al.*, 2006)
Cytosolic Phospholipase A2 ($cPLA_2$)	4-[2-[5-Chloro-1-(diphenylmethyl)-2-methyl-1*H*-indol-3-yl]-ethoxy] benzoic acid (CDIBA)	Vascular endothelial cells; mouse models of lung cancer and glioblastoma	(Linkous *et al.*, 2010)
Autotaxin (ATX) and Lysophosphatidic acid (LPA) receptors	BrP-LPA	Breast cancer and non-small cell lung cancer	(Prestwich *et al.*, 2008; Zhang *et al.*, 2009)
Enhancer of Zeste Homolog 2 (EZH2)	3-deazaneplanocin (DZNep)	Breast cancer, prostate cancer, and acute myeloid leukemia	(Chase and Cross, 2011; Fiskus *et al.*, 2009)
Cyclin-dependent kinases (CDKs)	Roscovitine	Vascular endothelial cells, breast cancer, non-small cell lung cancer, nasopharyngeal cancer	(Wesierska-Gadek *et al.*, 2011; Liebl *et al.*, 2011)

Table 1. Current angiogenic targets and their respective inhibitors.

Due to the overwhelming evidence of a pivotal role for VEGF-A in tumor angiogenesis, an array of therapeutic agents has been developed against the VEGF-A signaling pathway. In an initial study of glioma patients who received bevacizumab and a topoisomerase I inhibitor known as irinotecan, 19 out of 29 participants achieved at least a 50% reduction in maximal cross-sectional contrast-enhancing areas on magnetic resonance imaging (MRI) (Norden et al., 2009). Compared to a radiographic response rate of 5-8% in patients who received standard temozolomide treatment, this result was a marked improvement. Moreover, several large retrospective studies reported response rates of 25-74% and progression-free survival of 32-64%. These early studies also demonstrated an additional corticosteroid-sparing effect; the majority of patients were able to reduce their corticosteroid doses by 50% or more (Norden et al., 2009). Since it first entered routine clinical practice in the United States, however, bevacizumab treatment has provided only modest survival benefits overall. Furthermore, although a single infusion has been shown to decrease the density of existing microvasculature (Willett et al., 2004), bevacizumab primarily targets new blood vessel formation. Thus, bevacizumab monotherapy may lack long-term efficacy because it rarely targets the mature tumor vasculature that is already established at the time of diagnosis. Unfortunately, the molecular mechanism of bevacizumab failure is poorly understood, and the absence of effective post-bevacizumab salvage therapies only complicates treatment management. Currently, bevacizumab is approved for the treatment of metastatic colorectal cancer, non-squamous non-small cell lung cancer, metastatic breast cancer, glioblastoma, and metastatic renal cell carcinoma. In June of 2011, however, the FDA's Oncologic Drugs Advisory Committee recommended withdrawing approval of bevacizumab for breast cancer due to safety concerns and lack of proven efficacy. Pending the final decision of the committee, patients suffering from metastatic breast cancer may soon have to consider other therapeutic options (http://www.cancer.gov/cancertopics/druginfo/fda-bevacizumab, FDA Approval for Bevacizumab, National Cancer Institute, 2011).

3.1 Mechanisms of resistance

Emerging data from clinical and pre-clinical investigations indicate that the aggressive return to tumor growth after initial response to anti-VEGF-VEGFR therapies is due to a variety of drug resistance mechanisms. One mode of resistance to angiogenesis inhibitors is adaptive (evasive) resistance. Traditional models of drug resistance focus on the acquisition of genetic mutations within the gene that encodes the drug target. Such mutational alterations lead to reduced inhibition of the intended disease-promoting factor. In case of evasive resistance, the specific vascular target remains inhibited.

A possible explanation for adaptive resistance, even in the presence of continual drug blockade is that the tumor can activate or upregulate alternative pro-angiogenic signaling pathways. Evidence for this mechanism in cancer patients was demonstrated in a recent clinical investigation. In participants who received the VEGFR inhibitor cediranib, there was a temporary response phase followed by relapse. Upon analysis, patient blood levels of bFGF were significantly higher during the relapse phase than in the initial stage of response. Additional observations revealed increased serum levels of stromal cell-derived factor 1α (SDF1α) and elevated presence of circulating endothelial cells at the time of progression on cediranib (Batchelor et al., 2007; Norden et al., 2009). These findings support the hypothesis that anti-VEGF pathway inhibitors may be more effective when combined with drugs that target other pro-angiogenic factors.

In addition to the activation of other angiogenic targets, upregulation of VEGF-A itself can significantly enhance tumor resistance to therapy. Recent evidence has demonstrated that cytotoxic therapies such as chemotherapy and radiation can induce the production of VEGF-A in tumors of the lung, breast, colon, and kidney (Volk 2011; Volk 2008). This results in an autocrine positive feedback loop that promotes the survival of both tumor cells and endothelial cells. Thus, tumor cells can escape programmed cell death through the activation of angiogenic signaling *in vivo* (Volk et al., 2008; Volk et al., 2011).

A second mechanism that facilitates evasive resistance is the recruitment of bone marrow-derived cells (BMDCs). BMDCs are recruited in part through increased hypoxia. Hypoxia leading to necrosis is one of hallmarks of GBM (Chen et al., 2009), and hypoxic conditions often enhance tumor cell resistance to chemotherapy and ionizing radiation. Interestingly, the inhibition of VEGF-A with bevacizumab produced a substantial increase in hypoxia-inducible factor 1α (HIF1α) and CA9, another hypoxia marker (Iwamoto et al., 2009). HIF1α was shown to promote GBM neovascularization through the recruitment of pro-angiogenic bone marrow-derived $CD45^+$ myeloid cells and $F4/80^+$ tumor associated macrophages (Aghi et al., 2006; Bergers & Hanahan, 2008; Du et al., 2008). Tumors with little or no HIF1α expression displayed few BMDCs, and both angiogenesis as well as tumor growth were significantly impaired. Collectively, these observations suggest that anti-angiogenic therapy induces low oxygen conditions and accelerates blood vessel formation through BMDC recruitment.

Although pro-angiogenic BMDCs are important for progression after anti-VEGF-A therapy, other cell types, such as pericytes, also contribute to evasive resistance. Pericytes, structural support cells that envelop the microvasculature, serve a distinct role of maintaining the integrity and functionality of pre-existing blood vessels. Support for this concept is based on a variety of investigations which showed that increased PDGF signaling enhances the stabilization of tumor blood vessels by recruiting pericytes and promoting pericyte-endothelial cell interactions (Allt & Lawrenson, 2001; Bergers & Song, 2005; Norden et al., 2009). In light of these observations, therapeutic strategy of a combined VEGF-VEGFR and PDGF-PDGFR inhibition would reduce the resistance to anti-vascular therapy.

A fourth mechanism of adaptive resistance has gained considerable interest over recent years. This form of evasion involves increased invasiveness without the requirement of angiogenesis. Following a pharmaceutical blockade of angiogenesis in an orthotopic GBM mouse model, glioblastoma cells were able to co-opt the normal vasculature and disseminate deep into the brain (Bergers & Hanahan, 2008; Blouw et al., 2003; Du et al., 2008; Rubenstein et al., 2000). This phenotype is referred to as perivascular tumor invasion, and it allows cells to escape oxygen and nutrient deprivation. Consistent with results from animal studies, GBM patients who developed multi-focal recurrence after bevacizumab treatment exhibited pro-invasive adaptation as observed by MRI.

Not all modes of resistance are dependent on adaptation. Some tumors possess an intrinsic, pre-existing indifference to anti-angiogenic therapy. In a clinical trial of cediranib, one group of GBM patients exhibited transitory improvements while another subset of patients had no response. This differential reaction to the same therapy emphasizes the need for biomarkers that can accurately predict individual efficacy of anti-VEGF-A therapy from patient to patient.

3.2 Lack of predictive markers for therapeutic efficacy

The mechanistic evasion of anti-VEGF-A therapy is further complicated by the lack of indicators or predictive markers for therapeutic efficacy. The contrasting response to anti-angiogenic monotherapy suggests that individual tumors may possess unique angiogenic profiles (Jain, 2005). These profiles consist of informative parameters such as vascular permeability, blood flow, interstitial fluid pressure, and the upregulation or downregulation of key angiogenic factors. Deciphering these phenotypic codes on an individualized basis may allow physicians to better predict and monitor a patient's response to various anti-vascular agents. Until this approach of personalized medicine can be achieved, however, a growing number of efforts are focused on improving the potency and selectivity of VEGFR tyrosine kinase inhibitors.

4. Modified approach to inhibit the VEGF-VEGFR pathway

Although targeting the VEGF family presents a range of challenges, the evidence still suggests that the VEGF-VEGFR axis is the dominant signal transduction pathway in tumor vascularization. Thus, the rationale for using VEGF-A blockade remains quite valid for a variety of cancers. One potential obstacle to the therapeutic efficacy of VEGFR inhibition, however, is the lack of specificity for VEGFR tyrosine kinases. FDA-approved tyrosine kinase inhibitors (TKIs) such as sorafenib and sunitinib inhibit VEGFR TKIs **(Table 1)**, but they also potently block signaling through other targets including platelet-derived growth factor receptor (PDGFR), stem cell factor receptor (c-kit), and colony-stimulating factor 1 receptor (CSF1R) (Bhargava & Robinson, 2011). Due to the low selectivity of these multi-targeted inhibitors, higher dose administration is required to achieve maximal VEGFR inhibition. As a result, optimal blockade of VEGF-A receptors is often accompanied by increased off-target effects and enhanced toxicity. Adverse events associated with reduced target selectivity include hand-foot skin reactions, fatigue, vomiting, diarrhea, hypertension, cardiac ischemia, and thyroid dysfunction (Bhargava & Robinson, 2011). Consequently, the combined use of TKIs with conventional chemotherapeutic drugs is severely limited.

4.1 Second-generation VEGFR tyrosine kinase inhibitors

To circumvent the problems associated with off-target toxicities, a new initiative is underway to develop second-generation VEGFR TKIs that exhibit extreme potency and elevated selectivity. One of the most promising candidates is a pan-VEGFR antagonist known as tivozanib **(Table 1)**. Demonstrating picomolar potency to VEGFR-1, VEGFR-2, and VEGFR-3, tivozanib significantly increased progression-free survival from 6.2 months to 12.1 months in patients with renal cell carcinoma (Bhargava & Robinson, 2011). Furthermore, it is the first TKI to be safely combined with a mammalian target of rapamycin (mTOR) inhibitor and is currently involved in phase I studies with other therapeutic agents in both metastatic breast cancer and advanced colorectal cancer.

Tivozanib is not alone in this subset of novel, selective TKIs. Axitinib **(Table 1)**, a small molecule inhibitor of all known VEGFRs, also demonstrates increased efficacy as both monotherapy and in combination with chemotherapy. Further clinical evaluation is being performed to assess the effects of axitinib in lung cancer, metastatic breast cancer, pancreatic cancer, and advanced gastric cancers (Bhargava & Robinson, 2011). Overall, collective data generated from clinical studies indicate that second-generation TKIs are generally associated with lower off-target toxicities, more potent and less toxic than traditional inhibitors of receptor tyrosine kinases.

4.2 Inhibition of the protein kinase D family

Since the tolerability of novel TKIs is still unknown for multiple tumor types, another potential approach to control the angiogenic process is to target the VEGF-VEGFR pathway through indirect mechanisms of action. In this modified approach to vascular inhibition, therapeutic strategies are designed to block the downstream effectors of VEGF-A-induced angiogenic signaling. Recent investigation of tumor blood vessel formation revealed a key role for protein kinase D1 (PKD1) in VEGF-A signaling (LaValle et al., 2010).

A novel serine/threonine protein kinase, PKD1 mediates VEGFR-2-stimulated endothelial cell proliferation through the activation of extracellular signal-regulated kinases 1 and 2 (ERK 1/2) (Ha & Jin, 2009). Moreover, the subcutaneous implantation of matrigel plugs *in vivo* showed that functional PKD1 activity was necessary for VEGF-A-induced angiogenesis. The ability of PKD1 to promote angiogenesis is due in part to class IIa histone deacetylase (HDAC) activity. Important for chromatin modifications and repression of gene expression, HDAC5 and HDAC7 enzymes are direct targets of PKD1-dependent phosphorylation in endothelial cells stimulated with VEGF-A. Upon phosphorylation of Ser259/498 in HDAC5 and Ser178, Ser344, and Ser479 in HDAC7, HDAC translocation from the nucleus to the cytoplasm promotes the expression of myocyte enhancer factor-2 (MEF2)-dependent genes (Ha & Jin, 2009). Through an unidentified mechanism, the PKD1-HDAC pathway eventually leads to angiogenic gene expression, endothelial cell migration, tubule formation, and microvascular sprouting.

As a frequently upregulated isoform in pancreatic and prostate cancer, PKD1 has understandably become an attractive target for chemical inhibition. Perhaps the most promising compound of PKD inhibitors is CRT0066101 **(Table 1)** (LaValle et al., 2010). A pan-inhibitor of PKD1, PKD2, and PKD3, CRT0066101 is orally available and substantially suppresses the growth of pancreatic tumors in an orthotopic mouse model. Unfortunately, information regarding the three-dimensional (3D) structure of PKD is incomplete. Therefore, the present lack of structure-based drug design hinders the optimization of current anti-PKD compounds.

4.3 Rho GTPase signaling

Other downstream mediators of VEGF-VEGFR signaling are also generating interest as proponents of tumor angiogenesis. One particular signaling cascade, the Rho GTPase pathway, has recently been implicated in several phases of angiogenesis such as vascular permeability, endothelial cell migration, proliferation, and lumen formation. Functioning as molecular gatekeepers, this subfamily of the Ras superfamily of small GTPases is activated by VEGF-A binding to VEGFR-2 in endothelial cells (van der Meel et al., 2011).

This ligand-receptor interaction initiates the recruitment of proteins like c-Src or phospholipase C beta 3 (PLCβ3) to the phosphorylated tyrosine residues of the VEGF-A receptors. Following this initial recruitment, Rho GTPases like Rac1, RhoA, and Cdc42 become active and subsequently promote tumor vascularization through destabilization of endothelial barrier integrity, enhanced migration, proliferation, and tubule formation (van der Meel et al., 2011).

Attempts to disrupt Rho GTPase signal transduction frequently involve the use of Rho-associated coiled-coil-forming kinase (ROCK) inhibitors. One such inhibitor, HA1077 (fasudil) **(Table 1)**, can effectively block migration, cellular viability, and tubule formation in VEGF-A-stimulated vascular endothelial cells. Interestingly, treatment with fasudil attenuates the anchorage-dependent growth of breast cancer cells and significantly reduces tumor burden in an experimental model of murine lung metastasis (van der Meel et al., 2011).

Another compound, NSC23766 **(Table 1)**, is a small-molecule inhibitor of Rac1. Similar to ROCK inhibitors, NSC23766 attenuates cell proliferation as well as tumor growth. In contrast to the effects of pharmacological inhibition of Rac1, however, depletion of Rac1 in the tumor endothelium of adult wild-type mice had no effect on angiogenesis and revealed a complete lack of tumor growth suppression (van der Meel et al., 2011). In order to reconcile such conflicting outcomes, more information is needed regarding the regulation and downstream signaling of Rho GTPases. Unraveling the intricate relationships between different members of this signaling family may uncover the necessary combinations of druggable targets that will be most effective for clinical use.

5. Novel molecular targets for anti-angiogenesis therapy

For years, the VEGF-A signaling pathway has been the primary target of vascular inhibition. Due to the emerging complications of resistance, however, efforts to discover new molecular targets have increased. We have previously described the role of cytosolic phospholipase A2 ($cPLA_2$) in radiation-induced signal transduction in human lung cancer and ovarian carcinoma (Linkous et al., 2009; Schulte et al., 2011; Yazlovitskaya et al., 2008). Following the observation that $cPLA_2$ promotes the survival of vascular endothelium, we have also identified this cytoplasmic enzyme as a fundamental component of tumor angiogenesis (Linkous et al., 2010).

5.1 Cytosolic phospholipase A2 promotes tumor angiogenesis

In $cPLA_2\alpha$-deficient mice, a syngeneic glioblastoma cell line (GL261) failed to form tumors even after 2 months post-injection. By contrast, their $cPLA_2\alpha$-wild type counterparts displayed a tumor take rate of 100% (**Figure 3**). In similar experiments, Lewis lung carcinoma (LLC) cells did form tumors in $cPLA_2\alpha$-deficient mice; however, they were dramatically smaller than tumors in $cPLA_2\alpha$-wild type mice.

To determine the effects of $cPLA_2$ deficiency on tumor vascularity, LLC tumors from $cPLA_2\alpha^{+/+}$ and $cPLA_2\alpha^{-/-}$ mice were sectioned and examined for microvascular density using an antibody against von Willebrand Factor (vWF), a known vascular endothelial cell marker. Immunohistochemical examination revealed decreased blood vessel formation and increased areas of necrosis in tumors from $cPLA_2\alpha^{-/-}$ mice, thus implicating $cPLA_2$ as an important factor for tumor formation, growth and maintenance (Linkous et al., 2010).

Tumor vascularization requires not only capillary formation, but also the maturation of endothelial-lined blood vessels. This process of vessel maturation is dependent on the functions of cells known as pericytes. Previously regarded as inactive scaffolding components, pericytes are now recognized for their ability to coordinate intercellular signaling with endothelial cells and other elements of the blood vessel wall to prevent leakage. As necessary components in vessel stabilization, pericytes maintain vessel integrity and aid in the assembly of extracellular matrix (ECM) components. To determine whether $cPLA_2$ is involved in tumor blood vessel maturation, LLC tumor sections were co-stained with antibodies to vWF and to two established pericyte markers (alpha-smooth muscle actin (α-SMA) and desmin) used to detect stages of vascular development (**Figure 4**). Results from α-SMA immunofluorescence demonstrated significant pericyte coverage of the tumor vasculature in LLC tumors from $cPLA_2\alpha^{+/+}$ mice. In tumors from $cPLA_2\alpha^{-/-}$ mice, however, vessel-encircling pericytes were undetectable. Since α-SMA expression may be dependent upon the maturation stage of pericytes, tumor sections were also examined for the presence of desmin, which is expressed by both mature and immature pericytes. Although desmin was detected in tumor vasculature from $cPLA_2\alpha^{+/+}$ mice, no desmin-positive cells were observed within tumor blood vessels from $cPLA_2\alpha^{-/-}$ mice (Linkous et al., 2010). These marked differences in pericyte coverage suggest that, in addition to its role in endothelial cell function, $cPLA_2$ may also be responsible for pericyte recruitment and required vessel maturation. Such findings implicate a novel pro-angiogenic role for $cPLA_2$ in the tumor microenvironment.

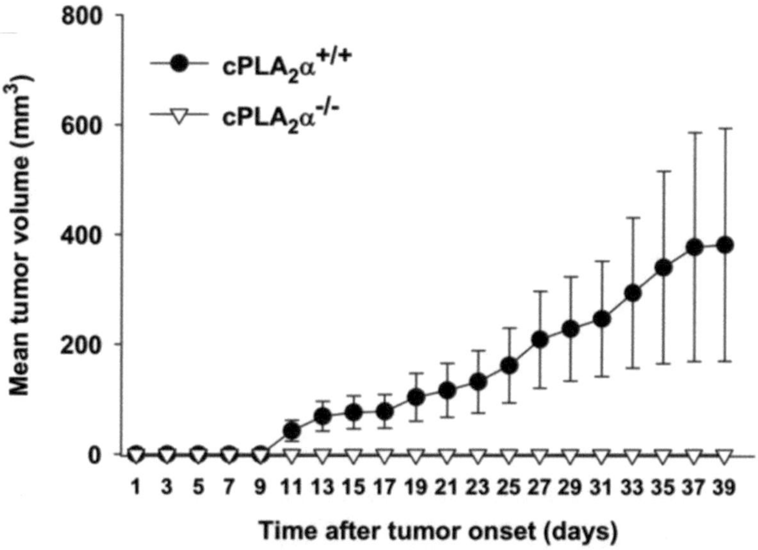

Fig. 3. GL261 tumor growth in $cPLA_2\alpha$-deficient mice (Linkous et al., 2010).
GL261 cells were injected subcutaneously into the hind limbs of $cPLA_2\alpha^{+/+}$ and $cPLA_2\alpha^{-/-}$ C57/BL6 mice (n = 6–7 mice per group). Tumor volume was measured using power Doppler sonography at 48-hour intervals beginning 1 week after injection and ending when tumors reached a volume of 700 mm^3 or a diameter of 15 mm). Shown are the mean GL261 tumor volumes. Days 11–39: $P < .001$ (longitudinal analysis of least squares means). Error bars correspond to 95% confidence intervals.

Since $cPLA_2$ is responsible for the production of bioactive lipid mediators, LPC, AA, and lysophosphatidic acid (LPA), we wanted to determine which of these products contributes to the promotion of vascular endothelial cell migration. Although the restoration of LPC, LPA, and AA alone resulted in increased migration, the most pronounced effect was observed with the addition of LPC + LPA or LPC + AA to primary endothelial cells isolated from $cPLA_2\alpha^{-/-}$ mice (Linkous et al., 2010). These results indicate that, in addition to AA and LPA, which regulate endothelial cell migration (Folkman, 2001; Herbert et al., 2009; Kishi et al., 2006; Ptaszynska et al., 2008), the less-characterized LPC pathway may also play a significant role in this process. In addition, the most pronounced increase in cellular proliferation was observed in $cPLA_2\alpha^{-/-}$ cells treated with a combination of LPC and LPA (Linkous et al., 2010). These data demonstrate a key role for $cPLA_2$ in endothelial cell proliferation and indicate that the lysophospholipids, LPC and LPA, may serve as effectors for this stage of angiogenesis.

Due to its functional responsibility in inflammation, radiation signaling, and angiogenesis, $cPLA_2$ has become an attractive target for chemical inhibition. Two of the most commonly

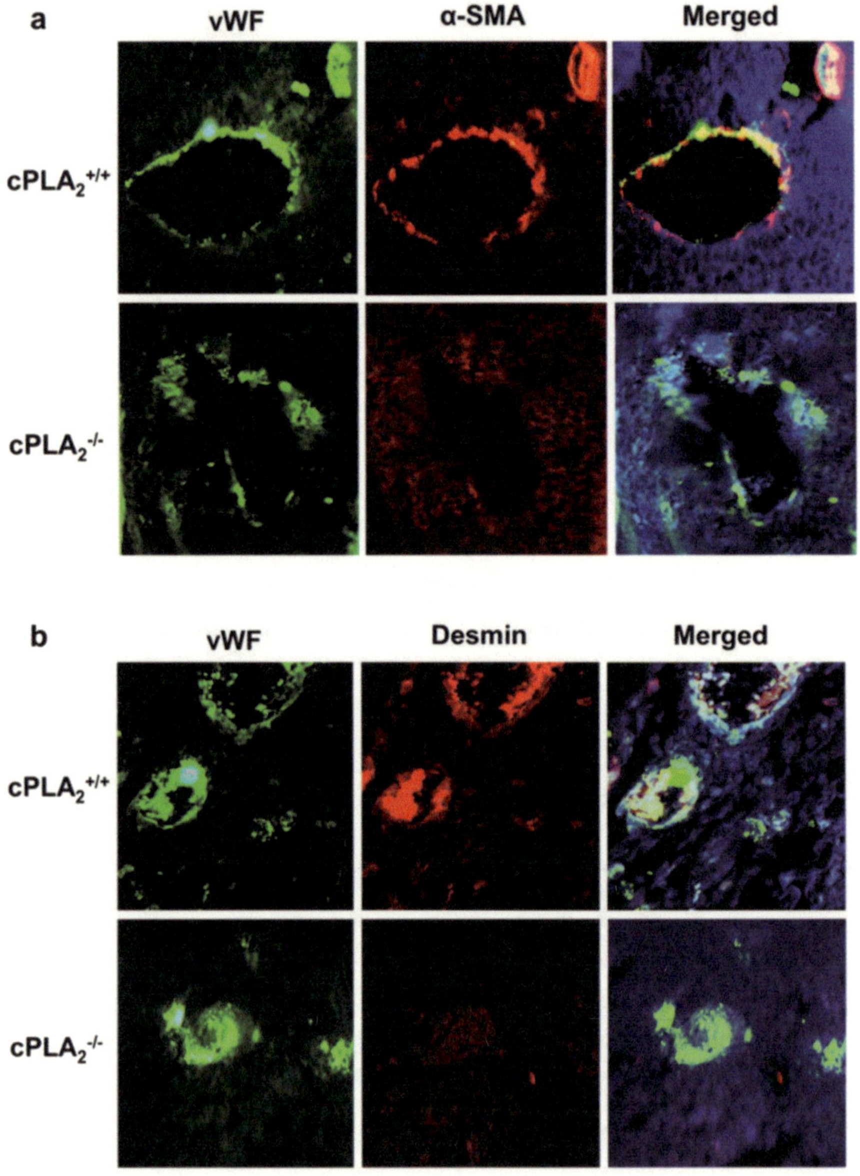

Fig. 4. Pericyte coverage of blood vessels in tumors from $cPLA_2\alpha^{+/+}$ and $cPLA_2\alpha^{-/-}$ mice (Linkous et al., 2010).
Formalin-fixed Lewis lung carcinoma (LLC) tumors from $cPLA_2\alpha^{+/+}$ (upper rows) and $cPLA_2\alpha^{-/-}$ (lower rows) were sectioned and co-stained with antibodies against von Willebrand factor (left panels) and either a-smooth muscle actin (middle panels, a) or desmin (middle panels, b) and counterstained with DAPI (4',6-diamidino-2-phenylindole). a) Representative micrographs of immunofluorescence staining for von Willebrand factor (green), a-smooth muscle actin (red), and DAPI (blue) in tumors from $cPLA_2\alpha^{+/+}$ and

$cPLA_2\alpha^{-/-}$ mice (at 40× magnification). Right panels present merged immunofluorescence staining of von Willebrand factor and cells positive for a–smooth muscle actin (yellow).
b) Representative micrographs of immunofluorescence staining for von Willebrand factor (green), desmin (red), and DAPI (blue) in tumors from $cPLA_2\alpha^{+/+}$ and $cPLA_2\alpha^{-/-}$ mice (at 40× magnification). Right panels present merged immunofluorescence staining of von Willebrand factor and cells positive for desmin (yellow).

used $cPLA_2$ inhibitors are arachidonyltrifluoromethyl ketone ($AACOCF_3$) and methyl arachidonyl fluorophosphonate (MAFP) **(Table 1)** (Yazlovitskaya et al., 2008). $AACOCF_3$ is a potent and cell-permeable trifluoromethyl ketone analog of arachidonic acid. Nuclear magnetic resonance studies have shown that the carbon chain of $AACOCF_3$ binds in a hydrophobic pocket of $cPLA_2$ and the carbonyl group of $AACOCF_3$ forms a covalent bond with serine 228 in the enzyme active site (Farooqui et al., 2006). This $cPLA_2$ inhibitor has been used to study the role of $cPLA_2$ in platelet aggregation, inflammation-associated apoptosis, and the radiosensitivity of vascular endothelial cells (Yazlovitskaya et al., 2008). Combined with radiation, $AACOCF_3$ was also demonstrated to significantly inhibit tumor growth and tumor vascularity in the mouse models of lung and ovarian cancers (Linkous et al., 2009; Schulte et al., 2011). Similar to $AACOCF_3$, MAFP is also a powerful inhibitory agent, however, this irreversible drug inhibits both the calcium-dependent and calcium-independent ($iPLA_2$) forms of the enzyme (Farooqui et al., 2006). Other agents including pyrrolidine-based inhibitors have also been used extensively to block PLA_2 enzymatic activity. Nevertheless, like other pyrrolidine-containing compounds, this class of drugs is non-specific and attenuates the activity of $cPLA_2$-γ and $iPLA_2$-β (Farooqui et al., 2006). Recent attempts to improve the specificity of these compounds have unveiled new indole-based candidates for $cPLA_2$-targeted therapy (McKew et al., 2006). Based on promising preliminary results, our laboratory synthesized a compound known as 4-[2-[5-Chloro-1-(diphenylmethyl)-2-methyl-1*H*-indol-3-yl]-ethoxy]benzoic acid (CDIBA) **(Table 1)** (Linkous et al., 2010). Shown to potently target $cPLA_2$-α and substantially attenuate arachidonic acid release in a wide variety of enzymatic and cell-based assays, CDIBA treatment inhibited capillary tubule formation, migration, and cellular proliferation in tumor vascular endothelial cells (Linkous et al., 2010). Furthermore, in heterotopic glioblastoma and lung cancer tumor models, mice treated with CDIBA exhibited delayed tumor growth and reduced tumor volume (Linkous et al., 2010). Accordingly, pharmaceutical companies are now focused on the continual optimization of these novel $cPLA_2$ inhibitors for clinical use.

5.2 Autotaxin and lysophosphatidic acid signaling

Advances in anti-angiogenic therapy are not solely dependent on the discovery of endothelial-associated targets, however. Indeed, as in the case of VEGF-A, tumor cells also secrete soluble inducers of angiogenesis. An excellent example of this paracrine effect can be found in the previously mentioned lipid second messenger, LPA. Shown to stimulate cell proliferation, migration, and survival, LPA has been implicated in the progression of many tumors including lung cancer, hepatocellular carcinoma, and epithelial ovarian cancer (Ptaszynska et al., 2008; Ren et al., 2006). LPA signaling is primarily mediated through classic G protein-coupled receptors that belong to the endothelial differentiation gene (EDG) family (LPA_1/EDG-2, LPA_2/EDG-4 and LPA_3/EDG-7). LPA can also exert its role through other receptors such as, LPA_4/GPR23, LPA_5/GPR92, GPR87 and P2Y5 (Aoki et al., 2008). There are two major pathways of LPA production: 1) phosphatidic acid generated by phospholipase D or diacylglycerol kinase is subsequently converted to LPA by $cPLA_2$; 2) lysophospholipids generated by $cPLA_2$ (such as LPC) are subsequently converted to LPA by lysophospholipase D, also known as autotaxin (ATX) (Aoki et al., 2008; Hama et al., 2004; Jansen et al., 2005; Tokumura et al., 1986; Umezu-Goto et al., 2002). Unlike other members of the ectonucleotide pyrophosphatase and phosphodiesterase (NPP) family of enzymes, ATX possesses robust lysophospholipase D activity (Jansen et al., 2005; Ptaszynska et al., 2008). Initially purified from melanoma cells as a potent chemoattractant (Stracke et al., 1992), this 103 kDa secreted protein is upregulated in a variety of malignancies and has been shown to stimulate cell proliferation and enhance tumor invasion and metastasis (Tanaka et al., 2006).

While ATX can be produced by endothelium, the majority of ATX is generated and secreted by a variety of tumor cells. As the primary enzyme involved in the production of LPA, ATX has recently sparked interest for its potential role in the development and progression of ovarian cancer. As the fifth leading cause of death in American women, ovarian tumors are known to produce larger quantities of LPA than nonmalignant cells (Fang et al., 2002) Due to the high substrate levels of LPC found in peritoneal fluids from patients with ovarian cancer, the observed increase in LPA is attributed to elevated ATX activity (Schulte et al., 2011; Tokumura et al., 2007). Moreover, expression of LPA receptors was found to determine tumorigenicity and aggressiveness of ovarian cancer cells. Our laboratory and others have recently demonstrated that ATX and LPA signaling may contribute to the resistance of ovarian carcinoma to cytotoxic therapies such as cisplatin and ionizing radiation (Schulte et al., 2011). Based on these results, it remains conceivable that LPA generated from LPC hydrolysis could bind to LPA receptors on vascular endothelium as well as those found on tumor cells.

Correspondingly, a cooperation of both VEGF-A and ATX was discovered in the regulation of endothelial cell migration (Ptaszynska et al., 2010). Knockdown of ATX expression prevented endothelial cell migration in response to stimulation with LPC, LPA, and VEGF-A. Moreover, the genetic silencing of ATX resulted in a concomitant reduction in the mRNA levels of LPA receptors (Ptaszynska et al., 2010). Taken together, these data suggest that ATX regulates the expression of LPA receptors that are necessary for VEGF-A- and lysophospholipid-induced angiogenesis. Thus, pharmacological inhibition of both ATX and LPA may serve as an effective method to reduce tumor vascularization.

Since ATX is a member of the alkaline phosphatase superfamily of metalloenzymes, initial medicinal chemistry efforts focused on metal chelaters as ATX inhibitors (Hoeglund et al., 2010). The chelaters reduce the metal-ion stimulation of ATX activity by competing with active site histidine and aspartic acid residues for divalent metal ions (Clair et al., 2005; Hoeglund et al., 2010; Tokumura et al., 1998). Not surprisingly, metal ion chelation is considered a relatively insensitive and non-specific method of ATX inhibition (Hoeglund et al., 2010). The library of ATX inhibitors has since expanded to include both non-lipid small-molecule inhibitors as well as analogs of bioactive lipids. Both categories of drugs are promising *in vitro*, although the non-lipid ATX inhibitors are more compliant with the characteristic parameters often found in orally bioavailable drugs (Hoeglund et al., 2010; Keller et al., 2006). Furthermore, these non-lipid compounds exhibit enhanced specificity for ATX without affecting other members of the NPP family (Hoeglund et al., 2010). Despite the identification of new inhibitory agents, the lack of information regarding the three-dimensional structure of ATX is impeding drug discovery (Parrill & Baker, 2010). Until the structural details of the enzyme are publicly disclosed, current medicinal chemistry efforts are focused on other ATX-associated targets such as LPA and the subsequent LPA receptors. One of the most common approaches to disrupt LPA signaling is to use LPA derivatives as selective receptor antagonists (Im, 2010). Many of these individual derivatives can exert a combined antagonistic effect against more than one LPA receptor. A primary example of this can be found in the α–bromomethylene phosphonate analog of LPA known as BrP-LPA **(Table 1)**. As a pan-antagonist of LPA_{1-4}, BrP-LPA has been shown to significantly reduce the migration, invasion, vascularity and tumor volume in mouse models of breast cancer and non-small cell lung cancer (Im, 2010; Prestwich et al., 2008; Xu & Prestwich, 2010; Zhang et al., 2009). Moreover, this potent and efficacious inhibitor also blocks over 98% of ATX activity at micromolar concentrations (Zhang et al., 2009). Such results suggest that the use of multi-target antagonists may provide the best strategy for the abrogation of ATX-LPA signal transduction.

5.3 Enhancer of Zeste homolog 2

The combined approach to anti-vascular therapy is becoming increasingly attractive as the tumor-endothelial cell interaction is deciphered. For instance, a paracrine relationship between VEGF-A and the enhancer of Zeste homolog 2 (EZH2) was just identified (Lu et al., 2010). EZH2 is a member of the polycomb-group (PcG) proteins and has intrinsic histone methyl transferase activity. Histone methylation is a common method of epigenetic gene regulation and is typically associated with transcriptional repression. Armed with this ability to inhibit transcription, EZH2 is frequently implicated in tumor progression and metastatic disease. A recent investigation revealed that VEGF secreted from human epithelial ovarian cancer cells could directly increase EZH2 mRNA levels in vascular endothelial cells (Lu et al., 2010). Elevated tumoral and endothelial EZH2 was also observed in more than 60% of available epithelial ovarian cancer samples. Furthermore, heightened levels of EZH2 were associated with high-grade disease and were predictive of poor overall survival. In a study to determine the mechanism behind such a dismal clinical outcome, Lu and colleagues investigated the relationship between EZH2 and the secreted protein, vasohibin1 (VASH1). Induced by VEGF-A stimulation, VASH1 is a newly identified negative regulator of angiogenesis. Interestingly, increased EZH2 resulted in the methylation and subsequent inactivation of VASH1 (Lu et al., 2010). Considering the complications of intrinsic or acquired resistance to anti-VEGF-A monotherapy, a combinatorial strategy that focuses on vascular and tumor-specific targets may provide the greatest efficacy.

Despite growing evidence of the relationship between EZH2 and tumorigenesis, there are currently no clinically available therapies that directly target histone methylation (Chase & Cross, 2011). Some experimental studies on the inhibition of EZH2 activity have been performed, however. Using a carbocyclic adenosine analog known as 3-deazaneplanocin (DZNep) **(Table 1)**, several groups have demonstrated depletion of EZH2 levels and reduced proliferation in breast cancer and prostate cancer cells (Chase & Cross, 2011). Futhermore, treatment with DZNep induced apoptosis in acute myeloid leukemia (AML) cells and significantly prolonged the survival of mice implanted with AML cells (Fiskus et al., 2009). Similar to other non-specific inhibitors, DZNep affects targets other than EZH2

(Chase & Cross, 2011; Fiskus et al., 2009; Yamaguchi et al., 2010). Although EZH2 is the catalytic subunit of the polycomb repressive complex 2 (PRC2), it is accompanied by other components including SUZ12, EED, and YY1. Consequently, treatment with DZNep results in the depletion of each of these PRC2 complex proteins and blocks the associated histone H3 lysine 27 methylation (Chase & Cross, 2011; Fiskus et al., 2009; Yamaguchi et al., 2010). Therefore, DZNep may interfere with normal physiological processes that require methyl transfer.

5.4 Cyclin-dependent kinases

Cyclin-dependent kinases (CDKs) have long been recognized for their involvement in the regulation of cell cycle transitions and cellular proliferation. As members of the serine-threonine kinase family, CDKs bind to regulatory proteins called cyclins and phosphorylate protein substrates on serine and threonine amino acid residues. Given the importance of cell cycle management in the prevention of uncontrolled cell growth, studies that shed light on the function of CDKs in tumorigenesis have gained recent momentum. A number of small-molecule inhibitors have been developed to alter the CDK deregulation that is frequently observed in human cancers (Baker, 2010; Liebl et al., 2011; Liebl et al., 2010). Success with one of the earliest CDK inhibitors, olomoucine, led to the widespread search for more specific compounds that would preclude aberrant CDK activity in tumors. To date, multiple CDK inhibitors have demonstrated anti-proliferative effects in cultured and xenografted myeloma, leukemia, colon cancer, lung cancer, and breast cancer cells (Baker, 2010; Liebl et al., 2011; Liebl et al., 2010). Recently, the CDK inhibitor roscovitine **(Table 1)**, was shown to arrest human estrogen receptor alpha (ER-α) positive MCF-7 breast cancer cells in the G(2) phase of the cell cycle and induce p53-dependent apoptosis (Wesierska-Gadek et al., 2011). Based on its anti-cancer activity both *in vitro* and *in vivo*, roscovitine is being evaluated in phase 2 clinical trials for the treatment of non-small cell lung cancer and nasopharyngeal cancer (Baker, 2010; Liebl et al., 2011; Liebl et al., 2010). Aside from its ability to impede tumor cell division, anti-angiogenic properties have also been discovered for this CDK inhibitor. Surprisingly, only a few prior reports have denoted a role for CDKs in tumor angiogenesis. To understand the molecular basis of these cell cycle and transcriptional regulators in tumor blood vessel formation, Liebl et al., assessed the effects of CDK inhibition in human umbilical vein endothelial cells (HUVEC) (Liebl et al., 2011; Liebl et al., 2010). In response to treatment with roscovitine, endothelial migration and tubule formation was significantly reduced. Furthermore, the chemical inhibition of CDKs greatly impaired endothelial cell sprouting from mouse aortic rings and abolished VEGF-A-induced vessel formation in the chorioallantoic membrane assay (Liebl et al., 2011; Liebl et al., 2010). While roscovitine does not selectively inhibit one specific CDK, the knockdown of cyclin-dependent kinase 5 (CDK5) revealed that roscovitine might exert its anti-vascular properties through a CDK5-dependent pathway (Liebl et al., 2011; Liebl et al., 2010). Other CDKs such as CDK4 have also been reported as plausible contributors to tumor vascularization. In a murine model of intestinal tumors, constitutive activation of CDK4 was shown to enhance tumor blood vessel formation and increase the expression of E2F target proteins involved in angiogenesis and proliferation (Abedin et al., 2010; Baker, 2010). Taken together, these findings suggest that the pharmacological inhibition of CDKs, either alone or in combination, may provide a novel method of vascular destruction (Baker, 2010; Liebl et al., 2011; Liebl et al., 2010).

6. Conclusion

Current attempts to disrupt the complex process of tumor blood vessel formation are predominantly focused on the VEGF-VEGFR signaling pathway. Although clinically proven to inhibit VEGF-A and its receptors, these pharmacologic agents are selective, but not specific. Consequently, many of the approved inhibitors also impair other molecular targets, thus, leading to increased toxicity. To reduce toxicity complications and augment the destruction of the tumor vascular network, an active search for new inhibitory agents has begun. In recent years, the emergence of several VEGF-VEGFR angiogenesis inhibitors has enhanced the clinical outcome for multiple tumors. It is important to note, however, that many of these pharmacologic agents resulted in transitory improvements followed by increased tumor resistance and metastasis. The observed resistance may be partially explained by the complex network of signal transduction that constitutes the angiogenic process. The frequent interconnectivity of these signaling pathways often results in redundancy during the formation of tumor blood vessels. As a result, when one pro-angiogenic target is inhibited, other molecules can be activated so that the requirement for vascularization is once again fulfilled. Furthermore, therapeutic pressure from chemotherapy and ionizing radiation can promote a VEGF-A-dependent autocrine loop which protects tumor cells and endothelial cells from cytotoxicity. Thus, the most effective therapeutic strategy may be to combine conventional treatment regimens with therapies that target multiple angiogenic pathways.

7. References

Abedin, Z.R., Ma, Z., &Reddy, E.P. (2010). Increased angiogenesis in Cdk4 (R24C/R24C) :Apc (+/Min) intestinal tumors. *Cell Cycle,* Vol. 9, No. 12, (Jun 15), pp. (2456-2463), 1551-4005 (Electronic), 1551-4005 (Linking).

Aghi, M., Cohen, K.S., Klein, R.J., Scadden, D.T., &Chiocca, E.A. (2006). Tumor stromal-derived factor-1 recruits vascular progenitors to mitotic neovasculature, where microenvironment influences their differentiated phenotypes. *Cancer Res,* Vol. 66, No. 18, (Sep 15), pp. (9054-9064), 0008-5472 (Print), 0008-5472 (Linking).

Allt, G., &Lawrenson, J.G. (2001). Pericytes: cell biology and pathology. *Cells Tissues Organs,* Vol. 169, No. 1, (Aug 16), pp. (1-11), 1422-6405 (Print), 1422-6405 (Linking).

Aoki, J., Inoue, A., &Okudaira, S. (2008). Two pathways for lysophosphatidic acid production. *Biochim Biophys Acta,* Vol. 1781, No. 9, (Sep), pp. (513-518), 0006-3002 (Print), 0006-3002 (Linking).

Baker, S.J. (2010). A role for Cdk4 in angiogenesis. *Cell Cycle,* Vol. 9, No. 13, (Jul 1), pp. (2456-2463), 1551-4005 (Electronic), 1551-4005 (Linking).

Batchelor, T.T., Sorensen, A.G., di Tomaso, E., Zhang, W.T., Duda, D.G., Cohen, K.S., Kozak, K.R., Cahill, D.P., Chen, P.J., Zhu, M., *et al.* (2007). AZD2171, a pan-VEGF receptor tyrosine kinase inhibitor, normalizes tumor vasculature and alleviates edema in glioblastoma patients. *Cancer Cell,* Vol. 11, No. 1, (Jan), pp. (83-95), 1535-6108 (Print), 1535-6108 (Linking).

Bergers, G., &Hanahan, D. (2008). Modes of resistance to anti-angiogenic therapy. *Nat Rev Cancer,* Vol. 8, No. 8, (Aug), pp. (592-603), 1474-1768 (Electronic), 1474-175X (Linking).

Bergers, G., &Song, S. (2005). The role of pericytes in blood-vessel formation and maintenance. *Neuro Oncol,* Vol. 7, No. 4, (Oct), pp. (452-464), 1522-8517 (Print), 1522-8517 (Linking).

Bhargava, P., &Robinson, M.O. (2011). Development of second-generation VEGFR tyrosine kinase inhibitors: current status. *Curr Oncol Rep,* Vol. 13, No. 2, (Apr), pp. (103-111), 1534-6269 (Electronic), 1523-3790 (Linking).

Blouw, B., Song, H., Tihan, T., Bosze, J., Ferrara, N., Gerber, H.P., Johnson, R.S., &Bergers, G. (2003). The hypoxic response of tumors is dependent on their microenvironment. *Cancer Cell,* Vol. 4, No. 2, (Aug), pp. (133-146), 1535-6108 (Print), 1535-6108 (Linking).

Brock, M.V., Hooker, C.M., Ota-Machida, E., Han, Y., Guo, M., Ames, S., Glockner, S., Piantadosi, S., Gabrielson, E., Pridham, G., *et al.* (2008). DNA methylation markers and early recurrence in stage I lung cancer. *N Engl J Med,* Vol. 358, No. 11, (Mar 13), pp. (1118-1128), 1533-4406 (Electronic), 0028-4793 (Linking).

Chase, A., &Cross, N.C. (2011). Aberrations of EZH2 in cancer. *Clin Cancer Res,* Vol. 17, No. 9, (May 1), pp. (2613-2618), 1078-0432 (Print), 1078-0432 (Linking).

Chen, Z., Htay, A., Dos Santos, W., Gillies, G.T., Fillmore, H.L., Sholley, M.M., &Broaddus, W.C. (2009). In vitro angiogenesis by human umbilical vein endothelial cells (HUVEC) induced by three-dimensional co-culture with glioblastoma cells. *J Neurooncol,* Vol. 92, No. 2, (Apr), pp. (121-128), 1573-7373 (Electronic), 0167-594X (Linking).

Clair, T., Koh, E., Ptaszynska, M., Bandle, R.W., Liotta, L.A., Schiffmann, E., &Stracke, M.L. (2005). L-histidine inhibits production of lysophosphatidic acid by the tumor-associated cytokine, autotaxin. *Lipids Health Dis,* Vol. 4, No. pp. (5), 1476-511X (Electronic), 1476-511X (Linking).

Clamon, G., Herndon, J., Cooper, R., Chang, A.Y., Rosenman, J., &Green, M.R. (1999). Radiosensitization with carboplatin for patients with unresectable stage III non-small-cell lung cancer: a phase III trial of the Cancer and Leukemia Group B and the Eastern Cooperative Oncology Group. *J Clin Oncol,* Vol. 17, No. 1, (Jan), pp. (4-11), 0732-183X (Print).

DeAngelis, L.M. (2001). Brain tumors. *N Engl J Med,* Vol. 344, No. 2, (Jan 11), pp. (114-123), 0028-4793 (Print).

Dent, P., Yacoub, A., Contessa, J., Caron, R., Amorino, G., Valerie, K., Hagan, M.P., Grant, S., &Schmidt-Ullrich, R. (2003). Stress and radiation-induced activation of multiple intracellular signaling pathways. *Radiat Res,* Vol. 159, No. 3, (Mar), pp. (283-300), 0033-7587 (Print), 0033-7587 (Linking).

Dietz, A., Boehm, A., Mozet, C., Wichmann, G., &Giannis, A. (2008). Current aspects of targeted therapy in head and neck tumors. *Eur Arch Otorhinolaryngol,* Vol. 265 No. Suppl 1, (Jul), pp. (S3-12), 0937-4477 (Print), 0937-4477 (Linking).

Du, R., Lu, K.V., Petritsch, C., Liu, P., Ganss, R., Passegue, E., Song, H., Vandenberg, S., Johnson, R.S., Werb, Z., *et al.* (2008). HIF1alpha induces the recruitment of bone marrow-derived vascular modulatory cells to regulate tumor angiogenesis and invasion. *Cancer Cell,* Vol. 13, No. 3, (Mar), pp. (206-220), 1878-3686 (Electronic), 1535-6108 (Linking).

Ellis, L.M., &Hicklin, D.J. (2008). VEGF-targeted therapy: mechanisms of anti-tumour activity. *Nat Rev Cancer,* Vol. 8, No. 8, (Aug), pp. (579-591), 1474-1768 (Electronic), 1474-175X (Linking).

Fang, X., Schummer, M., Mao, M., Yu, S., Tabassam, F.H., Swaby, R., Hasegawa, Y., Tanyi, J.L., LaPushin, R., Eder, A., *et al.* (2002). Lysophosphatidic acid is a bioactive mediator in ovarian cancer. *Biochim Biophys Acta,* Vol. 1582, No. 1-3, (May 23), pp. (257-264), 0006-3002 (Print), 0006-3002 (Linking).

Farooqui, A.A., Ong, W.Y., &Horrocks, L.A. (2006). Inhibitors of brain phospholipase A2 activity: their neuropharmacological effects and therapeutic importance for the treatment of neurologic disorders. *Pharmacol Rev,* Vol. 58, No. 3, (Sep), pp. (591-620), 0031-6997 (Print).

Fiskus, W., Wang, Y., Sreekumar, A., Buckley, K.M., Shi, H., Jillella, A., Ustun, C., Rao, R., Fernandez, P., Chen, J., *et al.* (2009). Combined epigenetic therapy with the histone methyltransferase EZH2 inhibitor 3-deazaneplanocin A and the histone deacetylase inhibitor panobinostat against human AML cells. *Blood,* Vol. 114, No. 13, (Sep 24), pp. (2733-2743), 1528-0020 (Electronic), 0006-4971 (Linking).

Folkman, J. (1971). Tumor angiogenesis: therapeutic implications. *N Engl J Med,* Vol. 285, No. 21, (Nov 18), pp. (1182-1186), 0028-4793 (Print).

Folkman, J. (2001). A new link in ovarian cancer angiogenesis: lysophosphatidic acid and vascular endothelial growth factor expression. *J Natl Cancer Inst,* Vol. 93, No. 10, (May 16), pp. (734-735), 0027-8874 (Print).

Forastiere, A.A., Trotti, A., Pfister, D.G., &Grandis, J.R. (2006). Head and neck cancer: recent advances and new standards of care. *J Clin Oncol,* Vol. 24, No. 17, (Jun 10), pp. (2603-2605), 1527-7755 (Electronic), 0732-183X (Linking).

Fujita, Y., Yoshizumi, M., Izawa, Y., Ali, N., Ohnishi, H., Kanematsu, Y., Ishizawa, K., Tsuchiya, K., &Tamaki, T. (2006). Transactivation of fetal liver kinase-1/kinase-insert domain-containing receptor by lysophosphatidylcholine induces vascular endothelial cell proliferation. *Endocrinology,* Vol. 147, No. 3, (Mar), pp. (1377-1385), 0013-7227 (Print), 0013-7227 (Linking).

Garcia-Barros, M., Paris, F., Cordon-Cardo, C., Lyden, D., Rafii, S., Haimovitz-Friedman, A., Fuks, Z., &Kolesnick, R. (2003). Tumor response to radiotherapy regulated by endothelial cell apoptosis. *Science,* Vol. 300, No. 5622, (May 16), pp. (1155-1159), 1095-9203 (Electronic), 0036-8075 (Linking).

Ha, C.H., &Jin, Z.G. (2009). Protein kinase D1, a new molecular player in VEGF signaling and angiogenesis. *Mol Cells,* Vol. 28, No. 1, (Jul 31), pp. (1-5), 0219-1032 (Electronic), 1016-8478 (Linking).

Haimovitz-Friedman, A., Kan, C.C., Ehleiter, D., Persaud, R.S., McLoughlin, M., Fuks, Z., &Kolesnick, R.N. (1994). Ionizing radiation acts on cellular membranes to generate ceramide and initiate apoptosis. *J Exp Med,* Vol. 180, No. 2, (Aug 1), pp. (525-535), 0022-1007 (Print).

Hama, K., Aoki, J., Fukaya, M., Kishi, Y., Sakai, T., Suzuki, R., Ohta, H., Yamori, T., Watanabe, M., Chun, J., *et al.* (2004). Lysophosphatidic acid and autotaxin stimulate cell motility of neoplastic and non-neoplastic cells through LPA1. *J Biol Chem,* Vol. 279, No. 17, (Apr 23), pp. (17634-17639), 0021-9258 (Print), 0021-9258 (Linking).

Hanahan, D., &Folkman, J. (1996). Patterns and emerging mechanisms of the angiogenic switch during tumorigenesis. *Cell,* Vol. 86, No. 3, (Aug 9), pp. (353-364), 0092-8674 (Print), 0092-8674 (Linking).

Herbert, S.P., Odell, A.F., Ponnambalam, S., &Walker, J.H. (2009). Activation of Cytosolic Phospholipase A2-{alpha} as a Novel Mechanism Regulating Endothelial Cell Cycle Progression and Angiogenesis. *J Biol Chem,* Vol. 284, No. 9, (Feb 27), pp. (5784-5796), 0021-9258 (Print).

Hicklin, D.J., &Ellis, L.M. (2005). Role of the vascular endothelial growth factor pathway in tumor growth and angiogenesis. *J Clin Oncol,* Vol. 23, No. 5, (Feb 10), pp. (1011-1027), 0732-183X (Print), 0732-183X (Linking).

Hirabayashi, T., Kume, K., Hirose, K., Yokomizo, T., Iino, M., Itoh, H., &Shimizu, T. (1999). Critical duration of intracellular Ca2+ response required for continuous translocation and activation of cytosolic phospholipase A2. *J Biol Chem,* Vol. 274, No. 8, (Feb 19), pp. (5163-5169), 0021-9258 (Print), 0021-9258 (Linking).

Hirabayashi, T., Murayama, T., &Shimizu, T. (2004). Regulatory mechanism and physiological role of cytosolic phospholipase A2. *Biol Pharm Bull,* Vol. 27, No. 8, (Aug), pp. (1168-1173), 0918-6158 (Print), 0918-6158 (Linking).

Hirabayashi, T., &Shimizu, T. (2000). Localization and regulation of cytosolic phospholipase A(2). *Biochim Biophys Acta,* Vol. 1488, No. 1-2, (Oct 31), pp. (124-138), 0006-3002 (Print), 0006-3002 (Linking).

Hoeglund, A.B., Howard, A.L., Wanjala, I.W., Pham, T.C., Parrill, A.L., &Baker, D.L. (2010). Characterization of non-lipid autotaxin inhibitors. *Bioorg Med Chem,* Vol. 18, No. 2, (Jan 15), pp. (769-776), 1464-3391 (Electronic), 0968-0896 (Linking).

Hoffman, P.C., Mauer, A.M., &Vokes, E.E. (2000). Lung cancer. *Lancet,* Vol. 355, No. 9202, (Feb 5), pp. (479-485), 0140-6736 (Print), 0140-6736 (Linking).

Im, D.S. (2010). Pharmacological tools for lysophospholipid GPCRs: development of agonists and antagonists for LPA and S1P receptors. *Acta Pharmacol Sin,* Vol. 31, No. 9, (Sep), pp. (1213-1222), 1745-7254 (Electronic), 1671-4083 (Linking).

Iranzo, V., Bremnes, R.M., Almendros, P., Gavila, J., Blasco, A., Sirera, R., &Camps, C. (2009). Induction chemotherapy followed by concurrent chemoradiation for patients with non-operable stage III non-small-cell lung cancer. *Lung Cancer,* Vol. 63, No. 1, (Jan), pp. (63-67), 0169-5002 (Print), 0169-5002 (Linking).

Iwamoto, F.M., Abrey, L.E., Beal, K., Gutin, P.H., Rosenblum, M.K., Reuter, V.E., DeAngelis, L.M., &Lassman, A.B. (2009). Patterns of relapse and prognosis after bevacizumab failure in recurrent glioblastoma. *Neurology,* Vol. 73, No. 15, (Oct 13), pp. (1200-1206), 1526-632X (Electronic), 0028-3878 (Linking).

Jain, R.K. (2005). Normalization of tumor vasculature: an emerging concept in antiangiogenic therapy. *Science,* Vol. 307, No. 5706, (Jan 7), pp. (58-62), 1095-9203 (Electronic), 0036-8075 (Linking).

Jansen, S., Stefan, C., Creemers, J.W., Waelkens, E., Van Eynde, A., Stalmans, W., &Bollen, M. (2005). Proteolytic maturation and activation of autotaxin (NPP2), a secreted metastasis-enhancing lysophospholipase D. *J Cell Sci,* Vol. 118, No. Pt 14, (Jul 15), pp. (3081-3089), 0021-9533 (Print), 0021-9533 (Linking).

Keller, T.H., Pichota, A., &Yin, Z. (2006). A practical view of 'druggability'. *Curr Opin Chem Biol,* Vol. 10, No. 4, (Aug), pp. (357-361), 1367-5931 (Print), 1367-5931 (Linking).

Kerbel, R.S. (1991). Inhibition of tumor angiogenesis as a strategy to circumvent acquired resistance to anti-cancer therapeutic agents. *Bioessays,* Vol. 13, No. 1, (Jan), pp. (31-36), 0265-9247 (Print), 0265-9247 (Linking).

Kishi, Y., Okudaira, S., Tanaka, M., Hama, K., Shida, D., Kitayama, J., Yamori, T., Aoki, J., Fujimaki, T., &Arai, H. (2006). Autotaxin is overexpressed in glioblastoma multiforme and contributes to cell motility of glioblastoma by converting lysophosphatidylcholine to lysophosphatidic acid. *J Biol Chem,* Vol. 281, No. 25, (Jun 23), pp. (17492-17500), 0021-9258 (Print).

LaValle, C.R., George, K.M., Sharlow, E.R., Lazo, J.S., Wipf, P., &Wang, Q.J. (2010). Protein kinase D as a potential new target for cancer therapy. *Biochim Biophys Acta,* Vol. 1806, No. 2, (Dec), pp. (183-192), 0006-3002 (Print), 0006-3002 (Linking).

Lee, J.H., Machtay, M., Kaiser, L.R., Friedberg, J.S., Hahn, S.M., McKenna, M.G., &McKenna, W.G. (1999). Non-small cell lung cancer: prognostic factors in patients treated with surgery and postoperative radiation therapy. *Radiology,* Vol. 213, No. 3, (Dec), pp. (845-852), 0033-8419 (Print).

Liebl, J., Krystof, V., Vereb, G., Takacs, L., Strnad, M., Pechan, P., Havlicek, L., Zatloukal, M., Furst, R., Vollmar, A.M., *et al.* (2011). Anti-angiogenic effects of purine inhibitors of cyclin dependent kinases. *Angiogenesis,* Vol. No. Apr 13), pp. 1573-7209 (Electronic), 0969-6970 (Linking).

Liebl, J., Weitensteiner, S.B., Vereb, G., Takacs, L., Furst, R., Vollmar, A.M., &Zahler, S. (2010). Cyclin-dependent kinase 5 regulates endothelial cell migration and angiogenesis. *J Biol Chem,* Vol. 285, No. 46, (Nov 12), pp. (35932-35943), 1083-351X (Electronic), 0021-9258 (Linking).

Linkous, A., Geng, L., Lyshchik, A., Hallahan, D.E., &Yazlovitskaya, E.M. (2009). Cytosolic Phospholipase A2: Targeting Cancer through the Tumor Vasculature. *Clin Cancer Res,* Vol. 15, No. 5, (Mar 1), pp. (1635-1644), 1078-0432 (Print).

Linkous, A.G., &Yazlovitskaya, E.M. (2011). Angiogenesis in Glioblastoma Multiforme: Navigating the Maze. *Anticancer Agents Med Chem,* Vol. No. Jun 27), pp. 1875-5992 (Electronic), 1871-5206 (Linking).

Linkous, A.G., Yazlovitskaya, E.M., &Hallahan, D.E. (2010). Cytosolic Phospholipase A2 and Lysophospholipids in Tumor Angiogenesis. *J Natl Cancer Inst,* Vol. 102, No. 18, (Aug 20), pp. (1398-1412), 1460-2105 (Electronic), 0027-8874 (Linking).

Lu, C., Han, H.D., Mangala, L.S., Ali-Fehmi, R., Newton, C.S., Ozbun, L., Armaiz-Pena, G.N., Hu, W., Stone, R.L., Munkarah, A., *et al.* (2010). Regulation of tumor angiogenesis by EZH2. *Cancer Cell,* Vol. 18, No. 2, (Aug 9), pp. (185-197), 1878-3686 (Electronic), 1535-6108 (Linking).

McGinn, C.J., Shewach, D.S., &Lawrence, T.S. (1996). Radiosensitizing nucleosides. *J Natl Cancer Inst,* Vol. 88, No. 17, (Sep 4), pp. (1193-1203), 0027-8874 (Print), 0027-8874 (Linking).

McKew, J.C., Foley, M.A., Thakker, P., Behnke, M.L., Lovering, F.E., Sum, F.W., Tam, S., Wu, K., Shen, M.W., Zhang, W., *et al.* (2006). Inhibition of cytosolic phospholipase A2alpha: hit to lead optimization. *J Med Chem,* Vol. 49, No. 1, (Jan 12), pp. (135-158), 0022-2623 (Print).

Norden, A.D., Drappatz, J., &Wen, P.Y. (2009). Antiangiogenic therapies for high-grade glioma. *Nat Rev Neurol,* Vol. 5, No. 11, (Nov), pp. (610-620), 1759-4766 (Electronic), 1759-4758 (Linking).

Parrill, A.L., &Baker, D.L. (2010). Autotaxin inhibitors: a perspective on initial medicinal chemistry efforts. *Expert Opin Ther Pat,* Vol. 20, No. 12, (Dec), pp. (1619-1625), 1744-7674 (Electronic), 1354-3776 (Linking).

Plate, K.H., Breier, G., Weich, H.A., Mennel, H.D., &Risau, W. (1994). Vascular endothelial growth factor and glioma angiogenesis: coordinate induction of VEGF receptors, distribution of VEGF protein and possible in vivo regulatory mechanisms. *Int J Cancer,* Vol. 59, No. 4, (Nov 15), pp. (520-529), 0020-7136 (Print), 0020-7136 (Linking).

Plate, K.H., Breier, G., Weich, H.A., &Risau, W. (1992). Vascular endothelial growth factor is a potential tumour angiogenesis factor in human gliomas in vivo. *Nature,* Vol. 359, No. 6398, (Oct 29), pp. (845-848), 0028-0836 (Print), 0028-0836 (Linking).

Prestwich, G.D., Gajewiak, J., Zhang, H., Xu, X., Yang, G., &Serban, M. (2008). Phosphatase-resistant analogues of lysophosphatidic acid: agonists promote healing, antagonists and autotaxin inhibitors treat cancer. *Biochim Biophys Acta,* Vol. 1781, No. 9, (Sep), pp. (588-594), 0006-3002 (Print), 0006-3002 (Linking).

Ptaszynska, M.M., Pendrak, M.L., Bandle, R.W., Stracke, M.L., &Roberts, D.D. (2008). Positive feedback between vascular endothelial growth factor-A and autotaxin in ovarian cancer cells. *Mol Cancer Res,* Vol. 6, No. 3, (Mar), pp. (352-363), 1541-7786 (Print).

Ptaszynska, M.M., Pendrak, M.L., Stracke, M.L., &Roberts, D.D. (2010). Autotaxin signaling via lysophosphatidic acid receptors contributes to vascular endothelial growth factor-induced endothelial cell migration. *Mol Cancer Res,* Vol. 8, No. 3, (Mar), pp. (309-321), 1557-3125 (Electronic), 1541-7786 (Linking).

Rastinejad, F., Polverini, P.J., &Bouck, N.P. (1989). Regulation of the activity of a new inhibitor of angiogenesis by a cancer suppressor gene. *Cell,* Vol. 56, No. 3, (Feb 10), pp. (345-355), 0092-8674 (Print), 0092-8674 (Linking).

Ren, J., Xiao, Y.J., Singh, L.S., Zhao, X., Zhao, Z., Feng, L., Rose, T.M., Prestwich, G.D., &Xu, Y. (2006). Lysophosphatidic acid is constitutively produced by human peritoneal mesothelial cells and enhances adhesion, migration, and invasion of ovarian cancer cells. *Cancer Res,* Vol. 66, No. 6, (Mar 15), pp. (3006-3014), 0008-5472 (Print), 0008-5472 (Linking).

Rubenstein, J.L., Kim, J., Ozawa, T., Zhang, M., Westphal, M., Deen, D.F., &Shuman, M.A. (2000). Anti-VEGF antibody treatment of glioblastoma prolongs survival but results in increased vascular cooption. *Neoplasia,* Vol. 2, No. 4, (Jul-Aug), pp. (306-314), 1522-8002 (Print), 1476-5586 (Linking).

Schmidt, N.O., Westphal, M., Hagel, C., Ergun, S., Stavrou, D., Rosen, E.M., &Lamszus, K. (1999). Levels of vascular endothelial growth factor, hepatocyte growth factor/scatter factor and basic fibroblast growth factor in human gliomas and their relation to angiogenesis. *Int J Cancer,* Vol. 84, No. 1, (Feb 19), pp. (10-18), 0020-7136 (Print), 0020-7136 (Linking).

Schulte, R.R., Linkous, A.G., Hallahan, D.E., &Yazlovitskaya, E.M. (2011). Cytosolic phospholipase A2 as a molecular target for the radiosensitization of ovarian cancer. *Cancer Lett,* Vol. 304, No. 2, (May 28), pp. (137-143), 1872-7980 (Electronic), 0304-3835 (Linking).

Stracke, M.L., Krutzsch, H.C., Unsworth, E.J., Arestad, A., Cioce, V., Schiffmann, E., &Liotta, L.A. (1992). Identification, purification, and partial sequence analysis of autotaxin, a novel motility-stimulating protein. *J Biol Chem,* Vol. 267, No. 4, (Feb 5), pp. (2524-2529), 0021-9258 (Print), 0021-9258 (Linking).

Stratford, I.J. (1992). Concepts and developments in radiosensitization of mammalian cells. *Int J Radiat Oncol Biol Phys,* Vol. 22, No. 3, (Jul 19), pp. (529-532), 0360-3016 (Print), 0360-3016 (Linking).

Strijbos, M.H., Gratama, J.W., Kraan, J., Lamers, C.H., den Bakker, M.A., &Sleijfer, S. (2008). Circulating endothelial cells in oncology: pitfalls and promises. *Br J Cancer,* Vol. 98, No. 11, (Jun 3), pp. (1731-1735), 1532-1827 (Electronic).

Suh, J.H., &Barnett, G.H. (1999). Brachytherapy for brain tumor. *Hematol Oncol Clin North Am,* Vol. 13, No. 3, (Jun), pp. (635-650, viii-ix), 0889-8588 (Print).

Tanaka, M., Okudaira, S., Kishi, Y., Ohkawa, R., Iseki, S., Ota, M., Noji, S., Yatomi, Y., Aoki, J., &Arai, H. (2006). Autotaxin stabilizes blood vessels and is required for embryonic vasculature by producing lysophosphatidic acid. *J Biol Chem,* Vol. 281, No. 35, (Sep 1), pp. (25822-25830), 0021-9258 (Print).

Tokumura, A., Harada, K., Fukuzawa, K., &Tsukatani, H. (1986). Involvement of lysophospholipase D in the production of lysophosphatidic acid in rat plasma. *Biochim Biophys Acta,* Vol. 875, No. 1, (Jan 3), pp. (31-38), 0006-3002 (Print), 0006-3002 (Linking).

Tokumura, A., Kume, T., Fukuzawa, K., Tahara, M., Tasaka, K., Aoki, J., Arai, H., Yasuda, K., &Kanzaki, H. (2007). Peritoneal fluids from patients with certain gynecologic tumor contain elevated levels of bioactive lysophospholipase D activity. *Life Sci,* Vol. 80, No. 18, (Apr 10), pp. (1641-1649), 0024-3205 (Print), 0024-3205 (Linking).

Tokumura, A., Miyake, M., Yoshimoto, O., Shimizu, M., &Fukuzawa, K. (1998). Metal-ion stimulation and inhibition of lysophospholipase D which generates bioactive lysophosphatidic acid in rat plasma. *Lipids,* Vol. 33, No. 10, (Oct), pp. (1009-1015), 0024-4201 (Print), 0024-4201 (Linking).

Tokuuye, K., Akine, Y., Sumi, M., Kagami, Y., Ikeda, H., Oyama, H., Inou, Y., Shibui, S., &Nomura, K. (1998). Reirradiation of brain and skull base tumors with fractionated stereotactic radiotherapy. *Int J Radiat Oncol Biol Phys,* Vol. 40, No. 5, (Mar 15), pp. (1151-1155), 0360-3016 (Print), 0360-3016 (Linking).

Umezu-Goto, M., Kishi, Y., Taira, A., Hama, K., Dohmae, N., Takio, K., Yamori, T., Mills, G.B., Inoue, K., Aoki, J., *et al.* (2002). Autotaxin has lysophospholipase D activity leading to tumor cell growth and motility by lysophosphatidic acid production. *J Cell Biol,* Vol. 158, No. 2, (Jul 22), pp. (227-233), 0021-9525 (Print), 0021-9525 (Linking).

Valerie, K., Yacoub, A., Hagan, M.P., Curiel, D.T., Fisher, P.B., Grant, S., &Dent, P. (2007). Radiation-induced cell signaling: inside-out and outside-in. *Mol Cancer Ther,* Vol. 6, No. 3, (Mar), pp. (789-801), 1535-7163 (Print).

van der Meel, R., Symons, M.H., Kudernatsch, R., Kok, R.J., Schiffelers, R.M., Storm, G., Gallagher, W.M., &Byrne, A.T. (2011). The VEGF/Rho GTPase signalling pathway: a promising target for anti-angiogenic/anti-invasion therapy. *Drug Discov Today,* Vol. 16, No. 5-6, (Mar), pp. (219-228), 1878-5832 (Electronic), 1359-6446 (Linking).

Videtic, G.M., Gaspar, L.E., Zamorano, L., Fontanesi, J., Levin, K.J., Kupsky, W.J., &Tekyi-Mensah, S. (1999). Use of the RTOG recursive partitioning analysis to validate the benefit of iodine-125 implants in the primary treatment of malignant gliomas. *Int J Radiat Oncol Biol Phys,* Vol. 45, No. 3, (Oct 1), pp. (687-692), 0360-3016 (Print).

Volk, L.D., Flister, M.J., Bivens, C.M., Stutzman, A., Desai, N., Trieu, V., &Ran, S. (2008). Nab-paclitaxel efficacy in the orthotopic model of human breast cancer is significantly enhanced by concurrent anti-vascular endothelial growth factor A therapy. *Neoplasia,* Vol. 10, No. 6, (Jun), pp. (613-623), 1476-5586 (Electronic), 1476-5586 (Linking).

Volk, L.D., Flister, M.J., Chihade, D., Desai, N., Trieu, V., &Ran, S. (2011). Synergy of nab-paclitaxel and bevacizumab in eradicating large orthotopic breast tumors and preexisting metastases. *Neoplasia,* Vol. 13, No. 4, (Apr), pp. (327-338), 1476-5586 (Electronic), 1476-5586 (Linking).

Wagner, H., Jr. (2000). Postoperative adjuvant therapy for patients with resected non-small cell lung cancer: still controversial after all these years. *Chest,* Vol. 117, No. 4 Suppl 1, (Apr), pp. (110S-118S), 0012-3692 (Print).

Wesierska-Gadek, J., Gritsch, D., Zulehner, N., Komina, O., &Maurer, M. (2011). Roscovitine, a selective CDK inhibitor, reduces the basal and estrogen-induced phosphorylation of ER-alpha in human ER-positive breast cancer cells. *J Cell Biochem,* Vol. 112, No. 3, (Mar), pp. (761-772), 1097-4644 (Electronic), 0730-2312 (Linking).

Willett, C.G., Boucher, Y., di Tomaso, E., Duda, D.G., Munn, L.L., Tong, R.T., Chung, D.C., Sahani, D.V., Kalva, S.P., Kozin, S.V., *et al.* (2004). Direct evidence that the VEGF-specific antibody bevacizumab has antivascular effects in human rectal cancer. *Nat Med,* Vol. 10, No. 2, (Feb), pp. (145-147), 1078-8956 (Print), 1078-8956 (Linking).

Xu, X., &Prestwich, G.D. (2010). Inhibition of tumor growth and angiogenesis by a lysophosphatidic acid antagonist in an engineered three-dimensional lung cancer xenograft model. *Cancer,* Vol. 116, No. 7, (Apr 1), pp. (1739-1750), 0008-543X (Print), 0008-543X (Linking).

Yamaguchi, J., Sasaki, M., Sato, Y., Itatsu, K., Harada, K., Zen, Y., Ikeda, H., Nimura, Y., Nagino, M., &Nakanuma, Y. (2010). Histone deacetylase inhibitor (SAHA) and repression of EZH2 synergistically inhibit proliferation of gallbladder carcinoma. *Cancer Sci,* Vol. 101, No. 2, (Feb), pp. (355-362), 1349-7006 (Electronic), 1347-9032 (Linking).

Yazlovitskaya, E.M., Linkous, A.G., Thotala, D.K., Cuneo, K.C., &Hallahan, D.E. (2008). Cytosolic phospholipase A2 regulates viability of irradiated vascular endothelium. *Cell Death Differ,* Vol. 15, No. 10, (Oct), pp. (1641-1653), 1350-9047 (Print).

Zhan, M., &Han, Z.C. (2004). Phosphatidylinositide 3-kinase/AKT in radiation responses. *Histol Histopathol,* Vol. 19, No. 3, (Jul), pp. (915-923), 0213-3911 (Print).

Zhang, H., Xu, X., Gajewiak, J., Tsukahara, R., Fujiwara, Y., Liu, J., Fells, J.I., Perygin, D., Parrill, A.L., Tigyi, G., *et al.* (2009). Dual activity lysophosphatidic acid receptor pan-antagonist/autotaxin inhibitor reduces breast cancer cell migration in vitro and causes tumor regression in vivo. *Cancer Res,* Vol. 69, No. 13, (Jul 1), pp. (5441-5449), 1538-7445 (Electronic), 0008-5472 (Linking).

Zingg, D., Riesterer, O., Fabbro, D., Glanzmann, C., Bodis, S., &Pruschy, M. (2004). Differential activation of the phosphatidylinositol 3'-kinase/Akt survival pathway by ionizing radiation in tumor and primary endothelial cells. *Cancer Res,* Vol. 64, No. 15, (Aug 1), pp. (5398-5406), 0008-5472 (Print).

13

Molecular Mechanisms of Tumor Angiogenesis

Kelly Burrell and Gelareh Zadeh
University of Toronto
Toronto Western Hospital, University Health Network
Canada

1. Introduction

It is well established that progression from a pre-malignant to malignant invasive tumor phenotype is dependent on angiogenesis[1-7]. As such, a hallmark of all solid cancers is their ability to induce the formation of their own blood supply thereby sustaining their growth and is characterized by increases in endothelial cell (EC) proliferation and blood vessel heterogeneity[8-10]. The 'angiogenic switch', is a complex balance of multiple pro- and anti-angiogenic factors secreted by both host and tumor cells, which when balanced in favor of pro-angiogenic factors will trigger new vessel formation (**Figure 1**)[1-7]. The expression of these pro- and anti- angiogenic regulators is dependent on various physiological and pathological factors in addition to the tumor type, stage and microenvironment[2,8]. It has been shown previously that although tumor angiogenesis to some extent recapitulates the normal process of angiogenesis, it is not well organized and leads to the majority of solid cancers having tortuous and dilated vessels that have abnormal physiological function. This commonly leads to insufficient blood flow, poor delivery of oxygen and nutrients, inadequate removal of waste, increased vessel permeability and tumor edema due to alteration in EC tight junctions and contacts[2,11-15]. These inefficiencies in blood flow result in changes within tumor microenvironment that can trigger further expression of a battery of angiogenic factors, setting up a continuous cycle of dysfunctional vessel formation[1,2,8,9]. The precise mechanisms governing expression of pro- or anti-angiogenic factors are still not fully understood. In response to oncogene activation and/or metabolic stress, such as that seen in solid tumors, tumor cells can directly secrete growth factors including vascular endothelial growth factor (VEGF) and Angiopoietin-1 (Ang-1) stimulating the angiogenic switch to enhance vessel formation[17-23] (**Figure 1**), or attracting macrophages that can indirectly promote release of angiogenic factors[10]. Multiple candidate factors that signal tumor cells to initiate this cascade have been proposed[1,2,11-14]. The main contributors include hypoxia and increased physical forces, both generated in rapidly growing tumors, that disrupt the EC connections within the extracellular matrix (ECM), and the products of oncogenes and mutated tumor suppressor genes[1,2,11-14]. The relative contribution of various angiogenic pathways, their interactions and combinatorial impact on tumor angiogenesis is not precisely known and requires further characterization in order to establish a comprehensive picture of tumor angiogenesis.

Principles of anti-angiogenic therapy

Originally, the knowledge that tumor angiogenesis was vital for solid tumor growth held much promise for designing efficacious treatments for cancer, with the hope of arresting tumor growth and progression, therefore maintaining a patients health in a stable

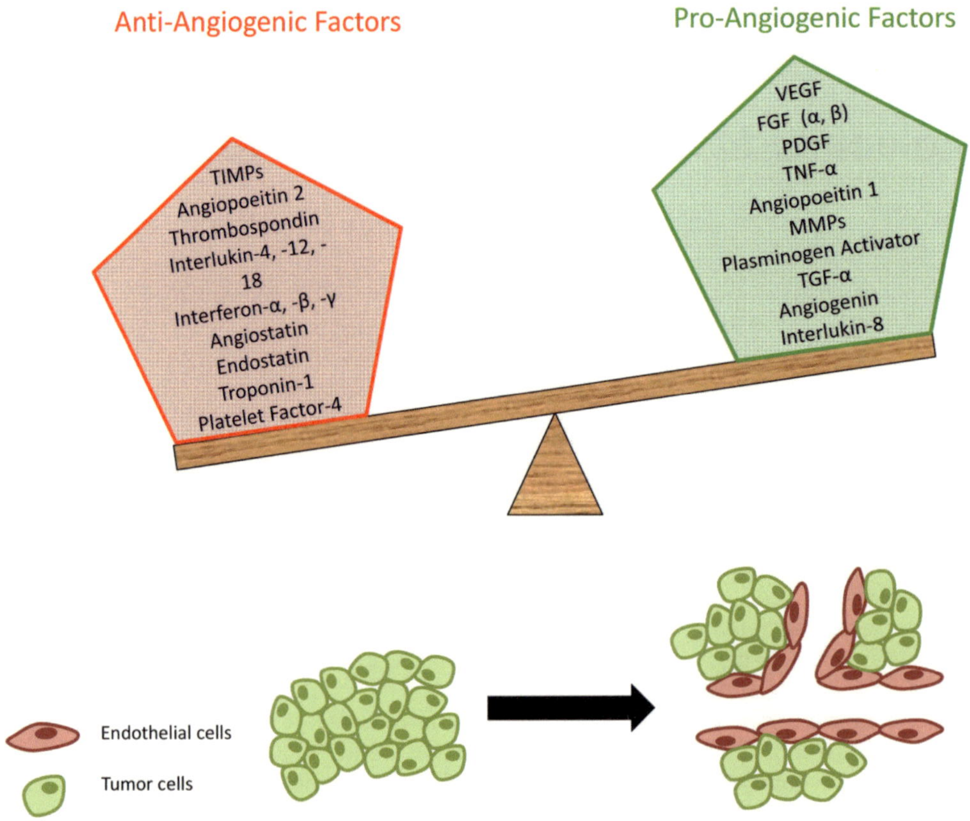

Fig. 1. The Angiogenic Switch
A complex balance between pro- and anti- angiogenic factors exists in all microenvironments and is instrumental in the enhancement or decrease in vessel formation. The main angiogenic factors that have so far been elucidated are listed, not all of their mechanisms are fully understood.

asymptomatic state. Anti-angiogenic cytostatic agents were thought to have several advantages over the traditional cytotoxic chemotherapeutic agents[7,13,15-18]. First, it was hypothesized that regardless of the extent of tumor heterogeneity, tumor angiogenesis is a non-neoplastic homogenous process; hence anti-angiogenic strategies would be efficacious against a variety of human solid cancers. Second, the issue of resistance to chemo- or radiation therapy (CT or RT) of tumor cells would not apply to the angiogenic component of a solid cancer. Third, the vascular compartment is readily accessible and no interstitial pressure would be required to reach the targeted ECs. Fourth, the presence of up-regulated and altered EC receptors in tumor vasculature, would permit specific targeting of therapeutic molecules to tumor vasculature, while normal blood vessels would not be targeted.

Overall the results of anti-angiogenic based clinical trials, however, have been somewhat disappointing[12,19]. With increased understanding and experience using anti-angiogenic treatment, certain limitations and causes for failure of anti-angiogenic therapy have come to light [8,12,19]. One of the principle realizations being that the process of tumor angiogenesis is as heterogeneous as tumor cells, and the dynamics of tumor vessel biology alters with tumor type, tumor stage and phase of tumor growth. Other reasons are that these trials have either targeted only one angiogenic pathway, or in several instances the exact anti-angiogenic mechanism is not known. We therefore need to expand our knowledge of the qualitative differences in tumor vessel formation that are specific to each tumor and individualize the therapeutic approach. We also need a more detailed understanding of the relevant angiogenic regulators in specific tumors, which differ according to tumor microenvironment, in order to generate target specific agents for testing in clinical trials Additional reasons why there has been some disappointment in the efficacy of translation of pre-clinical results to clinical trials include: (1) a lack of appropriate pre-clinical tumor models. To date, primarily xenograft models have been used where tumors are grown in an ectopic microenvironment in an immune deficient mouse. (2) There has been a lack of end-points of treatment and surrogate markers of response to anti-angiogenic therapy. To date, the primary method for establishing response has been measurement of tumor size in xenograft models, extent of EC apoptosis, number of EC progenitor cell (EPC) circulators and changes in EC signaling. Dynamic imaging of tumor characteristics in response to treatment would be of significant clinical and translational value. The future direction of tumor angiogenesis and anti-angiogenic therapy will focus on designing small animal imaging modalities that will best identify the extent of effective and functional blood flow within a tumor vascular network and the impact of treatment on the dynamic blood supply of a tumor. By establishing these methodologies we can then translate end-points of therapeutic response to drug more accurately that can be applied to clinical therapy.

An important evolution in anti-angiogenic therapy is the use of combinatorial therapy. Combinatorial therapy takes advantage of using anti-angiogenic strategies together with RT in order to improve the clinical efficacy of both treatment modalities. The principle of combinatorial therapy in large part relies on the concept of 'vascular normalization', which was introduced and popularized primarily by Rakesh Jain over the past decade. Vascular normalization states that abnormal pathological tumor vasculature, in response to anti-angiogenic therapy, becomes normalized and results in a window of opportunity during which more efficient tumor blood flow can be delivered to the tumor, improving delivery of tumor oxygenation and therapeutics, and ultimately response to RT [20-22]. Improvement in tissue oxygenation in particular the centre of tumor increases the functionality of RT ad CT in the tumor.

The precise timing of this window of opportunity and extent by which 'vascular normalization' improves response to RT however remains unknown. There are some pre-clinical studies and early clinical trials that have explored the therapeutic benefits of combining anti-angiogenesis with RT, but results have been inconsistent[34,37-48] and the optimal scheduling of these adjuvant treatments has to be established. Moreover, individual tumor type plays a significant role in determining the correct combinatorial scheduling and very few studies have focused on brain tumors.

1.1 Normal vessel formation: Vasculogenesis and angiogenesis

Our understanding of the molecular mechanisms of tumor angiogenesis heavily relies and derives from studies of the mechanisms of normal vessel development. Vascularization is critical for embryonal development and normal physiological functions in large multi-cellular organisms. It is also pivotal for the progression of a multitude of pathological processes.[6,7,23-27]. The primitive vascular network is modified by the process of angiogenesis, leading to maturation, branching and formation of a complex vascular network[6,7,9,23,28].

During physiological angiogenesis new vessels are formed from pre-existing ones via sprouting and non-sprouting mechanisms[6,7,9,23,28] concomitant with an increased interaction between EC and the pericytes (PC) and smooth muscle cells (SMC) of the ECM, creating a stabilized vascular network (**Figure 2 and 3**)[9,28]. The main organs that are vascularized primarily by angiogenesis are mesodermal organs such as the kidney and brain that do not contain angioblasts[6,7,9,23,28]. In addition to maturation of the vasculature into a complex network, determination of vessel fate is also a crucial aspect of normal vessel development[29,30]. Vessel fate was originally thought to be regulated by hemodynamic factors such as blood flow, extent of blood oxygenation, blood pressure and alteration in other blood and microenvironmental characteristics [29,30]. However, recent evidence suggests that it is primarily governed by genetic regulation and cytokines such as Ephrins and the Notch signaling pathway [29,30]. Normal angiogenesis is vital for wound healing and for the development of the endometrium during the uterine cycle. Angiogenesis is prevelant in pathological conditions such as tumor growth, ischemia, vascular malformations and inflammatory reactions however, the process is particularly abberant leading to the

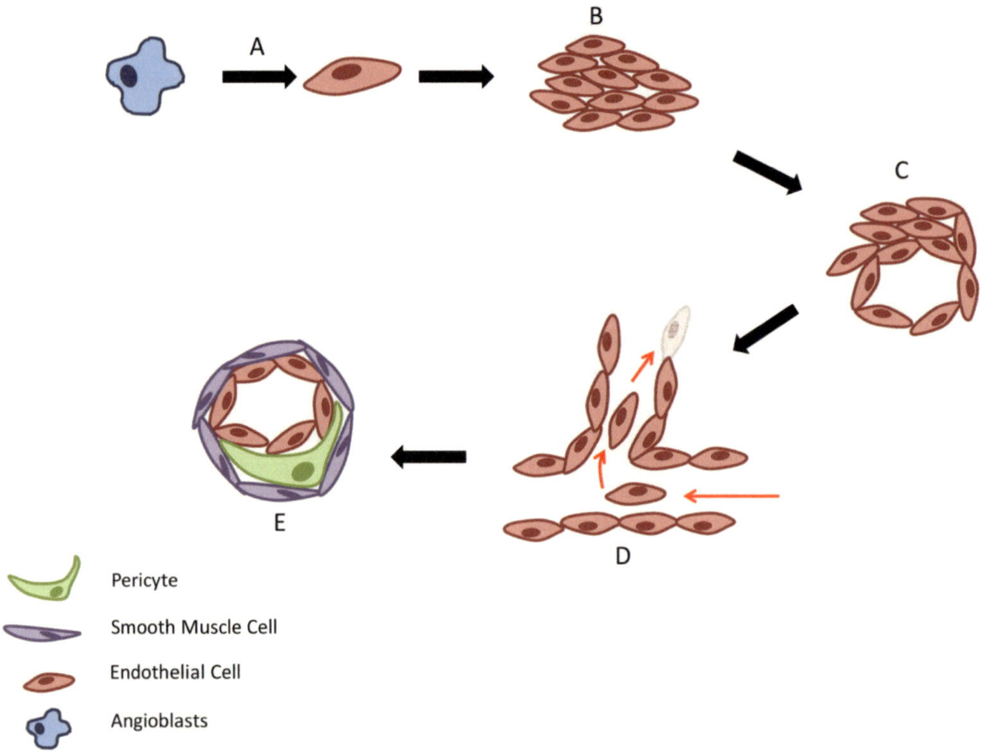

Fig. 2. The process of Physiological New Vessel Formation
A. Angioblasts differentiate to form endothelial cells ***B.*** Endothelial cells proliferate to form blood islands ***C.*** Blood islands coalesce to form hollow lumen vessels or primitive vascular tubes that subsequently form a primary vascular network ***D.*** Maturation of the vessel leads to new vessels sprouting through migration and proliferation of ECs with reassembly into new lumens ***E.*** The last step in the process of angiogenesis is stabilization of the vessels through recruitment of PC and SMC surrounding the vessel.

torturous heterogeneic vessels that have come to be associated with tumor vascular networks[19,31]. In some disease processes such as cerebral ischemia the angiogenic response is deficient, while in other disease processes, such as tumor angiogenesis or vascular malformation, there is excessive angiogenesis resulting in vessels that are abnormal in structure and function[19,31].

An alternative pathway for vessel formation is vasculogenesis, a process whereby mesenchymal progenitors migrate from the bone marrow (BM) and differentiate into ECs[6]. In turn, mesenchymal derived ECs then proliferate to form a *de-novo* primitive vascular network in an a vascular tissue in the process of in-situ angiogenesis (**Figure 3 and 4**)[6,7,23]. The main organs that are vascularized by means of vasculogenesis include the heart, great vessels, spleen and other endodermal organs[6,7,23]. Vasculogenesis has long been thought of as a pre-natal stage vessel formation occurring exclusively in the developing embryo. However, recent data has speculated that neovascularization in adult life, both in pathological and physiological conditions, can also occur by vasculogenesis[58-61], and is particularly prevalent in large-solid cancers[62].

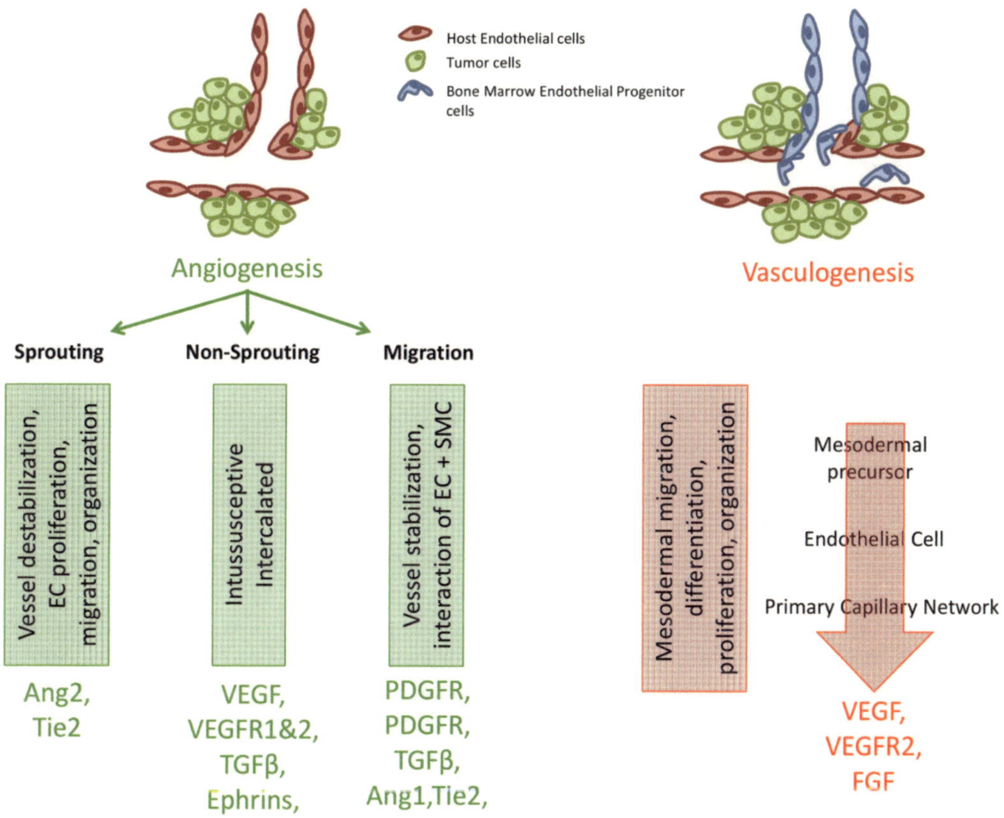

Fig. 3. Regulators of neo-angiogenesis

Although not fully understood the various Pro- and Anti- angiogenic factors can be broadly linked to specific mechanisms underlying neo-angiogenesis. As there is a high level of redundancy within this system many of the factors have multiple functions and multiple factors can be involved in each step.

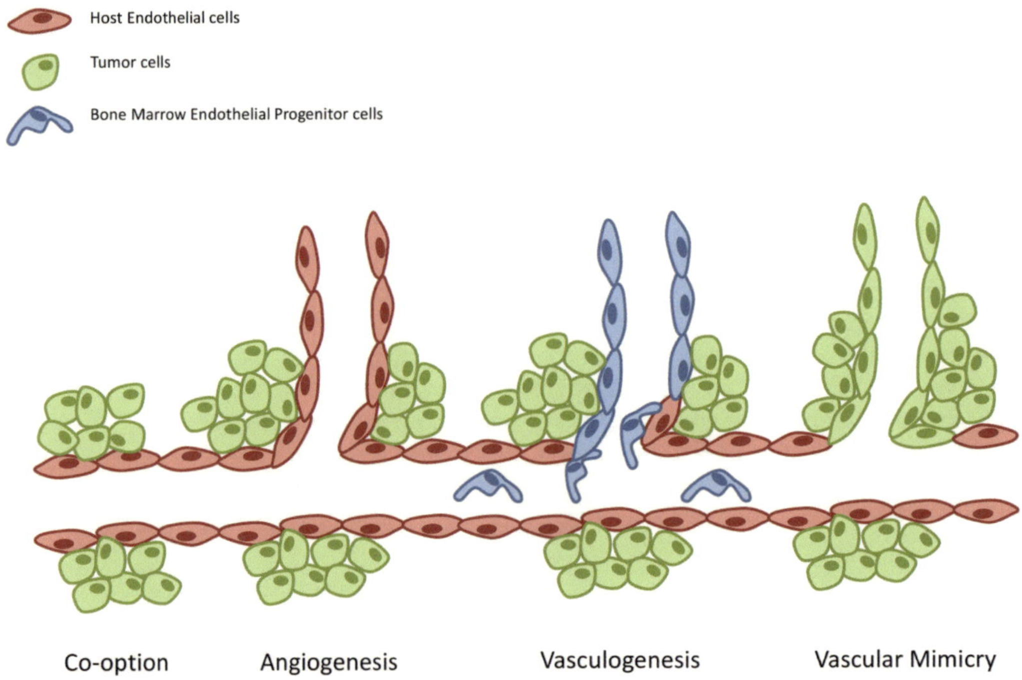

Fig. 4. Mechanisms of Tumor Neo-angiogenesis
Tumor angiogenesis is thought to arise from 4 mechanisms:
Co-option - the colonization of existing vessels
Angiogenesis - the branching and colonization of existing vessels
Vasculogenesis - the formation of new vessels *de novo* from circulating EC progenitors migrating from the bone marrow
Vascular Mimicry - the newest suggested source of vessels whereby the tumor cells directly transdifferentiate into EC forming their own vessels

Circulating BM-derived endothelial progenitor cells (EPC), the adult counterpart of embryonic angioblasts, were first isolated over 15 years ago from the peripheral blood of patients with vascular trauma, septic shock, sickle cell anemia and cancer[63,64]. Accumulating evidence indicates that these EPCs can be mobilized from the BM to initiate *de novo* vessel formation in response to oncogenic mediators in solid cancers[65-67 6,7,23]. When isolated from circulation and exposed to angiogenic factors, they formed highly proliferative endothelial-like colonies[63,64]. However, there is controversy as to whether these BM derived cells (BMDCs) contribute directly to vessel endothelium as ECs or as perivascular cells (PVC) and whether this varies with tumor type, growth stage and potentially in response to treatment[58,63,68-72]. A variety of BMDCs have so far been linked to vasculogenesis, however conflicting results exist over the degree of these BMDCs influence on the vascular endothelium. In particular EPCs[73-78], CD11b+ myeloid cells[79], Tie2+ monocytes[80,81], VEGFR1+ hemangiocytes, and tumor associated macrophages (TAM) [82,83] have all been seen to come from the BM and incorporate into tumors and their vasculature both directly, through generation of endothelium and indirectly, by stabilizing the tumor vasculature through localizing around the perivascular regions[62-64,84].

On the basis of recent studies, it appears that some, but definitely not all, experimental tumors and types of ischemia utilize vasculogenesis in generating their blood vessel endothelium, emphasizing the need to identify factors that may promote vasculogenesis. Once these factors are identified, possible therapeutic applications are numerous, including: (1) enhancing the pharmacologic ability to stimulate neovascularization after ischemia or disrupt tumor vasculature by targeting all types of vessel formation and (2) a gene therapy approach in which BM or EPCs are utilized as cellular delivery vehicles to deliver therapeutic genes to ischemic areas or tumors [63,64].

Alternate mechanisms of tumor neovasculogenesis exist including Co-option, whereby the tumor cells will accumulate around existing vessels and colonize the already efficient vascular networks. Although less supporting evidence exists, it has also been suggested that tumor cells themselves transdifferentiate into EC which are then able to form functional vessels in the tumor **(Figure 4).**

1.2 Molecular regulators of angiogenesis

A large number of endogenous pro- and anti-angiogenic factors have been identified **(Figure 1)**[1,14,18,19,31] whose signaling pathways interact in a highly complex and coordinated manner in order to produce functional vessels **(Figure 3).** Each angiogenic factor can play multiple roles depending on the context in which it is expressed. The regulatory role of each molecule is dependent on the microenvironment, the temporal and spatial expression profile, and the combinatorial effect of other angiogenic factors[32]. Additionally, angiogenesis is indirectly regulated by many transcriptional factors, oncogenes and tumor suppressor genes, which regulate other aspects of cellular function such as proliferation, apoptosis and motility[1]. Among the angiogenic factors identified, there are three groups that are thought to have an endothelial specific role, because their receptors are found exclusively on ECs[32]. These three groups are: VEGF, which binds to its receptors VEGFR1/Flt-1 and VEGFR2/Flk-1/KDR, Angiopoetins (Ang1 and Ang2), which bind to their receptors Tie2/TEK, and the more recently identified EphrinA and EphrinB, which bind to EphA and EphB receptors[32]. All three classes make a critical contribution to mature vessel formation **(Figure 3 and 5)**.

1.2.1 Pleotropic angiogenic factors

Several cytokines are direct regulators of angiogenesis in addition to being indirect modulators of EC specific factors such as VEGF[26,33]. Acidic and Basic Fibroblastic Growth Factor (aFGF, bFGF), were amongst the first cytokines implicated closely in angiogenesis[26,34]. FGFs (aFGF and bFGF) induce EC proliferation, migration and tubule formation, in addition to providing a mitogenic signal to many other cell types[2,26]. However, in transgenic knock-out mice for FGFs vessel development is normal, suggesting a level of redundancy in the pathway. Platelet Derived Growth Factor (PDGF) activate their receptors, homo- or hetero-dimeric complexes of PDGF-α or PDGF–β ($\alpha\alpha$,$\alpha\beta$,$\beta\beta$) subunits[88-90] (**Figure** 5). Increased expression of PDGF-β is noted in these PVC both physiologically and in many solid tumors, and activation of PDGF receptors results in proliferation of many cell types including astrocytes. Transforming growth factor-β (TGF-β) is able to regulate EC biology directly, affecting proliferation, differentiation, adhesion and apoptosis, and indirectly by upregulating VEGF[26]. There is speculation that at low doses TGF-β stimulates, while at high doses it inhibits growth of ECs, with a similar effect on EC tubule formation[35,36].

Additionally, TGF-β is thought to regulate angiogenesis by acting as a chemotactic agent for monocytes, fibroblasts and other inflammatory agents important in angiogenesis [26].

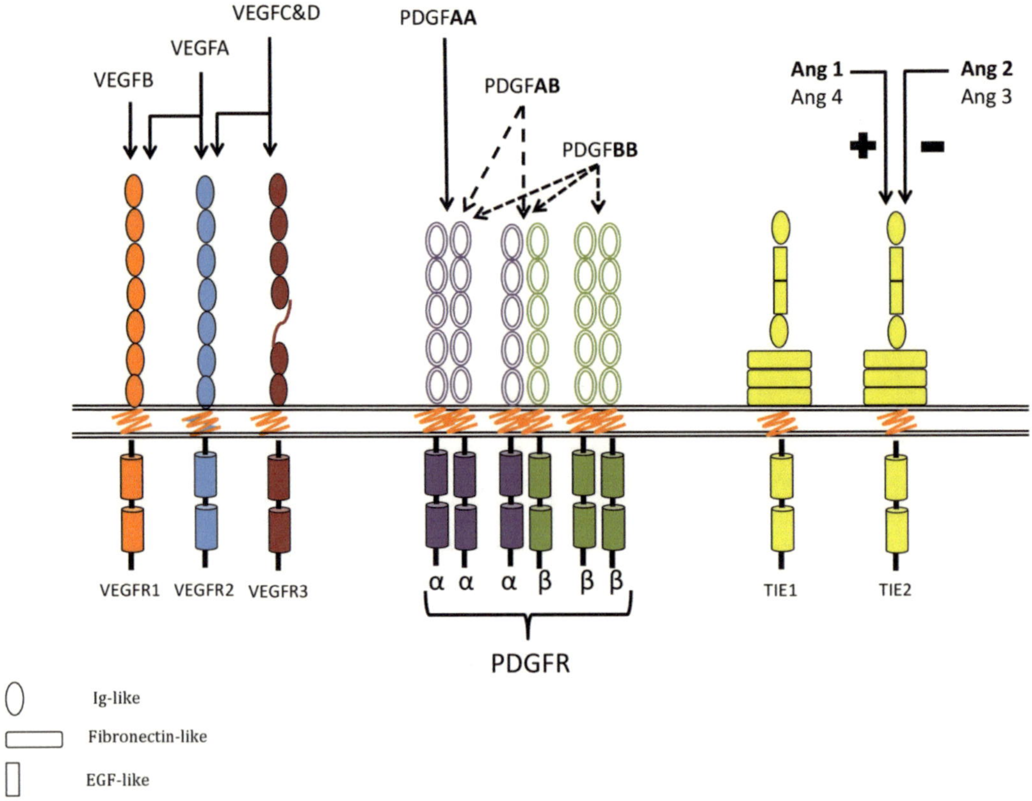

Fig. 5. Diagrammatic representation of VEGF, PDGF and Ang signaling
Schematic demonstrates the numerous interactions feasible amongst each signaling family, suggestive of the level of redundancy in these pathways determined by the microenvironment and so presence of signals and receptors.

1.2.2 Role of the extracellular matrix in tumor angiogenesis

Angiogenesis takes place in a complex ECM, which is critical for modulation of EC behavior. The ECM is composed of highly organized proteins and proteoglycans, and its composition effects EC shape, structure and proliferation, together with EC growth factor expression and interactions with blood vessels[37]. Remodeling of the ECM is a pre-requisite for formation of new blood vessels. The basement membrane provides structural support to the vasculature and is composed of type IV collagen, laminin and fibronectin[38]. Proteases such as Matrix Metalloproteinases (MMPs), and their tissue inhibitors, (TIMPs), regulate the breakdown of ECM and are associated with tissue destruction in many pathologic settings[38-40]. The relative contribution of individual MMPs to vessel formation is not precisely understood, however, certain MMPs are thought to have a more specific angiogenic regulatory role, in particular MMP-2 (gelatinaseA) and MMP-9 (gelatinaseB) both cleave collagen type IV, fibronectin and laminin, the major components of blood vessel basement membrane[41]. Various microenvironmental factors contribute to the regulation of MMPs including direct interactions of angiogenic factors. For instance, bFGF upregulates the expression of the gelatinases (MMP-2 and MMP-9), whereas VEGF markedly increases only the expression of MMP-2[42]. TIMPs tightly regulate the extent of MMPs activity in addition to directly inhibiting endothelial cell invasion, proliferation and migration. Therefore, identification of TIMPs holds great potential for designing effective anti-angiogenic treatment.

1.2.3 Role of Endothelial cell specific angiogenic factors

Vascular Endothelial Growth Factor

The best-characterized and most extensively studied EC-specific angiogenic factor is Vascular Endothelial Growth Factor-A, commonly referred to as VEGF, with the isoform VEGF-165 being the major secreted isoform and most abundant in human brains[27,43]. The various isoforms, which exist have distinct angiogenic roles, demonstrating organ specificity and making unique contributions to vessel development. VEGF through paracrine activation of its receptors VEGFR1 (Flt-1), VEGFR2 (Flk-1/KDR) that are predominantly expressed by ECs, triggers differentiation of EC precursors, promotes EC survival, mitogenesis and migration leading to the formation of tubule structures and neoangiogenesis[31] (**Figures 3 and 5**).

The critical role of VEGF in vessel development is demonstrated in knock-out mice, where deletions of a single allele of the VEGF gene is is embryonic lethal, due to lack of vessel formation in addition to deficient blood island formation in the yolk sac[44]. The biological response to VEGF is highly dose dependent, requiring strict control of *in vivo* VEGF expression for normal vessel formation[45,46]. Over-expression of VEGF in a dose dependent manner is also detrimental, leading to abnormal vessels characterized by an attenuated compact layer of myocardium, remodeling of the large vessels and tortuous and dilated epicardial vessels[100,102,103,].

During adult life, VEGF expression is low to absent in most organs, including the brain, other than at sites of physiological neo-angiogenesis[33,47,48] however, at sites where new vessel formation is required, VEGF is up-regulated. Various regulators of VEGF have been identified, the most prominent being hypoxia, which acts to regulate VEGF expression at both the transcriptional and post-transcriptional levels[49].

Although hypoxia is the most important physiological regulator of VEGF, other growth factors also play a role. Specific cytokines and receptors and their major downstream signaling pathways, are usually considered to be important mitogenic regulators, but also indirectly regulate expression of VEGF and VEGF receptors. In gliomas, some of these cytokine/receptors pathways include activated Epidermal Growth Factor Receptors (EGFR) or PDGFR and their signaling pathways such as those mediated by activation of p21-Ras or PI3-Kinase[33,49,50]. In specific, relating to tumor-mediated angiogenesis, VEGF is regulated by mutations in oncogenes and tumor suppressor genes, suggesting they act to initially trigger the signalling events involved in new vessel formation, thereby supporting further proliferation of tumor cells. It has been previously demonstrated that P53 and *ras* activating mutations result in a marked upregulation of VEGF expression. The cross talks between mitogenic and angiogenic signals, mediated by VEGF, are of high relevance, particularly in solid tumor vascularization.

Angiopoietins and Tie2/TEK Receptor

Angiopoietins, (Ang1/2) are important modulators of angiogenesis and are a second class of angiogenic factors to have their receptor expressed exclusively on ECs[31]. The two main family members are Ang1 and Ang2, with their cognate EC specific receptor being Tie2/TEK[51-53]. Ang1 is the activating ligand to Tie2/TEK[53], while Ang2 is the naturally occurring antagonist (**Figure 5**). The expression pattern for Ang1 and Ang2, and their isoforms, among variable tumor cell lines has been examined and suggests an as of yet undetermined role for the different isoforms in pathological scenarios [111,112].

Early in mouse development, Ang1 is found prominently in the myocardium and endocardium whilst later in development, it is primarily seen in the mesenchyme surrounding developing vessels, in close in close proximity to ECs[53,54]. This expression pattern suggested that Ang1 plays a role in the development of the heart and vascular structures[53,54]; however, a direct role in angiogenesis was not easily evident, since unlike the EC mitogenic signals of VEGF, Ang1 has no direct effect on EC proliferation[53,54]. Deletion of Tie2/TEK caused embryonic lethality due to defects in vascular development, characterized by a reduction in EC number, defect in the morphogenesis of microvessels, compromised heart development and internal hemorrhage[51].

Ang2 expression was primarily observed in the major vessels such as the dorsal aorta, but not in all vascular structures[55]. In adult life, Ang2 is present at sites of vascular remodeling such as in the ovary, placenta, uterus and other areas of active neo-vascularization[55]. Interestingly, transgenic mice over-expressing Ang2 died embryonically with a similar phenotype as the Ang1 and Tie2/TEK knock-out mice, suggesting that Ang2 is a natural antagonist for Ang1-mediated Tie2/TEK activation in EC, making Tie2/TEK the first known naturally occurring receptor tyrosine kinase (RTK) that is so precisely regulated *in vivo* [55].

Tie2/TEK expression persists throughout life in the quiescent endothelial cells including those in the normal brain, providing continuous stabilizing force to the mature adult vasculature through Ang1 activation[56,57]. Tie2/TEK is critical for normal embryonic vessel development and knock-out of Tie2/TEK or ablation with a dominant negative mutant causes embryonic lethality[58-60]. The abnormal vessels are characterized by a reduction in EC number and lack of recruitment of PVC[58-60]. There is a decrease in sprouting and remodeling of the primitive vascular network, leading to restricted growth of the head and heart, together with a loss of heart trabeculation[58-60]. During normal physiological processes such as wound healing and pathological angiogenic states such as tumor vascularization, Tie2/TEK expression and activation are increased[56,57,61,62], indicating a requisite role for this pathway in neo-angiogenesis.

A paradigm incorporating interactions of VEGF and Ang1/2 in the development of normal embryonal and adult vasculature has been proposed[63]. VEGF and VEGFRs are essential for the formation of the primitive vascular network, while Ang1/2 and Tie2/TEK interactions signal maturation of the primitive vessels[63]**(Figure 3).** During normal and pathological angiogenesis, a relative increase in Ang2 expression by the ECs inhibits Tie2/TEK activation, thereby destabilizing the vessels and sensitizing ECs to VEGF, which results in EC proliferation, sprouting and neo-angiogenesis [63]. However, this paradigm is an over-simplification as we are gradually deciphering the multiple areas of EC biology that Angs and Tie2/TEK play a role in[64-71]. Activation of Tie2/TEK by Ang1 modulates EC adhesion, motility and survival[67-71]. Additionally, Ang1/2 play a highly variable role in angiogenesis depending on the levels of VEGF expression, and the microenvironmental and tissue context in which they are expressed[64-69].

An important factor governing the functional role of Ang1/2 is their interactions with other angiogenic factors, with data suggesting that Ang1/2 can have a dual role in angiogenesis depending on the context in which they are expressed[32]. Recent biochemical research has focused on the collaborative functions that exist between Ang1, Ang2 and VEGF[72-75]. Transgenic mice over-expressing Ang1 in cardiac cells demonstrate no increase in angiogenesis, which is in contradiction to the findings of increased angiogenesis with Ang1 over-expression in skin[54]. Double transgenic mice over-expressing VEGF and Ang1 showed restricted angiogenesis and dampening of the potent angiogenic response Seen following VEGF signaling [65]. These findings highlight a very context specific role for Ang1 and how it can play both a positive or negative regulatory roles in normal physiological angiogenesis. Similarly, the role of Angs in tumor angiogenesis is proving to be context dependent, as demonstrated by our work in astrocytomas, described below.

Our current understanding of the Tie2/TEK-Ang pathway indicates that these cytokines have a multi-faceted role in promoting and maintaining normal vessels. The regulatory effects of Ang1/2 and Tie2/TEK can vary according to the organ and context in which they are expressed. Therefore, we postulate that this pathway potentially contributes in a similar context-dependent manner to the formation of the abnormal vasculature.

Ephrins

Eph receptors together with their EphrinA and EphrinB ligands were first identified in the nervous system for their role in neuronal patterning and axonal guidance [76,77]. Ephrins and Eph receptors are also postulated to play important functions in arterio-venous differentiation and maintenance. EphrinB2 is an early marker of arterial EC and the receptor EphB4 an early marker of venous EC[30,76-78]. Mice with a knock-out of EphrinB2 die embryonally due to lack of appropriate orchestration of arterial and venous ECs. EphB4 knock-out mice show similar phenotypic alterations such embryonal lethality with vascular changes that are identical to the EphrinB2 knock-out mice [30,76-78]. This suggests that EphB4 is the most important receptor interacting with EphrinB2 that regulates normal differentiation of the arterial and venous system. Furthermore, most recent evidence indicates that EphB4 along with Angiopoietin pathway are important not only in physiological but tumor vascular patterning [79,80]. Specifically it is thought that Ang1 and EphB4 interaction reduces the permeability of the tumor vasculature, potentially by altering EC and SMC interaction, in other words influencing vessel maturation [80].

1.3 Role of progenitor cells in tumor angiogenesis

The paradox of the sensitivity of the vasculature to irradiation and the resistance to RT could be resolved if, as postulated, circulating cells outside of the radiation field can re-colonize and/or stabilize the tumor vasculature after irradiation, thereby supporting any remaining viable tumor cells. This restoration of the vasculature facilitated by BMDCs is observed in ischemic normal tissues and in malignant tissues[73-75]. These BMDCs are also thought to create an environment for tumor growth and invasion, and metastasis [77,] **(Figure 6)**.

Whether EPCs are a true subpopulation of BMDC that are mobilized from the BM versus being present mainly in the circulation remains controversial and data supports that there may not be a clear distinction between angiogenesis and vasculogensis as traditionally proposed. One of the major limitations in the study of EPCs is the lack of exclusive cell-surface markers for these cells.

EPCs that are derived from BM can be mobilized during adult life to sites where new vessel formation is required[81,82]. It is also conceivable that they can reside in organs dormantly, become activated and differentiate into ECs in response to certain physiological and pathological triggers, thereby contributing to angiogenesis. EPCs express markers similar to

ECs, such as VEGFR2, Tie2/TEK, CD34, CD146, von Willebrand factor and PECAM[83,84]. Therefore, making a distinction between EC lining the vessel lumen and EPCs present within a vessel lumen can be difficult. Though their relative contribution to angiogenesis is not clear[85] very recent data suggests that EPCs within a specific vessel wall region, localized between smooth muscle and adventitial layer, act as a source of EPCs that will then trigger neo-vascularization in adult tumors[86]. The stem cell marker, CD133, with a yet to be determined function, stains EPCs[83,84]. Stem cells are $CD133^+$ / $VEGFR2^-$, but *in vitro* can be induced to become $CD133^-$/$VEGFR2^+$, and behave as a mature EC[83,84]. Until these recent observations it was thought that adult vessel formation relied solely on neo-angiogenesis however these recent results suggest that *de novo* vessel formation by EPCs to be potentially possible [86-88]. Recent studies using Id1&3 knock-out mice demonstrate an impaired VEGF induced EPCs mobilization and tumor vascularisation, suggesting bone marrow derived EPCs are incorporated to the vascular structures in both B6RV2 lymphoma and Lewis lung carcinoma tumors. The recruitment of EPCs occurs concurrently with myeloid cells, which are believed to stabilize the structure of newly formed vessels.

There is evidence that chemotactic factors expressed by injured tissue recruits hematopoetic stem cells and progenitor cells to aid in neoangiogenesis[85,89], however, their role and mechanism of activation in tumor angiogenesis is not known. The molecular mechanisms of

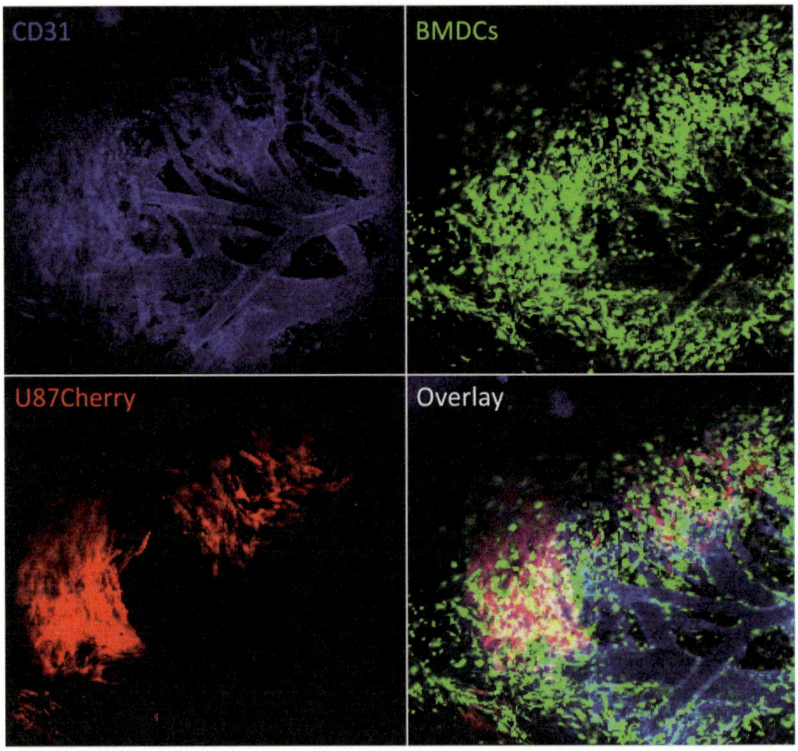

Fig. 6. BMDC recruitment to Tumor
Using *in vivo* 2-photon imaging it is possible to watch with time the recruitment of BMDCs to the site of tumor growth and ultimately their dynamic integration into the vasculature network. BMDCs distribution can be confirmed following end point histology looking at sections through the tumor.

activation, recruitment and differentiation of EPCs to tumor angiogenesis is beyond the scope of this chapter, but this is an exciting new direction for angiogenesis research, which will most likely result in significant advances and potentially yield therapeutic strategies for tumors.

1.4 Role of immuno-modulatory cells in tumor angiogenesis

In addition to EPCs, other subpopulations of BMDCs are thought to contribute to tumor neo-vascularization. It is well established that the role of macrophages extends beyond their originally recognized role as scavenger cells and as part of inflammatory cells they are proposed to play a crucial role in tumor neo-vascularization, though a specific role has not been definitively established. Recent studies demonstrate that monocytes derived from the bone marrow are recruited from the circulation and migrate into the tumor stroma where they differentiate to form macrophages. Several studies have shown tumor-associated macrophages (TAM) to promote tumor angiogenesis and metastases[90] and extent of TAM correlates with increased tumor angiogenesis. These TAMs can in turn promote neo-vascularization[61]. To date only a few studies have focused on this area in solid tumors, and it has been suggested that a small subpopulation of monocytes expressing an angiogenic specific receptor tyrosine kinase, TIE2 expressing Monocyte (TEM), also play a very specific role in neo-vascularization of tumors[91]. TEMs can be distinguished from TAMs by their surface markers (CD45,CD11b,TIE2,F4/80) and lack of mature EC cell surface markers (VEGF-R2/CD133/CD34)[92]. Depletion of the TEM population in mice results in altered endothelial staining, which indicates a dramatic reduction in vascular structures, suggesting that TEMs are important in the process of glioma tumor angiogenesis[93]. Another key subpopulation of BMDCs are BM derived myeloid cells or myeloid-derived suppressor cells (CD45/CD11b/Gr-1), which are thought to eventually differentiate into TAM, TEM and granuloctyes. The role of myeloid-cells in cancer progression, in particular vascular dependent growth, is becoming more recognized, and interest in using them as therapeutic targets is increasing as their depletion can prevent tumor recurrence post-RT[94].

Colony-stimulating factor (CSF-1) gene plays a critical role in macrophage growth and development. Inhbition of CSF-1 decreases tumor growth[95]. The paracrine loop signaling between macrophages and tumor cells is essential to the ability of tumor cells to invade within the primary tumor. TAMs are found to express a range of angiogenic regulating factors, most notable of which are epidermal growth factor (EGF), FGF-2, TGF-a and b and CSF-1[96]. A few studies have shown macrophages to be a source of EGF, which acts as a chemotactic for tumor cells in mammary tumors *in vivo* and *in vitro*. Another chemokine thought to be involved in macrophage recruitment is CCL2/monocyte chemotactic protein-1 (MCP-1), synthesized by ECs MCP-1 is seen to increase in both ischemia and malignancy.

1.5 Role of hypoxia in tumor angiogenesis

The responses to hypoxic condition are mostly mediated through activation of hypoxia inducible factor (HIF-1) and influenced by tumor microenvironment and underlying vessel density[97]. HIF-1 consists of a constituently active subunit, HIF-1β, and a secondary subunit, HIF-1α, which is not present under normoxia due to ubiquitin-mediated proteolysis. Hypoxia inhibits proteolytic degradation of HIF-1α, resulting in dimerization with HIF-1β and activation of many downstream targets through interaction with a 28-base sequence in the 5′ promoter region of the gene, termed the Hypoxia Response Element (HRE)[98,99]. The

critical regulation of HIF-1α by hypoxia is demonstrated during embryonal development, because whereby HIF-1α knock-out embryos die due to vascular defects.
Hypoxia induces the transcription of many key angiogenic signaling pathways including VEGF [100-105], through increasing the VEGF mRNA stability through binding of several RNA binding proteins [100,102,106-109].
Similarly it has been shown that in a tumor hypoxic environment, the activation of HIF1α induces Stromal Derived Factor-1 (SDF-1), a mobilizer of BMDCs, in turn recruiting EPCs, pericyte progenitor cells (PPCs) and CD45+ myeloid cells to the tumor contributing to neovascularisation. EPCs and PPCs directly contribute in vascular structure whilst myeloid cells have been shown to induce the bioavailability of VEGF, thus promoting the angiogenic potential of the tumor[63].
In addition to HIF-1α, a very recent study has identified the distinct upregulation of HIF-2α gene expression by glioma stem cells (GSCs) in response to hypoxia, potentially explaining the increased VEGF expression and highly angiogenic activity of tumors originating from GSC[110]. Therapeutic intervention such as RT will increase the hypoxic level of tumor and therefore contribute to the HIF-1 enhancement of the formation of new blood vessels. Kioi *et al* have shown that irradiation increases tumor hypoxic condition, which in turn enhances the number of BMDCs, such as myelomonocytes (CD11b+), recruited to the tumor environment, implying that vasculogenesis rather than angiogenesis contributes in RT induced tumor progression. Through the blockade of SDF-1, a downstream target of HIF1, the recruitment of BMDCs EPCs was completely inhibited demonstrating the specificity of the recruitment following RT[62].

1.6 Ionizing radiation and its affect on neo-vascularisation

A more comprehensive knowledge of the molecular mechanisms of angiogenesis in response to RT is required to allow more efficient targeting of angiogenic pathways. There is experimental evidence demonstrating that RT regulates tumor angiogenesis, both direct and indirectly. RT directly modulates EC biology, by inhibiting EC survival and proliferation, preventing EC invasion and tube formation and inducing EC apoptosis[111,112]. Some studies have shown a dose dependent response to RT, where at lower doses, RT can promote EC proliferation (<10 Gy)[113] while at higher doses (> 10 Gy) induce EC apoptosis[114,115]. EC apoptosis is promoted through inhibiting the main signaling pathway regulating EC survival, the PI3K/Akt pathway. Therefore, PI3K/Akt has been proposed as a strong candidate target for combinatorial therapy with RT[116,117]. In addition to regulating EC biology, RT also directly regulates expression of angiogenic factors and hence tumor angiogenesis. RT upregulates VEGF and VEGFR-2, in turn promoting EC proliferation and tumor angiogenesis, and overall tumor growth[45,46,111,118,119]. Levels of VEGF expression by ECs is suggested to be dependent on RT dose and fractionation schedule[120,121]. Other candidate angiogenic factors also found to modulate RT include Ang-1 and bFGF which protect ECs against RT damage[115,122], while bFGF enhance anti-tumor effect of RT[114,123]. Similarly, PECAM-1 elevation following RT increases anti-tumor effect of IR by upregulating vessel thrombosis and promoting anti-angiogenesis[124]. RT can regulate tumor angiogenesis indirectly as well, by generating hypoxia. Hypoxia in turn induces VEGF and VEGFR2 upregulation[125-127] and tumor angiogenesis. The tumor angiogenic response elicited post-RT is considered as a potential 'escape mechanism' that might provide an opportunity for tumor cells to avoid radiation cell kill and facilitates cancer recurrence. It is conceivable that inhibition of VEGF and other relevant angiogenic cytokines will eliminate the

angiogenic survival response post-RT, radiosensitizing ECs and potentiating the benefits of RT. The above results are supported to an extent by recent *in vivo* studies[120,121,123,128], however, unfortunately clinical trials involving combination of RT and anti-VEGF therapy have not proven beneficial, suggesting other mechanisms regulating tumor neo-vascularization in response to RT may be involved [34,37,39,48].
Recent evidence has demonstrated the specific migration and recruitment of BMDCs to the site of radiation specifically, although negates the process of differentiation following integration. The BMDCs instead are retained at the site of RT until a secondary signal, such as an oncogenic signal initiates their differentiation, possibly providing a vascular escape mechanism for the RT. The molecular mechanisms that regulate BMDC to site of cranial irradiation remains to be identified and their potential to be harnessed towards a therapeutic benefit further elucidated.

2. Abbreviations

EC - Endothelial Cell
VEGF - Vascular Endothelial Growth Factor
Ang 1&2 - Angiopoietin 1 & 2
ECM - Extracellular Matrix
CT - Chemotherapy
RT - Radiation Therapy
EPC - Endothelial Progenitor Cell
PC - Pericyte
SMC - Smooth Muscle Cell
BM - Bone Marrow
BMDC - Bone Marrow Derived Cell
PVC - Perivascular Cell
TAM - Tumor Associated Macrophage
GSC - Glioma stem Cells
PPC - Pericyte Progenitor Cells
HIF1 - Hypoxia Induced Factor 1
SDF-1 - Stromal Derived Factor 1
PDGF - Platelet Derived Growth Factor

3. References

[1] Carmeliet, P. & Jain, R.K. Angiogenesis in cancer and other diseases. *Nature* 407, 249-57. (2000).
[2] Darland D, D.A.P. *Tumor Angiogenesis and Microcirculation*, (Marcel Dekker Inc., New York, 2001).
[3] Folkman, J., Ed: Klein, G. & Weinhouse, S. Tumor Angiogenesis. "*Advances in Cancer Research*" New York, Academic Press, 43-52 (1974).
[4] Folkman, J. What is the evidence that tumors are angiogenesis-dependent? *J. Natl. Cancer Inst.* 82, 4-6 (1990).
[5] Holash, J., Wiegand, S.J. & Yancopoulos, G.D. New model of tumor angiogenesis: dynamic balance between vessel regression and growth mediated by angiopoietins and VEGF. *Oncogene* 18, 5356-62 (1999).

[6] Risau, W. & Flamme, I. Vasculogenesis. *Annu Rev Cell Dev Biol* 11, 73-91 (1995).
[7] Risau, W. Embryonic angiogenesis factors. *Pharmacol Ther* 51, 371-6 (1991).
[8] Bergers, G. & Benjamin, L.E. Tumorigenesis and the angiogenic switch. *Nat Rev Cancer* 3, 401-10 (2003).
[9] Wilting, J., Brand-Saberi, B., Kurz, H. & Christ, B. Development of the embryonic vascular system. *Cell Mol Biol Res* 41, 219-32 (1995).
[10] Polverini, P.J. & Leibovich, S.J. Induction of neovascularization in vivo and endothelial proliferation in vitro by tumor-associated macrophages. *Lab Invest* 51, 635-42 (1984).
[11] Lutsenko, S.V., Kiselev, S.M. & Severin, S.E. Molecular mechanisms of tumor angiogenesis. *Biochemistry (Mosc)* 68, 286-300 (2003).
[12] Kerbel, R.S. Tumor angiogenesis: past, present and the near future. *Carcinogenesis* 21, 505-15 (2000).
[13] Durairaj, A., Mehra, A., Singh, R.P. & Faxon, D.P. Therapeutic angiogenesis. *Cardiol Rev* 8, 279-87 (2000).
[14] Cavallaro, U. & Christofori, G. Molecular mechanisms of tumor angiogenesis and tumor progression. *J Neurooncol* 50, 63-70 (2000).
[15] Sipos, E.P., Tamargo, R.J., Weingart, J.D. & Brem, H. Inhibition of tumor angiogenesis. *Ann N Y Acad Sci* 732, 263-72 (1994).
[16] Muehlbauer, P.M. Anti-angiogenesis in cancer therapy. *Semin Oncol Nurs* 19, 180-92 (2003).
[17] Brem, S. Angiogenesis and Cancer Control: From Concept to Therapeutic Trial. *Cancer Control* 6, 436-458 (1999).
[18] Jain, R.K. & Carmeliet, P.F. Vessels of death or life. *Sci Am* 285, 38-45 (2001).
[19] Jain, R.K. Normalizing tumor vasculature with anti-angiogenic therapy: a new paradigm for combination therapy. *Nat Med* 7, 987-9 (2001).
[20] Jain, R.K. Normalization of tumor vasculature: an emerging concept in antiangiogenic therapy. *Science* 307, 58-62 (2005).
[21] Jain, R.K., Tong, R.T. & Munn, L.L. Effect of vascular normalization by antiangiogenic therapy on interstitial hypertension, peritumor edema, and lymphatic metastasis: insights from a mathematical model. *Cancer Res* 67, 2729-35 (2007).
[22] Risau, W. Mechanisms of angiogenesis. *Nature* 386, 671-4 (1997).
[23] Patan, S. Vasculogenesis and angiogenesis as mechanisms of vascular network formation, growth and remodeling. *J Neurooncol* 50, 1-15. (2000).
[24] Pardanaud, L., Altmann, C., Kitos, P., Dieterlen-Lievre, F. & Buck, C.A. Vasculogenesis in the early quail blastodisc as studied with a monoclonal antibody recognizing endothelial cells. *Development* 100, 339-49 (1987).
[25] Papetti, M. & Herman, I.M. Mechanisms of normal and tumor-derived angiogenesis. *Am J Physiol Cell Physiol* 282, C947-70 (2002).
[26] Houck, K.A. et al. The vascular endothelial growth factor family: identification of a fourth molecular species and characterization of alternative splicing of RNA. *Mol Endocrinol* 5, 1806-14 (1991).
[27] Wilting, J. & Christ, B. Embryonic angiogenesis: a review. *Naturwissenschaften* 83, 153-64 (1996).
[28] Hogan, K.A. & Bautch, V.L. Blood vessel patterning at the embryonic midline. *Curr Top Dev Biol* 62, 55-85 (2004).

[29] Adams, R.H. Molecular control of arterial-venous blood vessel identity. *J Anat* 202, 105-12 (2003).
[30] Yancopoulos, G.D. et al. Vascular-specific growth factors and blood vessel formation. *Nature* 407, 242-8. (2000).
[31] Patan, S. Vasculogenesis and angiogenesis. *Cancer Treat Res* 117, 3-32 (2004).
[32] Dunn, I.F., Heese, O. & Black, P.M. Growth factors in glioma angiogenesis: FGFs, PDGF, EGF, and TGFs. *J Neurooncol* 50, 121-37. (2000).
[33] Thomas, K.A. Fibroblast growth factors. *Faseb J* 1, 434-40 (1987).
[34] Muller, G., Behrens, J., Nussbaumer, U., Bohlen, P. & Birchmeier, W. Inhibitory action of transforming growth factor beta on endothelial cells. *Proc Natl Acad Sci U S A* 84, 5600-4 (1987).
[35] Merwin, J.R., Newman, W., Beall, L.D., Tucker, A. & Madri, J. Vascular cells respond differentially to transforming growth factors beta 1 and beta 2 in vitro. *Am J Pathol* 138, 37-51 (1991).
[36] Yurchenco, P.D. & Schittny, J.C. Molecular architecture of basement membranes. *Faseb J* 4, 1577-90 (1990).
[37] Madri, J.A., Pratt, B.M. & Tucker, A.M. Phenotypic modulation of endothelial cells by transforming growth factor-beta depends upon the composition and organization of the extracellular matrix. *J Cell Biol* 106, 1375-84 (1988).
[38] Romanic, A.M., White, R.F., Arleth, A.J., Ohlstein, E.H. & Barone, F.C. Matrix metalloproteinase expression increases after cerebral focal ischemia in rats: inhibition of matrix metalloproteinase-9 reduces infarct size. *Stroke* 29, 1020-30 (1998).
[39] Lukes, A., Mun-Bryce, S., Lukes, M. & Rosenberg, G.A. Extracellular matrix degradation by metalloproteinases and central nervous system diseases. *Mol Neurobiol* 19, 267-84 (1999).
[40] Bennett, S.-S. *Matrix Metalloproteinases and Their Inhibitors in Angiogenesis: Tumor Angiogenesis and Microcirculation*, (Marcel Dekker, New York, 2001).
[41] Burbridge, M.F. et al. The role of the matrix metalloproteinases during in vitro vessel formation. *Angiogenesis* 5, 215-26 (2002).
[42] Cohen, T. et al. VEGF121, a vascular endothelial growth factor (VEGF) isoform lacking heparin binding ability, requires cell-surface heparan sulfates for efficient binding to the VEGF receptors of human melanoma cells. *J Biol Chem* 270, 11322-6 (1995).
[43] Patan, S. Vasculogenesis and angiogenesis as mechanisms of vascular network formation, growth and remodeling. *Journal of neuro-oncology* 50, 1-15 (2000).
[44] Ferrara, N. et al. Heterozygous embryonic lethality induced by targeted inactivation of the VEGF gene. *Nature* 380, 439-42 (1996).
[45] Ferrara, N. VEGF: an update on biological and therapeutic aspects. *Curr Opin Biotechnol* 11, 617-24 (2000).
[46] Plate, K.H., Breier, G., Weich, H.A., Mennel, H.D. & Risau, W. Vascular endothelial growth factor and glioma angiogenesis: coordinate induction of VEGF receptors, distribution of VEGF protein and possible in vivo regulatory mechanisms. *Int J Cancer* 59, 520-9. (1994).
[47] Plate, K. & Risau, W. Angiogenesis in Malignant Gliomas. *Glia* 15, 339-347 (1995).
[48] Machein, M.R. & Plate, K.H. VEGF in brain tumors. *J Neurooncol* 50, 109-20. (2000).

[49] Guha, A., Feldkamp, M.M., Lau, N., Boss, G. & Pawson, A. Proliferation of human malignant astrocytomas is dependent on Ras activation. *Oncogene* 15, 2755-65. (1997).
[50] Dumont, D.J., Yamaguchi, T.P., Conlon, R.A., Rossant, J. & Breitman, M.L. tek, a novel tyrosine kinase gene located on mouse chromosome 4, is expressed in endothelial cells and their presumptive precursors. *Oncogene* 7, 1471-80. (1992).
[51] Dumont, D.J., Gradwohl, G.J., Fong, G.H., Auerbach, R. & Breitman, M.L. The endothelial-specific receptor tyrosine kinase, tek, is a member of a new subfamily of receptors. *Oncogene* 8, 1293-301. (1993).
[52] Davis, S. et al. Isolation of angiopoietin-1, a ligand for the TIE2 receptor, by secretion-trap expression cloning. *Cell* 87, 1161-9. (1996).
[53] Suri, C. et al. Requisite role of angiopoietin-1, a ligand for the TIE2 receptor, during embryonic angiogenesis. *Cell* 87, 1171-80. (1996).
[54] Maisonpierre, P.C. et al. Angiopoietin-2, a natural antagonist for Tie2 that disrupts in vivo angiogenesis. *Science* 277, 55-60. (1997).
[55] Korhonen, J. et al. Enhanced expression of the tie receptor tyrosine kinase in endothelial cells during neovascularization. *Blood* 80, 2548-55. (1992).
[56] Wong, A.L. et al. Tie2 expression and phosphorylation in angiogenic and quiescent adult tissues. *Circ Res* 81, 567-74. (1997).
[57] Dumont, D.J. et al. Dominant-negative and targeted null mutations in the endothelial receptor tyrosine kinase, tek, reveal a critical role in vasculogenesis of the embryo. *Genes Dev* 8, 1897-909. (1994).
[58] Sato, T.N., Qin, Y., Kozak, C.A. & Audus, K.L. Tie-1 and tie-2 define another class of putative receptor tyrosine kinase genes expressed in early embryonic vascular system. *Proc Natl Acad Sci U S A* 90, 9355-8 (1993).
[59] Sato, T.N. et al. Distinct roles of the receptor tyrosine kinases Tie-1 and Tie-2 in blood vessel formation. *Nature* 376, 70-4. (1995).
[60] Asahara, T. et al. Tie2 receptor ligands, angiopoietin-1 and angiopoietin-2, modulate VEGF-induced postnatal neovascularization. *Circ Res* 83, 233-40. (1998).
[61] Peters, K.G. et al. Expression of Tie2/Tek in breast tumour vasculature provides a new marker for evaluation of tumour angiogenesis. *Br J Cancer* 77, 51-6. (1998).
[62] Hanahan, D. Signalling Vascular Morphogenesis and Maintenance. *Science* 277, 48-50 (1997).
[63] Ward, N.L. & Dumont, D.J. The angiopoietins and Tie2/Tek: adding to the complexity of cardiovascular development. *Semin Cell Dev Biol* 13, 19-27 (2002).
[64] Visconti, R.P., Richardson, C.D. & Sato, T.N. Orchestration of angiogenesis and arteriovenous contribution by angiopoietins and vascular endothelial growth factor (VEGF). *Proc Natl Acad Sci U S A* 99, 8219-24 (2002).
[65] Papapetropoulos, A. et al. Direct actions of angiopoietin-1 on human endothelium: evidence for network stabilization, cell survival, and interaction with other angiogenic growth factors. *Lab Invest* 79, 213-23. (1999).
[66] Kwak, H.J., So, J.N., Lee, S.J., Kim, I. & Koh, G.Y. Angiopoietin-1 is an apoptosis survival factor for endothelial cells. *FEBS Lett* 448, 249-53. (1999).
[67] Kim, I. et al. Angiopoietin-2 at high concentration can enhance endothelial cell survival through the phosphatidylinositol 3'-kinase/Akt signal transduction pathway. *Oncogene* 19, 4549-52. (2000).

[68] Kim, I. et al. Angiopoietin-1 regulates endothelial cell survival through the phosphatidylinositol 3'-Kinase/Akt signal transduction pathway. *Circ Res* 86, 24-9. (2000).
[69] Gamble, J.R. et al. Angiopoietin-1 is an antipermeability and anti-inflammatory agent in vitro and targets cell junctions. *Circ Res* 87, 603-7. (2000).
[70] Carlson, T.R., Feng, Y., Maisonpierre, P.C., Mrksich, M. & Morla, A.O. Direct cell adhesion to the angiopoietins mediated by integrins. *J Biol Chem* 276, 26516-25. (2001).
[71] Thurston, G. Complementary actions of VEGF and angiopoietin-1 on blood vessel growth and leakage. *J Anat* 200, 575-80 (2002).
[72] Chae, J.K. et al. Coadministration of angiopoietin-1 and vascular endothelial growth factor enhances collateral vascularization. *Arterioscler Thromb Vasc Biol* 20, 2573-8 (2000).
[73] Saito, M., Hamasaki, M. & Shibuya, M. Induction of tube formation by angiopoietin-1 in endothelial cell/fibroblast co-culture is dependent on endogenous VEGF. *Cancer Sci* 94, 782-90 (2003).
[74] Moon, W.S. et al. Overexpression of VEGF and angiopoietin 2: a key to high vascularity of hepatocellular carcinoma? *Mod Pathol* 16, 552-7 (2003).
[75] Wang, H.U. & Anderson, D.J. Eph family transmembrane ligands can mediate repulsive guidance of trunk neural crest migration and motor axon outgrowth. *Neuron* 18, 383-96 (1997).
[76] Wang, X. et al. Multiple ephrins control cell organization in C. elegans using kinase-dependent and -independent functions of the VAB-1 Eph receptor. *Mol Cell* 4, 903-13 (1999).
[77] Gerety, S.S., Wang, H.U., Chen, Z.F. & Anderson, D.J. Symmetrical mutant phenotypes of the receptor EphB4 and its specific transmembrane ligand ephrin-B2 in cardiovascular development. *Mol Cell* 4, 403-14 (1999).
[78] Pfaff, D., Fiedler, U. & Augustin, H.G. Emerging roles of the Angiopoietin-Tie and the ephrin-Eph systems as regulators of cell trafficking. *J Leukoc Biol* 80, 719-26 (2006).
[79] Erber, R. et al. EphB4 controls blood vascular morphogenesis during postnatal angiogenesis. *Embo J* 25, 628-41 (2006).
[80] Rafii, S., Heissig, B. & Hattori, K. Efficient mobilization and recruitment of marrow-derived endothelial and hematopoietic stem cells by adenoviral vectors expressing angiogenic factors. *Gene Ther* 9, 631-41 (2002).
[81] Rafii, S. et al. Contribution of marrow-derived progenitors to vascular and cardiac regeneration. *Semin Cell Dev Biol* 13, 61-7 (2002).
[82] Hristov, M. & Weber, C. Endothelial progenitor cells: characterization, pathophysiology, and possible clinical relevance. *J Cell Mol Med* 8, 498-508 (2004).
[83] Hristov, M., Erl, W. & Weber, P.C. Endothelial progenitor cells: mobilization, differentiation, and homing. *Arterioscler Thromb Vasc Biol* 23, 1185-9 (2003).
[84] Zwaginga, J.J. & Doevendans, P. Stem cell-derived angiogenic/vasculogenic cells: possible therapies for tissue repair and tissue engineering. *Clin Exp Pharmacol Physiol* 30, 900-8 (2003).
[85] Zengin, E. et al. Vascular wall resident progenitor cells: a source for postnatal vasculogenesis. *Development* 133, 1543-51 (2006).

[86] Asahara, T. et al. Isolation of putative progenitor endothelial cells for angiogenesis. *Science* 275, 964-7 (1997).
[87] Gehling, U.M. et al. In vitro differentiation of endothelial cells from AC133-positive progenitor cells. *Blood* 95, 3106-12 (2000).
[88] Aghi, M., Cohen, K.S., Klein, R.J., Scadden, D.T. & Chiocca, E.A. Tumor stromal-derived factor-1 recruits vascular progenitors to mitotic neovasculature, where microenvironment influences their differentiated phenotypes. *Cancer Res* 66, 9054-64 (2006).
[89] Condeelis, J. & Pollard, J.W. Macrophages: Obligate Partners for Tumor Cell Migration, Invasion, and Metastasis. *Cell* 124, 263-266 (2006).
[90] De Palma, M., Murdoch, C., Venneri, M.A., Naldini, L. & Lewis, C.E. Tie2-expressing monocytes: regulation of tumor angiogenesis and therapeutic implications. *Trends Immunol* 28, 519-24 (2007).
[91] Lewis, C.E., De Palma, M. & Naldini, L. Tie2-expressing monocytes and tumor angiogenesis: regulation by hypoxia and angiopoietin-2. *Cancer Res* 67, 8429-32 (2007).
[92] De Palma, M., Murdoch, C., Venneri, M. & Naldini, L. Tie2-expressing monocytes: regulation of tumor angiogenesis and therapeutic implications. *Trends in …* (2007).
[93] H, G. Targetting inflammatory cells to improve abti-VEGF therapies in oncology. 1-17 (2009).
[94] Lin, E.Y. et al. Macrophages regulate the angiogenic switch in a mouse model of breast cancer. *Cancer research* 66, 11238-11246 (2006).
[95] Wyckoff, J. A Paracrine Loop between Tumor Cells and Macrophages Is Required for Tumor Cell Migration in Mammary Tumors. *Cancer research* 64, 7022-7029 (2004).
[96] Blouw, B. et al. The hypoxic response of tumors is dependent on their microenvironment. *Cancer Cell* 4, 133-146 (2003).
[97] Minet, E., Michel, G., Remacle, J. & Michiels, C. Role of HIF-1 as a transcription factor involved in embryonic development, cancer progression and apoptosis (review). *Int J Mol Med* 5, 253-9 (2000).
[98] Minet, E. et al. Hypoxia-induced activation of HIF-1: role of HIF-1alpha-Hsp90 interaction. *FEBS Lett* 460, 251-6 (1999).
[99] Stein, I. et al. Translation of vascular endothelial growth factor mRNA by internal ribosome entry: implications for translation under hypoxia. *Mol Cell Biol* 18, 3112-9. (1998).
[100] Oh, H. et al. Hypoxia and vascular endothelial growth factor selectively up-regulate angiopoietin-2 in bovine microvascular endothelial cells. *J Biol Chem* 274, 15732-9 (1999).
[101] Stein, I., Neeman, M., Shweiki, D., Itin, A. & Keshet, E. Stabilization of vascular endothelial growth factor mRNA by hypoxia and hypoglycemia and coregulation with other ischemia-induced genes. *Mol Cell Biol* 15, 5363-8 (1995).
[102] Shweiki, D., Neeman, M., Itin, A. & Keshet, E. Induction of vascular endothelial growth factor expression by hypoxia and by glucose deficiency in multicell spheroids: implications for tumor angiogenesis. *Proc Natl Acad Sci U S A* 92, 768-72 (1995).

[103] Shweiki, D., Itin, A., Soffer, D. & Keshet, E. Vascular endothelial growth factor induced by hypoxia may mediate hypoxia-initiated angiogenesis. *Nature* 359, 843-5 (1992).
[104] Flamme, I. et al. HRF, a putative basic helix-loop-helix-PAS-domain transcription factor is closely related to hypoxia-inducible factor-1 alpha and developmentally expressed in blood vessels. *Mech Dev* 63, 51-60 (1997).
[105] Semenza, G.L. & Wang, G.L. A nuclear factor induced by hypoxia via de novo protein synthesis binds to the human erythropoietin gene enhancer at a site required for transcriptional activation. *Mol Cell Biol* 12, 5447-54. (1992).
[106] Maxwell, P.H. et al. Hypoxia-inducible factor-1 modulates gene expression in solid tumors and influences both angiogenesis and tumor growth. *Proc Natl Acad Sci U S A* 94, 8104-9. (1997).
[107] Levy, A.P., Levy, N.S., Wegner, S. & Goldberg, M.A. Transcriptional regulation of the rat vascular endothelial growth factor gene by hypoxia. *J Biol Chem* 270, 13333-40. (1995).
[108] Ikeda, E., Achen, M.G., Breier, G. & Risau, W. Hypoxia-induced transcriptional activation and increased mRNA stability of vascular endothelial growth factor in C6 glioma cells. *J Biol Chem* 270, 19761-6. (1995).
[109] Li, Z., Bao, S., Wu, Q., Wang, H. & Eyler, C. Hypoxia-Inducible Factors Regulate Tumorigenic Capacity of Glioma Stem Cells. *Cancer Cell* (2009).
[110] Abdollahi, A. et al. SU5416 and SU6668 attenuate the angiogenic effects of radiation-induced tumor cell growth factor production and amplify the direct anti-endothelial action of radiation in vitro. *Cancer Res* 63, 3755-63 (2003).
[111] Li, M. et al. Small molecule receptor tyrosine kinase inhibitor of platelet-derived growth factor signaling (SU9518) modifies radiation response in fibroblasts and endothelial cells. *BMC Cancer* 6, 79 (2006).
[112] Gaugler, M.H. et al. Late and persistent up-regulation of intercellular adhesion molecule-1 (ICAM-1) expression by ionizing radiation in human endothelial cells in vitro. *Int J Radiat Biol* 72, 201-9 (1997).
[113] Langley, R.E., Bump, E.A., Quartuccio, S.G., Medeiros, D. & Braunhut, S.J. Radiation-induced apoptosis in microvascular endothelial cells. *Br J Cancer* 75, 666-72 (1997).
[114] Paris, F. et al. Endothelial apoptosis as the primary lesion initiating intestinal radiation damage in mice. *Science* 293, 293-7 (2001).
[115] Geng, L. et al. A specific antagonist of the p110delta catalytic component of phosphatidylinositol 3'-kinase, IC486068, enhances radiation-induced tumor vascular destruction. *Cancer Res* 64, 4893-9 (2004).
[116] Nakamura, J.L. et al. PKB/Akt mediates radiosensitization by the signaling inhibitor LY294002 in human malignant gliomas. *J Neurooncol* 71, 215-22 (2005).
[117] Gorski, D.H. et al. Blockage of the vascular endothelial growth factor stress response increases the antitumor effects of ionizing radiation. *Cancer Res* 59, 3374-8 (1999).
[118] Gospodarowicz, D., Abraham, J.A. & Schilling, J. Isolation and characterization of a vascular endothelial cell mitogen produced by pituitary-derived folliculo stellate cells. *Proc Natl Acad Sci U S A* 86, 7311-5 (1989).
[119] Williams, K.J. et al. ZD6474, a potent inhibitor of vascular endothelial growth factor signaling, combined with radiotherapy: schedule-dependent enhancement of antitumor activity. *Clin Cancer Res* 10, 8587-93 (2004).

[120] Williams, K.J. et al. Combining radiotherapy with AZD2171, a potent inhibitor of vascular endothelial growth factor signaling: pathophysiologic effects and therapeutic benefit. *Mol Cancer Ther* 6, 599-606 (2007).

[121] Cho, C.H. et al. Designed angiopoietin-1 variant, COMP-Ang1, protects against radiation-induced endothelial cell apoptosis. *Proc Natl Acad Sci U S A* 101, 5553-8 (2004).

[122] Abdollahi, A. et al. Inhibition of alpha(v)beta3 integrin survival signaling enhances antiangiogenic and antitumor effects of radiotherapy. *Clin Cancer Res* 11, 6270-9 (2005).

[123] Gaugler, M.H., Vereycken-Holler, V., Squiban, C. & Aigueperse, J. PECAM-1 (CD31) is required for interactions of platelets with endothelial cells after irradiation. *J Thromb Haemost* 2, 2020-6 (2004).

[124] Allalunis-Turner, M.J., Franko, A.J. & Parliament, M.B. Modulation of oxygen consumption rate and vascular endothelial growth factor mRNA expression in human malignant glioma cells by hypoxia. *Br J Cancer* 80, 104-9 (1999).

[125] Laderoute, K.R. et al. Opposing effects of hypoxia on expression of the angiogenic inhibitor thrombospondin 1 and the angiogenic inducer vascular endothelial growth factor. *Clin Cancer Res* 6, 2941-50 (2000).

[126] Veikkola, T., Karkkainen, M., Claesson-Welsh, L. & Alitalo, K. Regulation of angiogenesis via vascular endothelial growth factor receptors. *Cancer Res* 60, 203-12 (2000).

[127] Luo, X. et al. Radiation-enhanced endostatin gene expression and effects of combination treatment. *Technol Cancer Res Treat* 4, 193-202 (2005).